Artificial Intelligence in Radiology

Editor

DANIEL L. RUBIN

RADIOLOGIC CLINICS OF NORTH AMERICA

www.radiologic.theclinics.com

Consulting Editor
FRANK H. MILLER

November 2021 • Volume 59 • Number 6

ELSEVIER

1600 John F. Kennedy Boulevard ● Suite 1800 ● Philadelphia, Pennsylvania, 19103-2899

http://www.theclinics.com

RADIOLOGIC CLINICS OF NORTH AMERICA Volume 59, Number 6
November 2021 ISSN 0033-8389, ISBN 13: 978-0-323-81355-6

Editor: John Vassallo (j.vassallo@elsevier.com)
Developmental Editor: Karen Solomon

Radiologic Clinics of North America (ISSN 0033-8389) is published bimonthly by Elsevier Inc., 360 Park Avenue South, New York, NY 10010-1710. Months of issue are January, March, May, July, September, and November. Periodicals postage paid at New York, NY and additional mailing offices. Subscription prices are USD 518 per year for US individuals, USD 1309 per year for US institutions, USD 100 per year for US students and residents, USD 611 per year for Canadian individuals, USD 1368 per year for Canadian institutions, USD 703 per year for international individuals, USD 1368 per year for international institutions, USD 100 per year for Canadian students/residents, and USD 315 per year for international students/residents. To receive student and resident rate, orders must be accompanied by name of affiliated institution, date of term and the signature of program/residency coordinatior on institution letterhead. Orders will be billed at individual rate until proof of status is received. Foreign air speed delivery is included in all *Clinics* subscription prices. All prices are subject to change without notice. **POSTMASTER:** Send address changes to *Radiologic Clinics of North America*, Elsevier Health Sciences Division, Subscription Customer Service, 3251 Riverport Lane, Maryland Heights, MO63043. **Customer Service: Telephone: 1-800-654-2452** (U.S. and Canada); **1-314-447-8871** (outside U.S. and Canada). **Fax: 1-314-447-8029. E-mail: journalscustomerservice-usa@elsevier.com (for print support); journalsonlinesupport-usa@elsevier.com (for online support)**.

Reprints. For copies of 100 or more of articles in this publication, please contact the Commercial Reprints Department, Elsevier Inc., 360 Park Avenue South, New York, New York 10010-1710. Tel.: +1-212-633-3874; Fax: +1-212-633-3820; E-mail: reprints@elsevier.com.

Radiologic Clinics of North America also published in Greek Paschalidis Medical Publications, Athens, Greece.

Radiologic Clinics of North America is covered in *MEDLINE/PubMed (Index Medicus), EMBASE/Excerpta Medica, Current Contents/Life Sciences, Current Contents/Clinical Medicine, RSNA Index to Imaging Literature, BIOSIS, Science Citation Index,* and *ISI/BIOMED.*

Contributors

CONSULTING EDITOR

FRANK H. MILLER, MD, FACR
Lee F. Rogers MD Professor of Medical
Education, Chief, Body Imaging Section and
Fellowship Program, Medical Director, MRI,
Department of Radiology, Northwestern
Memorial Hospital, Northwestern University,
Feinberg School of Medicine, Chicago, Illinois,
USA

EDITOR

DANIEL L. RUBIN, MD, MS
Professor of Biomedical Data Science,
Radiology, and Medicine (Biomedical
Informatics) and, by courtesy, Computer
Science and Ophthalmology, Department of
Biomedical Data Science, Stanford University,
Director of Biomedical Informatics, Stanford
Cancer Institute, Stanford, California, USA

AUTHORS

NITAMAR ABDALA, MD, PhD
Adjunct Professor, Universidade Federal de
São Paulo, São Paulo, São Paulo, Brazil

CAGAN ALKAN, MS
Graduate Student, Department of Electrical
Engineering, Stanford University, Stanford,
California, USA

TARIK K. ALKASAB, MD, PhD
Department of Radiology, Massachusetts
General Hospital, Harvard Medical School,
Boston, Massachusetts, USA

RENATA R. ALMEIDA, MD, PhD
Department of Radiology, Brigham and
Women's Hospital, Harvard Medical School,
Boston, Massachusetts, USA

BERNARDO C. BIZZO, MD, PhD
Department of Radiology, Massachusetts
General Hospital, Harvard Medical School,
Boston, Massachusetts, USA

CHRISTOPHER BRIDGE, DPhil
Radiology, Martinos Center for Biomedical
Imaging, Massachusetts General Hospital,
Boston, Massachusetts, USA

KEN CHANG, PhD
Radiology, Martinos Center for Biomedical
Imaging, Massachusetts General Hospital,
Boston, Massachusetts, USA

AKSHAY S. CHAUDHARI, PhD
Assistant Professor, Department of Biomedical
Data Science, Department of Radiology,
Stanford University, Stanford, California, USA

ELIZABETH K. COLE, MS
Graduate Student, Department of Electrical
Engineering, Stanford University, Stanford,
California, USA

TESSA S. COOK, MD, PhD
Assistant Professor of Radiology, Perelman
School of Medicine, University of
Pennsylvania, Philadelphia, Pennsylvania, USA

JEREMY DAHL, PhD
Associate Professor, Department of Radiology,
Stanford University, Stanford, California, USA

JARED DUNNMON, PhD
Visiting Scholar, Department of Biomedical
Data Science, Stanford University, Stanford,
California, USA

BRADLEY J. ERICKSON, MD, PhD
Department of Radiology, Mayo Clinic,
Rochester, Minnesota, USA

SUELY FAZIO FERRACIOLLI, MD
Neuroradiologist, Dasalnova, Diagnósticos da
América SA (Dasa), São Paulo, São Paulo, Brazil

MARYELLEN L. GIGER, PhD
A. N. Pritzker Distinguished Service Professor
of Radiology and Committee on Medical
Physics, Department of Radiology, The
University of Chicago, Chicago, Illinois, USA

VRUSHAB GOWDA, JD
Petrie-Flom Fellow, Harvard Law School,
Cambridge, Massachusetts, USA

HARLAN BENJAMIN HARVEY, MD, JD
Assistant Professor, Radiology,
Massachusetts General Hospital, Harvard
Medical School, Boston, Massachusetts, USA

QIYUAN HU, BA
Committee on Medical Physics, Department of
Radiology, The University of Chicago, Chicago,
Illinois, USA

DONGWOON HYUN, PhD
Research Engineer, Department of Radiology,
Stanford University, Stanford, California, USA

ABDULLAH-AL-ZUBAER IMRAN, PhD
Postdoctoral Research Fellow, Radiological
Sciences Laboratory, Department of
Radiology, Stanford University, Stanford,
California, USA

JAYASHREE KALPATHY-CRAMER, PhD
Associate Professor, Radiology, Martinos
Center for Biomedical Imaging, Massachusetts
General Hospital, Boston, Massachusetts,
USA

**FELIPE CAMPOS KITAMURA, MD, MSc,
PhD**
Head of Innovation in Diagnostic Operations at
Dasalnova, Diagnósticos da América SA
(Dasa), Universidade Federal de São Paulo,
São Paulo, São Paulo, Brazil

SUNGWON LEE, MD, PhD
Imaging Biomarkers and Computer-Aided
Diagnosis Laboratory, Department of
Radiology and Imaging Sciences, National
Institutes of Health Clinical Center, Bethesda,
Maryland, USA

THOMAS W. LOEHFELM, MD, PhD
Associate Professor, UC Davis Medical Center,
Sacramento, California, USA

ANDREAS M. LOENING, MD, PhD
Assistant Professor, Department of Radiology,
Stanford University, Stanford, California, USA

MICHAEL MORRIS, MD, MS
Department of Radiology and Imaging
Sciences, Clinical Center, National Institutes of
Health, Bethesda, Maryland, USA; Department
of Computer Science and Electrical
Engineering, University of Maryland, Baltimore
County, Baltimore, Maryland, USA; Division of
Clinical Informatics, Networking Health, Glen
Burnie, Maryland, USA

SIMUKAYI MUTASA, MD
Thomas Jefferson University Medical Center,
Department of Diagnostic Radiology, Division
of Musculoskeletal Imaging, Philadelphia,
Pennsylvania, USA

IAN PAN, MD
Radiology Resident, Brigham and Woman's
Hospital, Boston, Massachusetts, USA;
Dasalnova, Diagnósticos da América SA
(Dasa), São Paulo, São Paulo, Brazil

JAY B. PATEL, BS
Radiology, Martinos Center for Biomedical Imaging, Massachusetts General Hospital, Boston, Massachusetts, USA

OLEG PIANYKH, PhD
Assistant Professor, Department of Radiology, Harvard Medical School, Massachusetts General Hospital, Boston, Massachusetts, USA

ERIK RANSCHAERT, MD, PhD
Elisabeth-Tweesteden Hospital, Tilburg, The Netherlands; Visiting Professor, Ghent University, Gent, Belgium

BABAK SABOURY, MD, MPH
Department of Radiology and Imaging Sciences, Clinical Center, National Institutes of Health, Bethesda, Maryland, USA; Department of Computer Science and Electrical Engineering, University of Maryland, Baltimore County, Baltimore, Maryland, USA; Department of Radiology, Hospital of the University of Pennsylvania, Philadelphia, Pennsylvania, USA

CHRISTOPHER M. SANDINO, PhD
Graduate Student, Department of Electrical Engineering, Stanford University, Stanford, California, USA

ELIOT SIEGEL, MD, FSIIM, FACR
Department of Diagnostic Radiology and Nuclear Medicine, University of Maryland School of Medicine, University of Maryland Medical Center, Department of Diagnostic Imaging, VA Maryland Healthcare System, Baltimore, Maryland, USA

JACKSON STEINKAMP, MD
Physician, Department of Medicine, Hospital of the University of Pennsylvania, Philadelphia, Pennsylvania, USA

RONALD M. SUMMERS, MD, PhD
Imaging Biomarkers and Computer-Aided Diagnosis Laboratory, Department of Radiology and Imaging Sciences, National Institutes of Health Clinical Center, Bethesda, Maryland, USA

LAURENS TOPFF, MD
Department of Radiology, Netherlands Cancer Institute, Amsterdam, the Netherlands

SHREYAS S. VASANAWALA, MD, PhD
Professor, Department of Radiology, Stanford University, Stanford, California, USA

ADAM S. WANG, PhD
Assistant Professor of Radiology and Electrical Engineering, Stanford University, Stanford, California, USA

KRISTEN W. YEOM, MD
Associate Professor, Department of Radiology, Stanford University, California, USA

PAUL H. YI, MD
University of Maryland Intelligent Imaging Center, Department of Diagnostic Radiology and Nuclear Medicine, University of Maryland School of Medicine, Baltimore, Maryland, USA

Contents

Natural language processing (NLP) is a subfield of computer science and linguistics that can be applied to extract meaningful information from radiology reports. Symbolic NLP is rule based and well suited to problems that can be explicitly defined by a set of rules. Statistical NLP is better situated to problems that cannot be well defined and requires annotated or labeled examples from which machine learning algorithms can infer the rules. Both symbolic and statistical NLP have found success in a variety of radiology use cases. More recently, deep learning approaches, including transformers, have gained traction and demonstrated good performance.

Machine learning is an important tool for extracting information from medical images. Deep learning has made this more efficient by not requiring an explicit feature extraction step and in some cases detecting features that humans had not identified. The rapid advance of deep learning technologies continues to result in valuable tools. The most effective use of these tools will occur when developers also understand the properties of medical images and the clinical questions at hand. The performance metrics also are critical for guiding the training of an artificial intelligence and for assessing and comparing its tools.

Automated approaches in health care have been transformed by machine learning. Although the use of pre-engineered features combined with traditional machine learning approaches has been popular, their implementation has been limited by the need to manually extract and design features. Interest in machine learning has been catalyzed by advancements in deep learning. Breakthrough performance across various tasks within computer science spurred interest in expanding the technique to the medical domain. The need for proper evaluation of these algorithms is an active area of research. The focus of this article is on current issues, techniques, and challenges of evaluating medical artificial intelligence.

The potential of artificial intelligence (AI) in radiology goes far beyond image analysis. AI can be used to optimize all steps of the radiology workflow by supporting a variety of nondiagnostic tasks, including order entry support, patient scheduling, resource allocation, and improving the radiologist's workflow. This article discusses several principal directions of using AI algorithms to improve radiological operations and workflow management, with the intention of providing a broader understanding of the value of applying AI in the radiology department.

Machine learning (ML) and Artificial intelligence (AI) has the potential to dramatically improve radiology practice at multiple stages of the imaging pipeline. Most of the attention has been garnered by applications focused on improving the end of the pipeline: image interpretation. However, this article reviews how AI/ML can be applied to improve upstream components of the imaging pipeline, including exam modality selection, hardware design, exam protocol selection, data acquisition, image reconstruction, and image processing. A breadth of applications and their potential for impact is shown across multiple imaging modalities, including ultrasound, computed tomography, and MRI.

Organ segmentation, chest radiograph classification, and lung and liver nodule detections are some of the popular artificial intelligence (AI) tasks in chest and abdominal radiology due to the wide availability of public datasets. AI algorithms have achieved performance comparable to humans in less time for several organ segmentation tasks, and some lesion detection and classification tasks. This article introduces the current published articles of AI applied to chest and abdominal radiology, including organ segmentation, lesion detection, classification, and predicting prognosis.

Radiologists have been at the forefront of the digitization process in medicine. Artificial intelligence (AI) is a promising area of innovation, particularly in medical imaging. The number of applications of AI in neuroradiology has also grown. This article illustrates some of these applications. This article reviews machine learning challenges related to neuroradiology. The first approval of reimbursement for an AI algorithm by the Centers for Medicare and Medicaid Services, covering a stroke software for early detection of large vessel occlusion, is also discussed.

We present an overview of current clinical musculoskeletal imaging applications for artificial intelligence, as well as potential future applications and techniques.

Harlan Benjamin Harvey and Vrushab Gowda

Artificial intelligence technology promises to redefine the practice of radiology. However, it exists in a nascent phase and remains largely untested in the clinical space. This nature is both a cause and consequence of the uncertain legaleregulatory environment it enters. This discussion aims to shed light on these challenges, tracing the various pathways toward approval by the US Food and Drug Administration, the future of government oversight, privacy issues, ethical dilemmas, and practical considerations related to implementation in radiologist practice.

Babak Saboury, Michael Morris, and Eliot Siegel

No one knows what the paradigm shift of artificial intelligence will bring to medical imaging. In this article, we attempt to predict how artificial intelligence will impact radiology based on a critical review of current innovations. The best way to predict the future is to anticipate, prepare, and create it. We anticipate that radiology will need to enhance current infrastructure, collaborate with others, learn the challenges and pitfalls of the technology, and maintain a healthy skepticism about artificial intelligence while embracing its potential to allow us to become more productive, accurate, secure, and impactful in the care of our patients.

PROGRAM OBJECTIVE
The objective of the *Radiologic Clinics of North America* is to keep practicing radiologists and radiology residents up to date with current clinical practice in radiology by providing timely articles reviewing the state of the art in patient care.

TARGET AUDIENCE
Practicing radiologists, radiology residents, and other healthcare professionals who provide patient care utilizing radiologic findings.

LEARNING OBJECTIVES
Upon completion of this activity, participants will be able to:
1. Describe foundational techniques and clinical applications of AI technologies in radiology.
2. Discuss Natural Language Processing, image pre-processing, machine learning and deep learning in radiology.
3. Recognize upstream and downstream clinical applications of AI in radiology.

ACCREDITATION
The Elsevier Office of Continuing Medical Education (EOCME) is accredited by the Accreditation Council for Continuing Medical Education (ACCME) to provide continuing medical education for physicians.

The EOCME designates this journal-based CME activity for a maximum of 14 *AMA PRA Category 1 Credit*(s)™. Physicians should claim only the credit commensurate with the extent of their participation in the activity.

All other healthcare professionals requesting continuing education credit for this enduring material will be issued a certificate of participation.

DISCLOSURE OF CONFLICTS OF INTEREST
The EOCME assesses conflict of interest with its instructors, faculty, planners, and other individuals who are in a position to control the content of CME activities. All relevant conflicts of interest that are identified are thoroughly vetted by EOCME for fair balance, scientific objectivity, and patient care recommendations. EOCME is committed to providing its learners with CME activities that promote improvements or quality in healthcare and not a specific proprietary business or a commercial interest.

The planning committee, staff, authors and editors listed below have identified no financial relationships or relationships to products or devices they or their spouse/life partner have with commercial interest related to the content of this CME activity:
Nitamar Abdala, MD, PhD; Cagan Alkan, MS; Tarik K. Alkasab, MD, PhD; Renata R. Almeida, MD, PhD; Bernardo C. Bizzo, MD, PhD; Christopher Bridge, DPhil; Ken Chang, PhD; Regina Chavous-Gibson, MSN, RN; Tessa S. Cook, MD, PhD; Jared Dunnmon, PhD; Suely Fazio Ferraciolli, MD; Vrushab Gowda, JD; Harlan Benjamin Harvey, MD, JD; Qiyuan Hu, BA; Jayashree Kalpathy-Cramer, PhD; Pradeep Kuttysankaran; Sungwon Lee, MD, PhD; Michael Morris, MD, MS; Simukayi Mutasa, MD; Jay B. Patel, BS; Oleg Pianykh, PhD; Erik Ranschaert, MD, PhD; Daniel L. Rubin, MD, MS; Babak Saboury, MD, MPH; Christopher M. Sandino, PhD; Eliot Siegel, MD, FSIIM, FACR; Jackson Steinkamp, MD; Laurens Topff, MD; John Vassallo; Kristen W. Yeom, MD; Paul H. Yi, MD

The planning committee, staff, authors, and editors listed below have identified financial relationships or relationships to products or devices they or their spouse/life partner have with commercial interest related to the content of this CME activity:
Akshay S. Chaudhari, PhD: Consultant/advisor: Chondrometrics GmbH, Culvert Engineering, Edge Analytics, Image Analysis Group, ICM, Skope, Subtle Medical; Stock ownership: Brain Key, Inc, LVIS Corp, Subtle Medical; Research support: GE Healthcare, Philips

Elizabeth K. Cole, MS: Research support: GE Healthcare

Jeremy Dahl, PhD: Research support: Siemens Healthcare; Consultant/advisor: Cephasonics Ultrasound, Vortex Imaging, Inc.
Bradley J. Erickson, MD, PhD: Founder, Stockholder: FlowSIGMA, Inc.

Maryellen L. Giger, PhD: Stockholder: Hologic, Inc.; Royalties: Hologic, GE Medical Systems, Median Technologies, Riverain Technologies, Mitsubishi, Toshiba; Co-founder: Qlarity Imaging

Dongwoon Hyun, PhD: Consultant/advisor: Exo Imaging, Inc.

Abdullah-Al-Zubaer Imran, PhD: Research support: GE Healthcare

Felipe Campos Kitamura, MD, MSc, PhD: Consultant/advisor: MD.ai

Thomas W. Loehfelm, MD, PhD: Founder: Panorad, LLC

Andreas M. Loening, MD, PhD: Research support: GE Healthcare

Ian Pan, MD: Consultant/advisor: MD.ai

Ronald M. Summers, MD, PhD: Royalties: iCAD, Inc., ScanMed, LLC, Philips, Translation Holdings, Ping An

Shreyas S. Vasanawala, MD, PhD: Research support: GE Healthcare; Consultant/advisor: Arterys, Inc., HeartVista, Inc.

Adam S. Wang, PhD: Research support: GE Healthcare, Siemens Healthineers, Varex Imaging

UNAPPROVED/OFF-LABEL USE DISCLOSURE
The EOCME requires CME faculty to disclose to the participants:
1. When products or procedures being discussed are off-label, unlabelled, experimental, and/or investigational (not US Food and Drug Administration [FDA] approved); and
2. Any limitations on the information presented, such as data that are preliminary or that represent ongoing research, interim analyses, and/or unsupported opinions. Faculty may discuss information about pharmaceutical agents that is outside of FDA-approved labelling. This information is intended solely for CME and is not intended to promote off-label use of these medications. If you have any questions, contact the medical affairs department of the manufacturer for the most recent pre-scribing information.

TO ENROLL
To enroll in the *Radiologic Clinics of North America* Continuing Medical Education program, call customer service at 1-800-654-2452 or sign up online at http://www.theclinics.com/home/cme. The CME program is available to subscribers for an additional annual fee of USD 356.00.

METHOD OF PARTICIPATION
In order to claim credit, participants must complete the following:
1. Complete enrolment as indicated above.
2. Read the activity.
3. Complete the CME Test and Evaluation. Participants must achieve a score of 70% on the test. All CME Tests and Evaluations must be completed online.

CME INQUIRIES/SPECIAL NEEDS
For all CME inquiries or special needs, please contact elsevierCME@elsevier.com.

RADIOLOGIC CLINICS OF NORTH AMERICA

RELATED SERIES

Advances in Clinical Radiology
Available at: https://www.advancesinclinicalradiology.com/
Magnetic Resonance Imaging Clinics
Available at: https://www.mri.theclinics.com/
Neuroimaging Clinics
Available at: www.neuroimaging.theclinics.com
PET Clinics
Available at: www.pet.theclinics.com

THE CLINICS ARE AVAILABLE ONLINE!
Access your subscription at:
www.theclinics.com

Preface
Artificial Intelligence in Radiology: Opportunities and Challenges

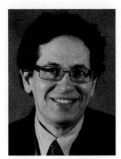

Daniel L. Rubin, MD, MS
Editor

Artificial Intelligence (AI) is currently one of the hottest topics in Radiology, with the potential to impact nearly every aspect of Radiologists' work. There are now many companies both large and small marketing AI tools to assist radiology practice broadly, such as exam ordering, scheduling, protocolling, image enhancement, image interpretation, and reporting. Increasingly, Radiologists will be called on to make or give input into decisions about adopting AI algorithms and will participate in their critical evaluation, deployment monitoring, and even application development. It is thus crucial for radiologists to have an understanding of this technology—not only the principles on which it works but also the broad range of clinical applications and regulatory issues underpinning it—in order to be educated consumers and future participants in its creation.

This issue of *Radiologic Clinics of North America* provides an overview of the foundational techniques and clinical applications of AI technologies.

Since text reports, clinical data, and images are the core data in radiology, there are articles on natural language processing, image preprocessing, machine learning, and deep learning in radiology. There is also an article on techniques for evaluation of AI tools, to equip Radiologists for assessment of the limitations of these tools and understand how they perform in their own patient populations.

Later articles provide a broad overview of clinical applications of AI, which can be divided into "upstream" and "downstream" applications. "Upstream" refers to all processing that happens up until the time the image is produced by the imaging device. This includes applications in the preliminary steps in the lifecycle of ordering of imaging exams, patient scheduling, choosing the suitable protocol for the imaging study, processing the image once it is acquired by the modality, and creating a prioritized study worklist. Once the image is produced, it flows "downstream" for the

Radiol Clin N Am 59 (2021) xv–xvi
https://doi.org/10.1016/j.rcl.2021.08.010
0033-8389/21/© 2021 Published by Elsevier Inc.

radiologic.theclinics.com

radiologist to interpret. Many clinical AI applications focus on this step, including those for disease detection, segmentation of structures or disease, diagnosis, and even clinical prediction. Articles in this issue focusing on the major clinical specialties in radiology summarize emerging applications for image preprocessing and enhancement as well as radiology workflow, including order entry, reporting, and quality improvement. This issue concludes with an article that looks forward to future directions for AI in radiology.

AI is the latest "modality" to enter radiology, and like all new modalities, radiologists need to understand its capabilities, clinical applications, and—importantly, since it is still a maturing field—its limitations and ways to assess them. AI will be unique, however, in being a true partner for radiologists, enhancing their practice in many ways. Providing the background to enable radiologists to understand these methods and how best to use them is the goal of this issue of *Radiologic Clinics of North America*.

Daniel L. Rubin, MD, MS
Department of Biomedical Data Science
Stanford University
Medical School Office Building
1265 Welch Road, Room X-335
Stanford, CA 94305-5479, USA

E-mail address:
dlrubin@stanford.edu

Basic Artificial Intelligence Techniques

Natural Language Processing of Radiology Reports

Jackson Steinkamp, MD[a], Tessa S. Cook, MD, PhD[b],*

KEYWORDS

• Natural language processing • Radiology reports • Transformers • Word embeddings • Radiology

KEY POINTS

- *Natural language processing* describes computer programming that aims to process or generate natural language data, and it is largely divided into symbolic (eg, rule-based) and statistical (eg, machine learning) approaches.
- Common tasks useful in radiology report NLP include document classification, sentence classification, named entity recognition, relation extraction, automatic summarization, question answering, and image captioning.
- Even the relatively restricted domain of radiology report text is complex and consists of phenomena that must be accounted for in task design, such as negation, uncertainty, and coreference.
- *Simple string matching* and *regular expressions* are useful techniques to gain initial familiarity with a dataset in advance of performing NLP and can provide quick baseline performance measures.
- *Word embeddings* are vector representations of tokens designed to capture notions of similarity and difference between them. Recurrent neural networks and attention-based networks, such as *transformers*, are common architectures that tend to perform well on NLP tasks.

INTRODUCTION

Natural language processing (NLP) is a subfield of computer science and linguistics. NLP involves the creation and study of computer programs that interact with human language data, including written, typed, or spoken language.[1] Specific NLP applications might extract relevant pieces of information from language data,[2–4] generate language data automatically,[5–7] or change the form of language data (eg, translation, text-to-speech software).[8,9] NLP drives real-world applications such as automatic translation systems, speech recognition or dictation software, search engines, conversational chatbots, question-answering systems, and digital assistants. NLP is considered a type of artificial intelligence (AI), which focuses on teaching computers to mimic human behavior. Machine learning (ML), which teaches computers to mimic human behavior without being explicitly programmed, and deep learning (DL), a subset of ML that uses deep neural networks, both overlap with NLP: NLP can be performed using neural networks; however, not all NLP uses ML or DL (**Fig. 1**).

Radiology reports are the final product of the radiology workflow and contain all the relevant information as parsed and interpreted by the radiologist. The format of the radiology report can vary greatly between individual radiologists, subspecialty groups, or larger practices.[10] The lack of a consistent structure or format necessitates the application of NLP to solve problems that require

a Department of Medicine, Hospital of the University of Pennsylvania, 3400 Spruce Street, Philadelphia, PA 19104, USA; b Perelman School of Medicine at the University of Pennsylvania, 3400 Spruce Street, 1 Silverstein Radiology, Philadelphia, PA 19104, USA
* Corresponding author.
E-mail address: Tessa.Cook@pennmedicine.upenn.edu

Radiol Clin N Am 59 (2021) 919–931
https://doi.org/10.1016/j.rcl.2021.06.003
0033-8389/21/Published by Elsevier Inc.

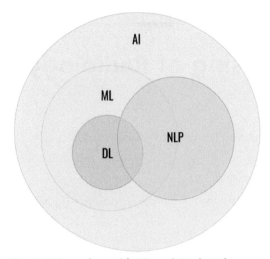

Fig. 1. NLP overlaps with ML and DL, but there are NLP techniques that do not use either ML or DL.

extraction of information concepts or even discrete data from radiology reports.[11–13] Radiology use cases of NLP have the potential to improve routine patient care,[13–15] clinician efficiency,[16] and by extension, even job satisfaction. In addition, NLP also enables novel uses of routinely generated radiology data—for research studies,[17] quality improvement initiatives,[18] and medical education.[19] This article discusses the major paradigms of NLP, common NLP tasks, and how these tasks map into the world of radiology. We discuss the differences between ML and non-ML approaches to NLP, as well as common linguistic phenomena that make NLP projects both interesting and uniquely difficult. Last, we discuss use cases of NLP for radiology reports and an end-to-end example of a radiology NLP project.

NATURAL LANGUAGE PROCESSING PARADIGMS

Like other domains of data science and AI, NLP can be divided into symbolic and statistical paradigms.[20] These differ fundamentally in how they approach language data and are typically not combined. Symbolic systems specify an exact algorithmic protocol for the system to follow using precise, human-designed rules.[21] For example, if trying to identify normal-appearing organs in a report one might prescribe the following rule: *if there is a word representing the name of an organ, followed by the phrase "appears X," where X is one of the words in the set ["normal", "unremarkable"], then the organ is normal-appearing.* Most of the work in a symbolic NLP algorithm goes into writing such rules. Regular expressions, which allow

flexible, elaborate text matching, are a valuable tool for implementing complex rules.[22]

Symbolic, or rule-based, systems can be useful for multiple reasons. First, they are relatively interpretable: the user knows exactly why a system produced a particular answer, including why it might make a particular incorrect decision. Symbolic systems are therefore also modifiable—it is relatively straightforward for the algorithm designer to add additional rules or exceptions, enabling simple incorporation of new knowledge or the correction of errors. Debugging or updating a symbolic system just requires carefully reading and editing the rules. In addition, symbolic approaches do not require labeling large amounts of training data to train a model, in the way that ML models do. However, given the complexity and variability of language, symbolic approaches tend to be difficult to scale to complex problems. Owing to their reliance on precisely specified rules, symbolic systems tend to be "brittle," that is, they break if the data are even slightly different from what was expected. Simple but common linguistic phenomena such as typographical errors, synonyms, indirect references (eg, pronouns), and variation in grammatical forms make specifying all possible instances of a rule extremely difficult. Furthermore, certain linguistic tasks are less amenable to rule-based approaches. Imagine, for example, specifying all the rules required to answer whether a sentence expresses a positive or negative emotional sentiment, or to answer arbitrary questions about a radiology report. By contrast, the statistical paradigm, which includes ML techniques, eschews specific linguistic knowledge and hand-crafted rules in favor of an "end-to-end" approach that relies on a set of expert-annotated examples of the desired task.[23] The system takes these examples, known as the *training set*, and uses an algorithm to convert that information into a general procedure for labeling unseen examples; this is considered the *training* process. To evaluate the performance of the system, a separate *test set*, which does not contain the same examples as the training set, is used to evaluate the resulting model's performance. Neural networks trained using gradient descent are one example of a statistical NLP approach.[24] For instance, one could train an algorithm to decide whether a radiology report contains findings that require immediate clinical action.[25] Under a supervised learning paradigm, the radiology reports could be annotated at the document level, where "1" indicates a finding requiring action and "0" does not, and then the system uses these data to create an algorithm for annotating the unseen reports accordingly.

There are many benefits to statistical NLP approaches. A statistical solution does not require painstakingly crafting hundreds of linguistic rules. In fact, it does not even require the developer to know *why* an answer might be correct; all that is required is training data annotated with correct answers. Many of these algorithms, including deep neural networks, are able to handle "complex" or "fuzzy" logic, which does not easily map to a narrow set of symbolic rules, and are often more robust to small changes than symbolic approaches. Some complex problems, including open domain question answering, seem to be tractable only under a statistical paradigm. Disadvantages include the following: although less work is required to specify rules, that work is channeled into creation of high-quality annotations and large training data sets. DL systems, in particular, require large amounts of annotated training examples to effectively learn from. Statistical NLP solutions also tend to be less interpretable—it may be impossible to know exactly *why* a system got an answer wrong—and difficult to modify in predictable ways. It is difficult to edit a single behavior of an ML algorithm in isolation without retraining it entirely, and even then there are no foolproof ways to ensure that the system changes in the desired direction.

Despite advances in ML in recent decades, there are still scenarios when a symbolic approach is preferable. To decide between a symbolic and statistical algorithm, one should consider the characteristics of the specific task at hand. If it would be easy to specify all the rules required to perform a task in a foolproof or near-foolproof way, a symbolic approach is generally faster and more reliable. Similarly, if it is important to be able to edit or augment your system in predictable ways (beyond just "acquiring more data"), or to know exactly *why* the system got something wrong, a symbolic approach is likely required. However, for more complex or fuzzy tasks, which may be difficult to specify due to the complexity of natural language, an ML or statistical approach is likely to perform better.

TYPES OF NATURAL LANGUAGE PROCESSING TASKS

NLP tasks range from the relatively simple (splitting a document into sentences) to the extremely complex (answering arbitrary natural language questions about a particular document). Some are better performed by certain types of algorithms; it is advisable to be guided by the recent general NLP literature to determine which systems best map to which tasks (**Table 1**). Here, we focus

Table 1
Common terms used in natural language processing

Term	Definition
Document	Single discrete body of text, eg, a radiology report
Corpus	A related set of documents, eg, all radiology reports generated between 2010 and 2020 at our hospital
Token	Small unit of text with meaning, eg, word, character, punctuation mark, or similar
Type	Class of tokens containing the same sequence of characters

on those tasks that are likely to be of interest to radiologists and data scientists working with radiology reports.

Tokenization is the process of splitting a document up into its corresponding tokens, which can be performed either using handwritten rules or with a trained ML model.[26] In languages that have spaces between words, such as English, simple algorithms using spaces and other punctuation marks to tokenize documents tend to work relatively well. In languages that do not use spaces to separate written words, tokenization may be a more difficult problem. Most freely available NLP software packages contain ready-made tokenization algorithms.

Information extraction (IE) refers to any NLP task that attempts to extract information from a text, instead of generating or translating text.[27] Most IE systems are designed to take messy, textual data and use it to answer a specific question.[28] There are many subtasks of information extraction, including document, sentence, or token classification; named-entity recognition (NER); relation extraction; coreference resolution; and free-text question answering.

Document classification is an umbrella term for any NLP task that classifies an entire text document into one of a set of categories and is usually applied to an entire corpus.[29,30] The input is typically a document or corpus, and the output is one or more category labels. In radiology, document classification might identify reports that (1) contain abnormal findings, (2) omit expected sections or required templates, (3) contain typographical errors, or (4) mention new or unexpected findings that require follow-up.

Similarly, *sentence classification* takes as input a single sentence and produces an answer (binary or categorical) for the sentence.[31] For example, one might wish to determine whether a sentence contains one or more follow-up recommendations, is part of the report impression, or mentions a specific organ. A sentence classification task requires preprocessing of the document into discrete sentences, which is called *sentence segmentation* or *sentence tokenization*. If the document is written with punctuation and spaces to clearly delineate sentence boundaries, sentence tokenization becomes straightforward and can be performed with many open source or free NLP packages. However, medical text sometimes contains lists, forms, tables, subheadings, nonprose text elements, and typographical errors, which can complicate the process.

Token classification produces a binary or categorical answer for each token in a document. For instance, one might ask which words in a radiology report represent the name of an organ, the beginning of the "impression" section, abnormal findings in the kidney, or the name of the clinician notified about a critical finding.

Named-Entity Recognition

Perhaps the most common token classification task is NER.[32] This task focuses on identifying which *tokens* in a document correspond to *entities* in a particular class. All the aforementioned token classification tasks are also examples of NER. NER tasks can be solved with either symbolic or statistical NLP. Generally, if the "answers" to the task can be defined, for example, identifying all the organs listed in a radiology report, a symbolic approach would be suitable. *Relation extraction* is the task of identifying conceptual relations between words, phrases, or entities in a document.[33]

To better understand these tasks, consider the sentence "There is a 2 cm lesion in the superior pole of the left kidney," that one might find in a radiology report. If the NER task is "which words specify the location of a radiologic finding?" there are multiple possible correct answers, depending on how the NER task is defined (**Fig. 2**). These

tasks require the NLP programmer to have domain-specific knowledge of the problem as well as knowledge of how the NER output is to be used. In addition, the output of the NER task does not specify the finding whose location is being described, unless the relation extraction task connects it back to the word "lesion." Relation extraction may be formulated to first identify all relevant entities, and then subsequently define their relationships, or to first perform the NER task and then extract the relationships to the entities.

Another important NLP operation is *coreference resolution*, by which an entity is mentioned more than once, sometimes with different words.[34] For example, in "There is a new lesion in the left kidney. It measures…," the words "lesion" and "it" refer to the same entity. Coreferent entity mentions may be spread across multiple sentences, paragraphs, or even multiple documents. In addition, the entity may be referenced in whole, in part, or in combination with other entities. For these reasons, coreference resolution, although innate to human language, remains a relatively difficult NLP task.

Text Generation

Some NLP applications are dedicated to producing natural language data, rather than extracting information from existing natural language data. These tasks are typically highly complex even with ML approaches. Perhaps the most obvious use case for text generation in radiology is automated report generation based on image data. Alternatively, *text summarization* might be useful in either extracting snippets of text verbatim from a document or summarizing the document by producing new text. Text summarization could be applied to autogenerate radiology report impressions or create versions of reports for different audiences, including patients and caregivers, primary care physicians, or specialists.[35]

Language Modeling

Language modeling predicts natural language data given surrounding context. For instance, a language model might assign a high probability that the word "cat" fills the blank in the sentence "the __ in the hat." Recent neural network-based language models such as Bidirectional Encoder Representations from Transformers (BERT)[36] and the Generative Pre-trained Transformer series[37] are trained on large corpora of existing natural language data to perform language modeling. Language models can also be repurposed to *produce* text, by having them repeatedly output

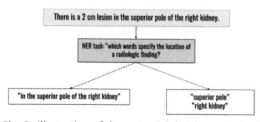

Fig. 2. Illustration of the potential decisions required in developing an NER task; "in the" and "of the" contain location information but may not have to be included in the output of the task.

the most likely next token given all the tokens that have come before. Entire documents can be built up from scratch by repeatedly applying this rule. Although the radiologic use cases for "spontaneous text generation" may not be readily apparent, well-trained language models are capable of performing certain tasks, such as question answering or automatic summarization, without explicitly being trained on them.

UNIQUE CONSIDERATIONS FOR RADIOLOGY REPORT NATURAL LANGUAGE PROCESSING

In building or evaluating NLP for radiology reports, it is worthwhile to consider the unique aspects of radiology report text that may degrade the performance of NLP developed and tested in other domains.

Structured Reporting

Structured data generally have predictable characteristics, including their form (eg, numeric, textual) or domain of acceptable values (positive real numbers). As such, they are generally easier for machines to consume, transform, and generate. Laboratory data and vital signs are highly structured, whereas natural language data are considered to be unstructured. However, some natural language data are more structured than others, simply by belonging to the same domain.

Radiology reports have inherent structure by virtue of being *radiology reports;* they will use a narrow set of words from the language, compared with a book or newspaper. Reports of abdominal imaging studies will tend to mention all the major abdominal organs. However, even within the domain of radiology reports, there is a wide spectrum of structure, depending on the imaging modality, indication, body region, and individual and institutional documentation preferences and culture.[10,38] Nevertheless, these forms of structure can all be helpful when designing an NLP task, algorithm, or model.

Negation is a common linguistic phenomenon that is extremely prevalent in radiology reports; it can take a simple form, for example, "No metastatic disease is seen in the chest," or make more oblique references to the absence of an entity or abnormality, for example, "The lungs are clear" or "There has been a prior hysterectomy." As negation is a relatively stereotyped linguistic phenomenon, and particularly if a radiology practice uses many templates, it lends itself to symbolic NLP approaches. Algorithms such as NegEx[39] have been designed for medical text, and other freely available software packages designed for general NLP applications contain explicit negation algorithms.

Statistical NLP requires negation be considered during task definition and data annotation.

Like negation, *uncertainty* is a common phenomenon in radiology reports.[40] Rarely does a radiology report contain a statement such as "this is X." More commonly, statements such as "an X cannot be excluded," "without evidence of Y," "finding suggestive of Z," or complex conditional statements such as "consider A if B" or "in light of C, D is favored" are found. These phenomena may make it difficult to define a task in terms of binary yes/no outcomes. Both symbolic and statistical approaches will need to consider these questions in their task design, data annotation, and performance assessment. Symbolic rule-based approaches will also need to include additional rules to handle the wide variety of ways to convey uncertainty in radiology reports.

USE CASES OF NATURAL LANGUAGE PROCESSING IN RADIOLOGY

As has been alluded to earlier, there are many applications for NLP in radiology. The vast majority deal with corpora of radiology reports, and more recently, use DL rather than symbolic NLP. Detection of follow-up recommendations, identification of critical findings, and characterization of disease progression are all frequent use cases.

Although earlier initiatives in radiology NLP focused almost exclusively on symbolic approaches, the more common paradigm is some combination of symbolic and statistical NLP, with the latter typically using conventional ML. There are many such examples in the literature: detecting critical findings[25] and follow-up recommendations,[41] quantifying oncologic response,[42] describing the degree of interval change in radiologic findings over time,[43] and identifying diseases such as pneumonia,[44] urinary tract calculi,[14] thromboembolism,[45] and peripheral arterial disease,[46] among others. Extraction of quantitative data from narrative reports, such as measurements,[47] BI-RADS categories,[48] and data that can predict downstream resource use,[49] are other practical applications. Report summarization, including automated generation of report impressions, has also been explored with conventional ML.[50] Radiology-pathology correlation, which has implications in quality improvement, peer learning, and resident education, leverages NLP of both radiology and pathology reports.[51]

DL radiology NLP approaches have become popular in recent years.[24] The use cases are similar to those for symbolic and non-DL statistical NLP and include quantifying oncologic response,[52] identifying pulmonary emboli,[13,30] flagging critical findings,[53,54] and detecting follow-up recommendations.[55] Broader information extraction from radiology reports has also been demonstrated.[56]

FRAMEWORK FOR PERFORMING RADIOLOGY NATURAL LANGUAGE PROCESSING

This section is intended to provide a general framework for performing radiology NLP (**Fig. 3**). Rather than focusing on specific NLP techniques or models, which may become obsolete, this discussion will present a high-level overview with a common sample use case in mind: detecting pulmonary nodules reported on computed tomography (CT).

Specify the Task in Detail

Defining the NLP task clearly and unequivocally with the use case in mind has major downstream implications, which is why it is the first step. Identifying which *reports* describe pulmonary nodules is very different from identifying the specific *sentence* and *word* tokens used in the descriptions. In other words, at what level is the classification task being performed: document, sentence, or token level?

Before data annotation can begin, multiple questions need to be considered. Is the task to identify the reports that contain the nodules, or the nodules themselves? What constitutes a nodule to be counted—any described nodule or only new nodules that are not already being followed? If the goal is to count the number of chest CTs on which nodules were diagnosed in 2020, each "document" (ie, report) would be labeled as "1" for containing a nodule and "0" otherwise,

and the output of the eventual NLP would be similar. Alternatively, if the goal is to notify the ordering physician of the need to follow-up an incidental pulmonary nodule, the NLP would also need to extract additional information about the nodules (size, location, severity, etc.). Specifying the task in detail will help the annotation process run smoothly and efficiently, while ensuring a consistent high-quality testing data set.

Select an Evaluation Metric

Once the task is defined, an appropriate metric or series of metrics for algorithmic performance must also be defined.[57] The most common metrics include precision, recall, accuracy, and F_1 score, which are defined in **Fig. 4**. *Precision* (or positive predictive value) measures the ability of the model to avoid false-positives. *Recall* (or sensitivity) measures the ability of the model to avoid false-negatives. *Accuracy* is the percentage of document labels the model correctly predicted; because it treats positive and negative examples equally, performance is equally affected by a false-positive as by a false-negative. The *F_1 score* is the harmonic mean of precision and recall. The metrics behave differently in the setting of class imbalance or situations where the different categories are not equally represented in the data. For example, there are likely going to be many more reports *without* pulmonary nodules than *with* them. Although recall and precision are useful in the setting of class imbalance, they can also become artificially elevated by algorithms and models that exploit the imbalance. F_1 score balances precision and recall and is often better than accuracy in such situations.

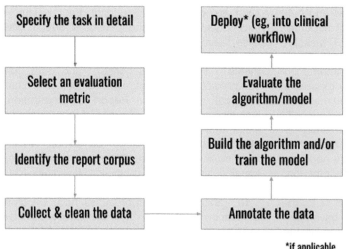

Fig. 3. Framework for radiology NLP implementation.

*if applicable

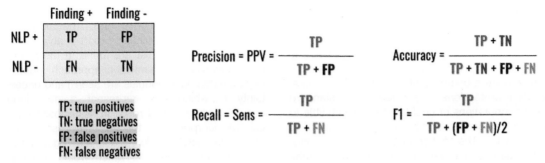

Fig. 4. Metrics for algorithmic performance.

Identifying the Corpus

Although task selection is presented as the first step, the availability of a particular dataset may dictate which tasks or projects are feasible. How will the reports for the project be identified—by modality, by text tag in the reports, or by patient criteria? How many reports are accessible—the practice's entire database, a subset of modalities, or an even smaller set of reports collected for a previous project? Will the data used to build the NLP be representative of the larger scope of data to which the NLP will be applied? These considerations are important as the corpus of reports to be processed is identified. In our example use case, choosing a corpus of chest CTs is appropriate; however, one might wish to decide between all outpatient chest CTs at a practice, all chest CTs at a particular practice location, or only lung cancer screening chest CTs; each of these corpora will likely necessitate a different NLP design with variability in performance.

The type of NLP also dictates the need for data. Symbolic NLP will require a single dataset to evaluate the algorithm. However, statistical NLP, that is, ML approaches, will require both a training set and a test set. The training set will need to be annotated or labeled, either manually by experts or in a semiautomated approach (which may involve extracting elements of a structured template from the reports).[56,58] In our practice, all chest CT templates contain a section for nodule follow-up, which is assigned to "none" if no nodules are detected. As a result, chest CTs are labeled for the presence of pulmonary nodules during routine clinical practice and become an easy dataset to which NLP can be applied. Practically, annotation is time and labor intensive, so the amount of person-time available for annotation may be what limits the size of the available datasets. When choosing the size of the dataset, the training set and the test set should not overlap, and the test set should only be used to evaluate algorithm/model performance. The size of the test set can be selected according to standard statistical principles regarding significance and power (ie, X reports would be required to detect effect size Y with power level Z).

Collecting and Cleaning the Data

Data aggregation and cleaning is not only important but also time-consuming. When doing statistical NLP, an added consideration is that ML systems are very good at learning from patterns and finding correlations, even if spurious or unintended; this can result in high performance due to peculiarities in the data, rather than use of the text data to make an appropriate prediction. For instance, if the ML-based NLP "learns" the styles of certain radiologists, that is, their templates, word choices, or grammatical preferences, the system may spuriously learn to correlate particular radiologists with the presence of pulmonary nodules in the report. Writing style and word choice are nearly impossible to effectively purge from a dataset. Instead, careful selection of a large, representative set of reports is the best strategy to mitigate an ML algorithm's potential to "cheat." Cleaning data of easily identified text elements, such as radiologists' names or structured templates that also serve as data labels, becomes additionally important. In our practice, pulmonary nodule follow-up recommendations are encapsulated in a standard template, from which the radiologist chooses the most appropriate recommendation. A symbolic NLP may identify the phrase "pulmonary nodule" in the recommendation and use that to signify the presence of a nodule in the report, whereas an ML system may learn that the presence of the template indicates that a nodule is being described elsewhere in the report. Formatting reports to remove unnecessary white space and consistently encode line breaks may also be helpful.

Annotating the Data

Data annotation is one of the most time- and labor-intensive parts of an NLP project. A variety of software packages for text annotation currently exist, both free and paid, open source and proprietary.[59] Besides the raw hours required to annotate the data, one should also consider the expertise required of the annotators. Does the task require a board-certified radiologist or other medical professional to provide a gold-standard set of annotations or could someone with little to no medical background be adequately trained to perform it?[60] The cost and time required to annotate a dataset may vary greatly depending on the required expertise as well as the raw size of the dataset. If person power is available, having multiple annotators label the same reports may be helpful, both for increasing the overall quality of the resulting dataset and to enable evaluation of individual-level human performance and interrater reliability. In this instance, it is important to prepare an annotation guide and to give the annotators the option to discuss ambiguous situations with each other or the project lead. Otherwise, if each annotator makes independent assumptions, the noise in the data labels will ultimately affect the performance of the algorithm/model. Very few publicly available radiology report datasets exist, and even fewer with labels.[61,62]

Build the Algorithm and/or Train the Model

Resource availability often determines the NLP approach that is chosen for a particular problem. In addition to the resources required for annotation, computing requirements can also limit the choice of NLP technique. To identify pulmonary nodules described in a corpus of chest CT reports, we might use either symbolic or statistical approaches.

Symbolic natural language processing: string matching

A *string* is defined as a series of characters. String matching is the simplest and fastest NLP approach and can often serve as a starting point for a more sophisticated approach. If nothing else, it is valuable in becoming familiar with the dataset and establishing a performance baseline against which more advanced methods can be benchmarked. **Fig. 5** illustrates a simple string

```
for document in corpus
    contains_nodule = False
    for expression in ["lung nodule", "pulmonary nodule"]
        If expression in document.text
            contains_nodule = True
    endfor
    document.answer = contains_nodule
endfor
```

Fig. 5. String matching algorithm to identify pulmonary nodules in reports.

matching algorithm (written in pseudocode) for the lung nodule detection task. The algorithm returns true for a particular report if any of the strings in the match list are found in the report text. However, this simplistic approach ignores negation ("No lung nodules are seen") and uncertainty ("...which may represent a new lung nodule"), which would result in false-positives. It fails to incorporate all the possible descriptions of a pulmonary nodule ("...a 5 mm right upper lobe nodule is seen..."), which would result in false-negatives. It neglects to consider the surrounding context of a word and would be susceptible to voice recognition errors. However, it is a quick starting point from which to build based on the limitations identified and can guide the next choice of NLP approach.

Symbolic natural language processing: regular expressions

A *regular expression* is a search pattern of characters designed to allow for matching of more complex text patterns than single strings. For instance, the pattern "a*b" matches any number of *a's*, followed by a single *b* and the pattern "favo?urite" matches either the US ("favorite") or UK ("favourite") spelling of the same word. Combinations of individual operators can result in matching of elaborate, complex text patterns. Regular expressions are a step up from simple string matching in flexibility while maintaining string matching's advantages (ease of implementation, interpretability, low computational cost). However, they suffer from many of the same limitations as string matching, and as with string matching can be valuable data exploration tools.

Statistical natural language processing: neural networks

An *artificial neural network* is an ML model loosely modeled off of concepts from the biological brain, whose atomic unit is the *artificial neuron,* and which are commonly trained via *backpropagation* with *gradient descent*. There are 2 major neural network architectures that have been particularly salient in NLP thus far and less commonly present in other subfields such as computer vision, which merit special mention.

Statistical natural language processing: word embeddings

Pixel data lend itself well to ML, which uses gradient descent to move *continuously* and *gradually* within a space of possible hypotheses; the similarity or difference between 2 pixel values is easily computed. However, word and subword tokens, which are the atomic elements of NLP, do not have the same properties. As a result, the notion of word similarity or difference requires that they be encoded in a different way. Representing words as categorical variables is one solution, but treats words as completely independent of one another, and equally "far apart" in vector space, which does not help the similarity problem. *Word embeddings* represent words as points, or vectors, in a high-dimensional vector space. This enables calculation of "distances" between words, such that similar words are "closer together" and different words are "further apart." Word embeddings can be learned based on large volumes of real natural language text and used to train ML algorithms on a downstream task, such as our pulmonary nodule detection task. Word embeddings are generally learned by predicting a word token based on surrounding tokens. Word2Vec, GloVe, and fasttext have become increasingly popular for creating word vector embeddings.[30,33,63–65] In some cases, custom word embeddings specific to medical or radiological text may lead to better model performance.[66,67]

Statistical natural language processing: recurrent neural networks

One of the most important design choices in a neural network is its connectivity pattern. Different connectivity patterns between artificial neurons in a network impose different *inductive biases.* An inductive bias refers to a set of assumptions baked into a learning algorithm that informs how the algorithm will generalize to unseen data. *Recurrent neural networks* (RNNs) were designed to mimic the inductive bias of sequentiality, the fact that we read or listen to text in sequence and update our understanding of the text token by token as more information is accumulated. In general, RNNs process an individual token, update their internal "state" (which reflects the information accumulated up until the current time point), and then process the next token in the sequence (**Fig. 6**). At present, the long short-term memory cell and gated recurrent unit are 2 of the most common atomic units used in RNNs for NLP.[30]

Statistical natural language processing: attention-based neural networks

Rather than a convolutional paradigm (neurons representing pixels or words are connected only to their neighbors), a recurrent paradigm (inputs are processed sequentially), or a fully connected paradigm (all neurons in a layer are connected to all neurons in the next layer), an attentional paradigm enables the network to essentially learn a connectivity pattern and have this connectivity pattern depend on the specific data point being processed at the time. *Transformers*, deep neural

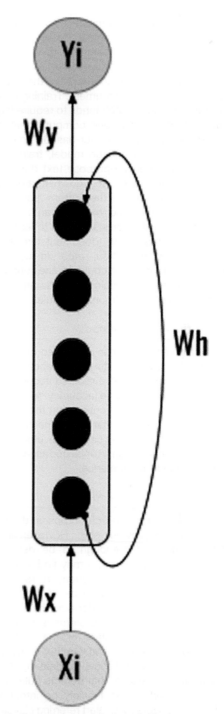

Fig. 6. Recurrent neural network diagram.

networks consisting primarily of attentional layers, operate by using successive self-attentional layers to form progressively "deeper" representations of each word token. At each layer of the network, the neural unit associated with each token calculates an attentional map to every other token in the document and uses the information from the tokens with high attention matches to update its representation of the original "query" token. Through successive application of this rule, the word representations get progressively more complex and can incorporate context from the related tokens in the rest of the document. Training transformer models from scratch tends to require large amounts of training data and computational power. However, transformer-based models including the BERT language model, trained on large volumes of general-purpose text data, can be effectively leveraged for downstream NLP tasks without retraining them from scratch.[36] Instead, these pretrained models can be fine-tuned using a smaller corpus of data to learn the specific downstream task (document classification, information extraction, etc.). In our use case, a BERT transformer could be fine-tuned on a corpus of chest CT radiology reports and used to detect mentions of pulmonary nodules.

Evaluate the Algorithm/Model

Once the algorithm has been developed or the ML model has been trained, its performance on the hold-out *test set* should be evaluated according to the metrics discussed above (accuracy, recall, precision, F1 score, etc.). It is critical that the test set contain labeled examples that are distinct from any data that have already been used to develop the algorithm or model, to obtain an unbiased assessment of algorithm/model performance.

Deploy the Algorithm/Model (if Applicable)

If the use case is for research purposes, the process ends at the previous step. However, if the system performs well enough to be deployed into the radiology workflow, it may find a role as an adjunct to clinical care, education, research, or quality improvement initiatives. If this is the case, it is important to consider how the application will integrate with other systems, such as the radiology information system or the dictation/voice recognition system, and whether those systems, if commercial, will allow for data input into the application. A system that detects pulmonary nodules in reports could feasibly be integrated with the medical record, to alert referring clinicians about the need for follow-up. It could also be integrated into a practice's quality and safety program to ensure that patients with recommended follow-up return for their care.

SUMMARY

Because of the inherent variety and variability in radiology reports, NLP has become a valuable technique for extracting discrete data and meaningful information from reports. Both symbolic and statistical approaches exist, and fundamental NLP tasks can often be applied to a radiology corpus. As with other kinds of ML, a great deal of attention must be paid to preparation of the data to be used. There are numerous use cases for radiology NLP, and ongoing efforts such as the development of standardized reporting templates and common data elements will only augment more powerful DL-based techniques that continue to be developed.

CLINICS CARE POINTS

- NLP has become a valuable technique for extracting discrete data and meaningful information from reports.
- Standardized reporting templates and common data elements will augment deep learning-based NLP for radiology in the future.

DISCLOSURE

The authors have no disclosures relevant to the submitted work.

REFERENCES

1. Chowdhury GG. Natural language processing. Annu Rev Inf Sci Technol 2005;37(1):51–89.
2. Glaser AP, Jordan BJ, Cohen J, et al. Automated Extraction of Grade, Stage, and Quality Information From Transurethral Resection of Bladder Tumor Pathology Reports Using Natural Language Processing. JCO Clin Cancer Inform 2018;(2):1–8.
3. Moon S, Liu S, Scott CG, et al. Automated extraction of sudden cardiac death risk factors in hypertrophic cardiomyopathy patients by natural language processing. Int J Med Inf 2019;128:32–8.
4. Si Y, Roberts K. A Frame-Based NLP System for Cancer-Related Information Extraction. AMIA Annu Symp Proc 2018;2018:1524–33.
5. Zeni Montenegro JL, Andre Da Costa C, Da Rosa Righi R, Roehrs A, Farias ER. A Proposal for Postpartum Support Based on Natural Language Generation Model. In: 2018 International Conference on Computational Science and Computational Intelligence (CSCI). IEEE. Las Vegas, NV, December 12-14, 2018. https://doi.org/10.1109/CSCI46756.2018.00151.
6. Dale R. Natural language generation: The commercial state of the art in 2020. Nat Lang Eng 2020; 26(4):481–7.

7. Gatt A, Krahmer E. Survey of the State of the Art in Natural Language Generation: Core tasks, applications and evaluation. J Artif Intell Res 2018;61:65–170.

8. Tootooni MS, Pasupathy KS, Heaton HA, et al. CCMapper: An adaptive NLP-based free-text chief complaint mapping algorithm. Comput Biol Med 2019;113:103398.

9. Weng W-H, Chung Y-A, Szolovits P. Unsupervised Clinical Language Translation. In: Proceedings of the 25th ACM SIGKDD International Conference on Knowledge Discovery & Data Mining. ACM. Anchorage, AK, July 2019. p. 3121–1. https://doi.org/10.1145/3292500.3330710.

10. European Society of Radiology (ESR). ESR paper on structured reporting in radiology. Insights Imaging 2018;9(1):1–7. https://doi.org/10.1007/s13244-017-0588-8.

11. Goldberg-Stein S, Chernyak V. Adding Value in Radiology Reporting. J Am Coll Radiol 2019;16(9):1292–8. https://doi.org/10.1016/j.jacr.2019.05.042.

12. Bozkurt S, Alkim E, Banerjee I, et al. Automated detection of measurements and their descriptors in radiology reports using a hybrid natural language processing algorithm. J Digit Imaging 2019;32(4):544–53.

13. Chen MC, Ball RL, Yang L, et al. Deep learning to classify radiology free-text reports. Radiology 2018;286(3):845–52.

14. Li AY, Elliot N. Natural language processing to identify ureteric stones in radiology reports. J Med Imaging Radiat Oncol 2019;63(3):307–10.

15. Trivedi G, Dadashzadeh ER, Handzel RM, et al. Interactive NLP in Clinical Care: Identifying Incidental Findings in Radiology Reports. Appl Clin Inform 2019;10(04):655–69.

16. Yetisgen-Yildiz M, Gunn ML, Xia F, et al. A text processing pipeline to extract recommendations from radiology reports. J Biomed Inform 2013;46(2):354–62.

17. Cai T, Giannopoulos AA, Yu S, et al. Natural Language Processing Technologies in Radiology Research and Clinical Applications. RadioGraphics 2016;36(1):176–91.

18. Kalra A, Chakraborty A, Fine B, et al. Machine Learning for Automation of Radiology Protocols for Quality and Efficiency Improvement. J Am Coll Radiol 2020;17(9):1149–58.

19. Tajmir SH, Alkasab TK. Toward Augmented Radiologists. Acad Radiol 2018;25(6):747–50.

20. Maruyama Y. Symbolic and Statistical Theories of Cognition: Towards Integrated Artificial Intelligence. In: Cleophas L, Massink M, editors. Software Engineering and formal methods. SEFM 2020 Collocated Workshops. Vol 12524. Lecture notes in computer science. Springer International Publishing; 2021. p. 129–46. https://doi.org/10.1007/978-3-030-67220-1_11.

21. Nguyen AN, Lawley MJ, Hansen DP, et al. Symbolic rule-based classification of lung cancer stages from free-text pathology reports. J Am Med Inform Assoc 2010;17(4):440–5.

22. Bui DDA, Zeng-Treitler Q. Learning regular expressions for clinical text classification. J Am Med Inform Assoc 2014;21(5):850–7.

23. Marcus M. New trends in natural language processing: statistical natural language processing. Proc Natl Acad Sci 1995;92(22):10052–9.

24. Sorin V, Barash Y, Konen E, et al. Deep Learning for Natural Language Processing in Radiology—Fundamentals and a Systematic Review. J Am Coll Radiol 2020;17(5):639–48.

25. Heilbrun ME, Chapman BE, Narasimhan E, et al. Feasibility of Natural Language Processing–Assisted Auditing of Critical Findings in Chest Radiology. J Am Coll Radiol 2019;16(9):1299–304.

26. Subhashini R, Kumar VJS. Shallow NLP techniques for noun phrase extraction, . Trendz in information sciences & computing(TISC2010). IEEE; 2010. p. 73–7. Available at: https://ieeexplore.ieee.org/stamp/stamp.jsp?tp=&arnumber=5714595.

27. Grishman R. Twenty-five years of information extraction. Nat Lang Eng 2019;25(06):677–92.

28. Datta S, Bernstam EV, Roberts K. A frame semantic overview of NLP-based information extraction for cancer-related EHR notes. J Biomed Inform 2019;100:103301.

29. Ferrario A, Naegelin M. The art of natural language processing: classical, modern and contemporary approaches to text document classification. SSRN Electron J Published Online 2020. https://doi.org/10.2139/ssrn.3547887.

30. Banerjee I, Ling Y, Chen MC, et al. Comparative effectiveness of convolutional neural network (CNN) and recurrent neural network (RNN) architectures for radiology text report classification. Artif Intell Med 2019;97:79–88.

31. Hassan A, Mahmood A. Convolutional Recurrent Deep Learning Model for Sentence Classification. IEEE Access 2018;6:13949–57.

32. Chen P-H. Essential Elements of Natural Language Processing: What the Radiologist Should Know. Acad Radiol 2020;27(1):6–12.

33. Lei M, Huang H, Feng C, et al. An input information enhanced model for relation extraction. Neural Comput Appl 2019;31(12):9113–26.

34. Névéol A, Zweigenbaum P. Making Sense of Big Textual Data for Health Care: Findings from the Section on Clinical Natural Language Processing. Yearb Med Inform 2017;26(01):228–34.

35. Lourenco AP, Baird GL. Optimizing Radiology Reports for Patients and Referring Physicians: Mitigating the Curse of Knowledge. Acad Radiol 2020;27(3):436–9.

36. Devlin J, Chang M-W, Lee K, et al. BERT: Pre-training of Deep Bidirectional Transformers for Language Understanding. *ArXiv181004805 Cs*. 2019. Available at: http://arxiv.org/abs/1810.04805. Accessed February 2, 2021.

37. Brown TB, Mann B, Ryder N, et al. Language Models are Few-Shot Learners. *ArXiv200514165 Cs*. 2020. Available at: http://arxiv.org/abs/2005.14165. Accessed February 2, 2021.

38. Langlotz CP. Structured radiology reporting: are we there yet? Radiology 2009;253(1):23–5.

39. Chapman WW, Bridewell W, Hanbury P, et al. A Simple Algorithm for Identifying Negated Findings and Diseases in Discharge Summaries. J Biomed Inform 2001;34(5):301–10.

40. Audi S, Pencharz D, Wagner T. Behind the hedges: how to convey uncertainty in imaging reports. Clin Radiol 2021;76(2):84–7.

41. Lou R, Lalevic D, Chambers C, et al. Automated Detection of Radiology Reports that Require Follow-up Imaging Using Natural Language Processing Feature Engineering and Machine Learning Classification. J Digit Imaging 2020;33(1):131–6.

42. Chen P-H, Zafar H, Galperin-Aizenberg M, et al. Integrating Natural Language Processing and Machine Learning Algorithms to Categorize Oncologic Response in Radiology Reports. J Digit Imaging 2018;31(2):178–84.

43. Hassanpour S, Bay G, Langlotz CP. Characterization of Change and Significance for Clinical Findings in Radiology Reports Through Natural Language Processing. J Digit Imaging 2017;30(3):314–22.

44. Dublin S, Baldwin E, Walker RL, et al. Natural Language Processing to identify pneumonia from radiology reports: NLP FOR PNEUMONIA. Pharmacoepidemiol Drug Saf 2013;22(8):834–41.

45. Pham A-D, Névéol A, Lavergne T, et al. Natural language processing of radiology reports for the detection of thromboembolic diseases and clinically relevant incidental findings. BMC Bioinformatics 2014;15(1):266.

46. Savova GK, Fan J, Ye Z, et al. Discovering peripheral arterial disease cases from radiology notes using natural language processing. AMIA Annu Symp Proc 2010;2010:722–6.

47. Sevenster M, Buurman J, Liu P, et al. Natural language processing techniques for extracting and categorizing finding measurements in narrative radiology reports. Appl Clin Inform 2015;06(03):600–10.

48. Sippo DA, Warden GI, Andriole KP, et al. Automated Extraction of BI-RADS Final Assessment Categories from Radiology Reports with Natural Language Processing. J Digit Imaging 2013;26(5):989–94.

49. Brown AD, Kachura JR. Natural Language Processing of Radiology Reports in Patients With Hepatocellular Carcinoma to Predict Radiology Resource Utilization. J Am Coll Radiol 2019;16(6):840–4.

50. Goff DJ, Loehfelm TW. Automated Radiology Report Summarization Using an Open-Source Natural Language Processing Pipeline. J Digit Imaging 2018;31(2):185–92.

51. Filice RW. Radiology-Pathology Correlation to Facilitate Peer Learning: An Overview Including Recent Artificial Intelligence Methods. J Am Coll Radiol 2019;16(9):1279–85.

52. Kehl KL, Elmarakeby H, Nishino M, et al. Assessment of Deep Natural Language Processing in Ascertaining Oncologic Outcomes From Radiology Reports. JAMA Oncol 2019;5(10):1421.

53. Jnawali K, Arbabshirani MR, Ulloa AE, Rao N, Patel AA. Automatic Classification of Radiological Report for Intracranial Hemorrhage. In: 2019 IEEE 13th International Conference on Semantic Computing (ICSC). IEEE. Newport Beach, CA, January 30-February 1, 2019. p. 187–0. https://doi.org/10.1109/ICOSC.2019.8665578.

54. Bressem KK, Adams LC, Gaudin RA, et al. Highly accurate classification of chest radiographic reports using a deep learning natural language model pretrained on 3.8 million text reports. Bioinformatics 2021;36(21):5255–61.

55. Carrodeguas E, Lacson R, Swanson W, et al. Use of Machine Learning to Identify Follow-Up Recommendations in Radiology Reports. J Am Coll Radiol 2019;16(3):336–43.

56. Steinkamp JM, Chambers C, Lalevic D, et al. Toward Complete Structured Information Extraction from Radiology Reports Using Machine Learning. J Digit Imaging 2019;32(4):554–64.

57. Powers DMW. Evaluation: from precision, recall and F-measure to ROC, informedness, markedness and correlation. ArXiv201016061 Cs Stat. 2020. Available at: http://arxiv.org/abs/2010.16061. Accessed February 2, 2021.

58. Smit A, Jain S, Rajpurkar P, et al. CheXbert: Combining Automatic Labelers and Expert Annotations for Accurate Radiology Report Labeling Using BERT. *ArXiv200409167 Cs*. 2020. Available at: http://arxiv.org/abs/2004.09167. Accessed February 2, 2021.

59. Stenetorp P, Pyssalo S, Topic G, Ohta T, Ananiadou S, Tsujii J. BRAT: a web-based tool for NLP-assisted text annotation. In: Demonstrations at the 13th Conference of the European Chapter of the Association for Computational Linguistics. Avignon, France, April 2012.

60. Ye C, Coco J, Epishova A, et al. A crowdsourcing framework for medical data sets. AMIA Jt Summits 2018;2017:273–80.

61. Demner-Fushman D, Kohli MD, Rosenman MB, et al. Preparing a collection of radiology examinations for distribution and retrieval. J Am Med Inform Assoc 2016;23(2):304–10.

62. Johnson AEW, Pollard TJ, Berkowitz SJ, et al. MIMIC-CXR, a de-identified publicly available

database of chest radiographs with free-text reports. Sci Data 2019;6(1):317.

63. Ong CJ, Orfanoudaki A, Zhang R, et al. Machine learning and natural language processing methods to identify ischemic stroke, acuity and location from radiology reports. PLoS One 2020;15(6): e0234908.

64. Nunes N, Martins B, André da Silva N, et al. A Multimodal Deep Learning Method for Classifying Chest Radiology Exams. In: Moura Oliveira P, Novais P, Reis LP, editors. *Progress in artificial intelligence.* Vol 11804. Lecture notes in computer science. Springer International Publishing; 2019. p. 323–35. https://doi.org/10.1007/978-3-030-30241-2_28.

65. López-Úbeda P, Díaz-Galiano MC, Martín-Noguerol T, et al. Detection of unexpected findings in radiology reports: A comparative study of machine learning approaches. Expert Syst Appl 2020; 160:113647.

66. Banerjee I, Madhavan S, Goldman RE, et al. Intelligent Word Embeddings of Free-Text Radiology Reports. AMIA Annu Symp Proc 2017;2017:411–20.

67. Banerjee I, Chen MC, Lungren MP, et al. Radiology report annotation using intelligent word embeddings: Applied to multi-institutional chest CT cohort. J Biomed Inform 2018;77:11–20.

Basic Artificial Intelligence Techniques
Machine Learning and Deep Learning

Bradley J. Erickson, MD, PhD

KEYWORDS

• Deep learning • Convolutional neural network • U-net • Feature engineering

KEY POINTS

- There has been and will continue to be rapid advances in deep learning technology that will have a positive impact on medical imaging.
- It is critical to understand the unique properties of medical images and the performance metrics when building a training set and training a network.
- Medical images have some unique properties compared to photographic images which require adaptation of models built for photographic imaging.

MEDICAL IMAGES

An important starting point in the application of machine learning and deep learning, particularly for those unfamiliar with medical imaging, is to recognize some of the special properties of medical images. Compared with photographic images, medical images typically have lower spatial resolution but higher contrast resolution. For instance, MR images typically are 256 × 256 and computed tomography (CT) images are 512 ×512. CT images have at least 12 bits of grayscale information, which is more than what the eye can perceive; therefore, perceiving all the information present in a CT image requires that multiple contrast and brightness settings be used. In the radiology world, these are referred to as the window width and window center. Essentially, the intensity ranges from center—width/2 up to the center + width/2. CT images have a constant intensity meaning, such that water has a value of 0 and air is −1000. And the units are Hounsfield units, honoring the inventor of the CT scanner, Sir Godfrey Hounsfield. On the other hand, other medical imaging types typically do not have a reproducible intensity scale; therefore, intensity normalization is a critical early step in the image processing pipeline.

It was recognized in the late 1980s that an open standard for representing and transmitting medical images was critical to the advance of the medical imaging sciences. That led to the development of the American College of Radiology (ACR) National Electrical Manufacturer Association (NEMA) standard, which subsequently became known as Digital Imaging and Communications in Medicine (DICOM) rather than ACR-NEMA, version 3. DICOM images consist of a header and a body, where the actual pixels of the image are the body. The header consists of several keys and values, where the keys are a set of standard and coded tags and the values are encoded in a prescribed way. DICOM tags typically are referred to as having a group and an element, each consisting of 4 hexadecimal digits. The NEMA Web site[1] contains the entire dictionary of legal DICOM tags. Thaicom does permit manufacturers to insert proprietary information in any tag where the group number is an odd number. This allows storage of information of interest to the image generator and/or not yet standardized by DICOM.

Department of Radiology, Mayo Clinic, Mayo Building East 2, 200 First Street Southwest, Rochester, MN 55905, USA
E-mail address: bje@mayo.edu

Radiol Clin N Am 59 (2021) 933–940
https://doi.org/10.1016/j.rcl.2021.06.004

HOW IMAGES ARE STORED

The original focus of DICOM was focused on the transfer of image data between 2 devices; therefore, a file format was not included in the original specification. Even today, much of the DICOM standard focuses on transfer of the image data rather than storage. There is a DICOM standard, however, for how image data should be stored, which essentially is a serialization of the header and body. Most of the time, each 2-dimensional image is stored as a separate DICOM file although standards do exist for both multidimensional and multi–time point images. Adoption of these letter formats has been slow.

Particularly before these multidimensional formats existed, medical imaging researchers developed their own formats for storing images. One of the early popular formats is referred to as the analyze[2,3] format. it had 1 file for the header information, which described the image data, whereas the other file was the actual pixel data. The Neuroimaging Informatics Technology Initiative (NIfTI) format extends the analyze format to provide more information in the header and also to join the 2 components into 1 file. There are other formats, such as mhd and nrrd, which are similar to NIfTI and supported by some specific software packages.

ELEMENTS OF MACHINE LEARNING
Features

A machine learning system requires features that are numerical values computed from the image(s). When several such values for 1 example are put together, they are called a feature vector. For a system to learn, it must be given the answer for each of these examples, and it must be given a reasonable number of examples. The number required depends on how strong the signal is in the features as well as the machine learning method used.

Features are the real starting point for machine learning. In cases of medical images, features may be the actual pixel values, edge strengths, variation in pixel values in a region, or other values computable from the pixels. Nonimage features, such as the age of the patient and whether a laboratory test has positive or negative results, also can be used. When all these features are combined for an example, this is referred to as a feature vector or input vector.

Feature engineering
Although these features might make it sound like the native pixel values simply could be used as the features, this actually is rare. The intensity often is 1 part of the vector, but other features, such as edge strength, regional intensity, regional texture, and many others, routinely are used. Determining what should be used and how to calculate those from medical images is feature engineering. Good feature engineering requires knowledge of the medical image properties (eg, how to normalize intensities and whether pixel dimensions are fixed, calculable, or unknown) and knowledge of image processing algorithms that can extract the features likely to be useful.

Feature reduction
In general, machine learning benefits from having more data for each example (as well as having more examples) in order to learn the task. It also is the case, however, that including features that either do not help in making the prediction (the feature is not informative) or that overlap with other features can result in poorer performance. Therefore, it generally is desirable to remove noncontributory features and also those that do not contribute significantly, a process known as feature reduction and as feature selection. Feature reduction has the additional benefit of reducing the computational cost at inference time.

There are 3 categories of methods used to achieve feature reduction: filter methods, wrapper methods, and embedding methods. Filter-based methods use some metric to determine how independently predictive a given feature is, and those features that are most predictive while also being independent of others are selected. Pearson correlation and chi-square are 2 popular filter methods.

Wrapper methods search for those features that result in the least reduction in performance when some feature is removed. As a wrapper method proceeds, it continually tries removing features, removing those that either are not predictive or that overlap significantly with other features.

Some learning methods have feature reduction built into them, and thus the term, *embedded*. Examples of embedded methods include lasso and random forests, where the process of training includes removal of features that do not significantly improve performance.

Machine Learning Models

Before discussing the actual machine learning techniques, the use of the term model should be addressed. A model can refer to the general shape of the machine learning method, such as a decision tree or support vector machine (SVM), and also to the specific form of a deep learning network, such as ResNet50 or DenseNet121. Model also can refer to the trained version of the machine learning tool, so readers must infer from context which meaning of model is meant by an investigator. Because this article does not describe any trained versions, model always refers to the architecture and not to a trained version.

Logistic regression
Logistic regression is a well-established technique which, despite its name, is used more generally as a classifier. Logistic regression models have a fixed number of parameters that depend on the number of input features, and they output categorical prediction. It is similar to linear regression, where several points are fitted to a line, minimizing a function like the mean squared error (MSE). Logistic regression instead fits the data to a sigmoid function from 0 to 1, and, when the output is less than 0.5, the example is assigned to a class, else it is the other.

Decision trees and random forests
Decision trees get their name because they make a series of binary decisions until they make a final decision. In the simplest case, a range of values is tried and the best threshold is the one that gets the most cases right. Just 1 such branch usually is too simple for practical uses. The training process consists of determining which feature to make a decision on (eg, age of the subject) and what the criterion is (eg, Is age >68?). The metric used for selecting the feature usually is the Gini index or the entropy (also called information gain) for categorical decision trees or the mean error or MSE for regression trees. These metrics all focus on finding the feature that improves the most in making a prediction. Once that feature is determined, the threshold/decision criteria are computed. This process of finding the feature and criterion is applied recursively to each of the groups that result from applying the split until some stopping criterion is met (eg, no more than X decisions or until there are fewer than Y examples after a decision is applied).

An important advantage of decision trees is how easy they are to interpret. Although other machine learning models are close to black boxes, decision trees provide a graphical and intuitive way to understand what the ML model does.

Support vector machines
SVMs are based on the idea of finding a hyperplane that best divides the set of training examples into 2 classes. Support vectors are the examples nearest to the hyperplane, the points of a data set that, if removed, would alter the position of the dividing hyperplane. A hyperplane is a line that linearly separates and classifies a set of data. The goal then is to determine the formula for a plane that best separates the examples.

This is called a hyperplane because the dimensionality of the plane is the dimension of the examples (and remember each example is a vector of features). It is common to remap the points from simple n-dimensional space to a different type of space if that can produce a better separation of points. There also are hyperparameters (a variable that is external to the model and whose value cannot be estimated from data) that have an impact on how a model develops. For instance, in cases of SVMs, a penalty must be assigned to an example that is on the wrong side of the decision plane. The hyperparameter is the weighting of that penalty—the weighting of no examples really wrong (therefore, assigning a high power to the error) versus fewer examples wrong, even if those are really wrong.

Neural networks
Neural networks get their name because they are modeled on how it is believed the neurons of the brain work. A neural network has an input layer, an output layer, and a variable number of middle (hidden) layers. The input layer of course receives the example vector—each entry in the vector goes to one neuron (hereafter referred to as a node). Each node then applies an activation function, similar to how a biological neuron fires given a strong enough input. The output of each node then is passed to every node of the next layer, but there is a weight for each of these connections that alters the strength of that signal. Each node in this layer applies its activation function and in turn passes their outputs to the next layer after applying a weight. This continues until the output layer. Although earlier versions used sigmoidal functions because they were similar to biological neurons, it is common to use simpler functions like rectified linear functions (eg, values below a threshold become 0, and values above the threshold are passed through).

Although the activation function is predetermined, the weights are actively learned. A common way those weights are learned (that is, altered until the network makes good predictions) is by applying back propagation. Back propagation repeatedly adjusts the weights of the connections in the network so as to minimize a measure of the difference between the actual output vector of the net and the desired output vector.[4] When the prediction is very wrong and getting worse compared with prior example, the weights are altered more and in the opposite direction, and, when the prediction is getting better, the weights are altered less and in the same direction as before. An important challenge is deciding which weights should be adjusted, because adjust all weights probably should not be adjusted the same amount.

DEEP LEARNING

As discussed previously, neural networks are a machine learning technique that has been around for many years, but they were never successful. Attempts to have more than 1 hidden layer resulted in not just significant computing demands, but algorithmic challenges in how to update the weights. As a result, they fell into disfavor with SVMs and decision tree methods becoming much more popular.

Some scientists did continue to work on them, however, and made a splash in 2012 when they crushed the competition with their deep network system.[5,6] There appear to be a few factors that came together that contributed to this accomplishment. Although computers were benefiting from Moore's law, deep learning in particular benefitted from speed improvements much greater than Moore's law because the deep learning computations were mapped onto graphical processing units, which had hundreds to thousands of cores, versus the 4 to 8 cores present in a typical central processing unit. Perhaps more important were theoretic advances that made these calculations work. These included better back propagation methods, which was a critical element of updating the weights in a multilayer neural network. It also was the combination of convolutional layers with the traditional neural network as well as other specialized layers that also made a difference.

Convolutional Neural Networks

These first winning deep learning networks were convolutional networks, and they still enjoy much success today, albeit with some modifications. Although there are many variants of convolutional neural networks (CNN)s , such as AlexNet, VGGNet, GoogLeNet, and so on, all of these start with the first layers consisting of convolutions that are passed over the image. The size of the kernel varies, although more modern architectures usually use 3 × 3 kernels. The next layer after the convolution is a pooling layer, where the output of the kernel typically is reduced in size (eg, a 2 × 2 is reduced to a single pixel), most often by using the maximum value of the output is taken (MaxPool). This reduced resolution image then has another kernel applied, again followed by a MaxPool. These layers typically are finding low-level features (eg, lines and edges) in early layers and as pooling reduces resolution and combines these low-level features together to find higher-

level features (eg, complete circles, eyes, or noses). After a few of these convolution and pooling layers, the output typically is flattened to a 1-dimensional vector, and that vector then is passed into a fully connected network—the familiar neural network structure (**Fig. 1**).

Fig. 2 provides a visualization of the actual content passing from layer to layer. Each output node usually maps to a class, so that if trying to predict an image as 1 of 5 classes, there are 5 output nodes. The output of the fully connected network then often is passed through a softmax function, which adjusts the output values so that they sum to 1.0, thus making the output of each node in the output layer akin to a probability.

A critical element of making such a network useful is that the weights must be adjusted so that the predictions are accurate. The most common way of doing this is by a process called back propagation. Before a network is trained, and an example is passed into the CNN (or any neural network), the output most likely is wrong. Wrong is defined as the sum of the outputs of the nodes: for the node that was the correct class, the output should have been 1 and all others 0. The error thus is the sum of 1 minus the output of the correct node plus the outputs of all the other nodes. This error then is used to guide the adjustment of the weights in the network.

Another critical element of success in training a network is normalization of the input, It can be imagined that if some images are very bright, and others are very dark, that this could confuse a machine learning tool, because it might focus on global intensity as signal rather than the other aspects that are more important. Although a few medical modalities like CT have a reproducible intensity scale, most do not. That means that normal brain tissue could have an intensity of 100 for 1 scan and 1000 on another. A common approach to normalization is to set the mean value to 0 and the range set such that 1 would has a magnitude of 1. This can work for CT as well, although it might mean that important information is lost.

Normalization also may be applied within a network, sometimes at the layer level and sometimes at the batch level. This can help avoid cases where values spiral to very high or very low levels that can exceed the numerical accuracy of the processors used, and thus produce less predictable training.[7]

Another important advance in network training that is less intuitive is dropout.[7,8] Dropout is the random removal of nodes from a network. This can substantially reduce the chance of overfitting,[7–9] apparently because the removal of nodes

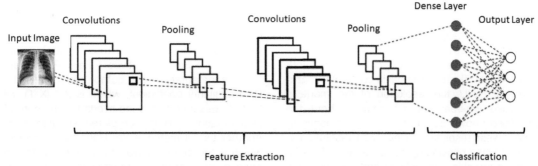

Fig. 1. A simple CNN applies convolutions to small regions of an input image, typically pooling the output of the convolution to select the important features and reduce resolution, until the last pooling layer where the output is flattened into a 1-dimensional vector that is used as input to a dense layer. There may be more that 1 of these densely connected layers, but, ultimately, there is an output layer for the prediction of the CNN.

forces the remaining nodes to maximize the contribution to the prediction.

Another technique that can reduce the chance of overfitting is the application of residual blocks (also called residual networks).[10,11] Residual blocks essentially force each layer of a network to learn—to contribute to reducing error—by having a skip connection around that layer that is the identity function. If the skipped layer(s) do worse than identity, they are ignored, and the identity function output is used. This emphasizes the point

that layers cannot keep being added and performance improved out to infinity—there is a point where adding layers becomes counterproductive, but residual blocks help reduce sensitivity to this situation.

Although most of this discussion is focused more on the problem of classification, deep learning also can be useful for performing image segmentation—the assignment of labels to pixels within an image to indicate what they are (eg, pixels of the liver or brain or lung tumor). The

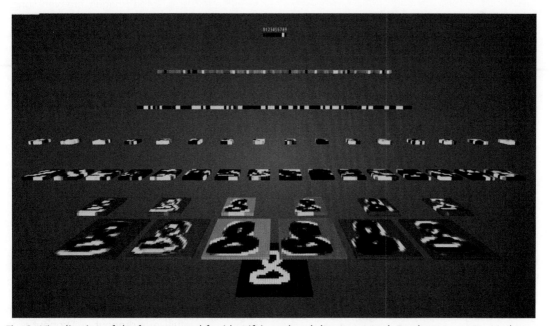

Fig. 2. Visualization of the features used for identifying a hand-drawn numeral. Readers are encouraged to access the Web site used to generate this figure and interactively see the features recognized and ultimately flattened to a 1-dimensional vector used to predict the numeral. The Web site is https://www.cs.ryerson.ca/~aharley/vis/conv/.

U-net is an important technique for image segmentation, because it performs better than most other machine learning techniques. It first was described in 2015 by Ronneberger and colleagues[12] and gets its name because the network diagram looks like a U. The basic concept is that in 1 arm of the U, the resolution of the image is decreased whereas the information about the layer (also known as filters) usually increases to some lowest resolution level. Then resolution is restored when passing up the other arm of the U, but there are skip connections that help produce a high-quality segmentation. Since the original description, many variations of U-Net have been described, including a volumetric (3-dimensional) version called a V-Net.[2]

Assessing Performance

There are many ways to measure the performance of an artificial intelligence (AI) tool. A simple one is accuracy—which percentage of cases are predicted accurately? But accuracy is sometimes misleading. For instance, if trying to determine whether there are any images of a giraffe in some collection of images, and if the number of giraffe images is quite small (say <1%), an algorithm that says there are no giraffe images would be greater than 99% accurate. For this reason, the author usually reports multiple measure,

including sensitivity (true positives/all positives) or specificity (true negatives/all negatives) or metrics like the F1 statistic that try to capture more of what is going on, such that F1 = (2*True Positives [TP])/(2*TP + False Negatives + False Positives).

For segmentation, the author often uses the Dice similarity coefficient, which is 2 * (X ∩ Y)/ (X + Y). Essentially, it is the overlap of the correct segmentation and the predicted segmentation. Another useful metric is the Hausdorff distance, which is the perpendicular distance between the edge of the correct segmentation and the predicted segmentation.

There are many more performance metrics used in AI, depending on the nature of the task and the data. It is important to select the correct metric when evaluating the performance of an AI tool.

Saliency maps and their relatives provide an indication of which parts of an image were important in making a prediction (Fig. 3). This serves at least 2 important purposes. First, it is a sanity check that the AI is making a decision based on a medically relevant part of an image. There now are several examples where saliency maps have shown AI tools making predictions using irrelevant portions of an image, such as the nature of a patient identification marker reflected a facility with a higher incidence of the disease being predicted. In other cases, the AI tool found that detecting chest tubes was a good way to detect

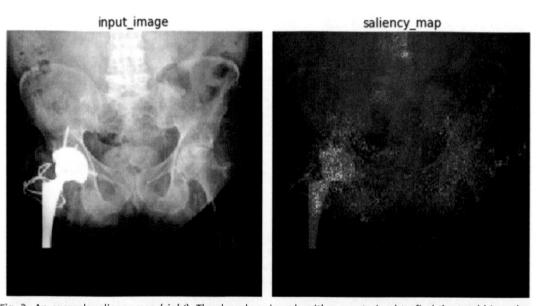

Fig. 3. An example saliency map (*right*). The deep learning algorithm was trained to find the total hip arthroplasty (*left*). Many activations overlying the implant that make sense can be seen. The other activations are not necessarily wrong and may reflect localization of the implant relative to the pelvis. There are some low-intensity activations outside the pelvis, and it is common to have such spurious hits as well. Most, however, should be in locations that make sense.

pneumothorax, but that is not clinically useful because the presence of a chest tube indicates the pneumothorax that already had been detected.

Adaptations of Neural Networks for Deep Learning in Medical Images

All the descriptions to this point are general and not specific to medical images. There are a few important distinctions between medical images and photographic images that should be considered when designing and training a network. First, there are advantages, such as the fact that the size of pixels and the orientation of the images usually are well known, and this can mean that fewer examples are required than with photographs of the real world. Second, in cases like CTs, the intensity scale is quite reproducible, whereas for most other imaging modalities, the intensity scale is not known, and some type of intensity normalization must be applied. There also can be shading in the image, where the intensity varies as a function of location, such as in MR imaging and field heterogeneity. Knowledge of the imaging modality, the anatomy, and the problem at hand is important in selecting the best approach to handling intensity.

Medical images also can have lots of other important associated information, and this still is a rather unexplored area. The simplest is that there can be images of the same anatomy but acquired with different properties—for example T1-weighted and T2-weighted images or images without and with intravenous contrast. There also may be old imaging examinations and the task may be to detect changes over time. Nonpixel information, such as age, gender, blood test results, and other information, can improve AI performance significantly. A description of how to apply these is beyond scope of this introduction but it is important to keep these factors in mind when planning an AI tool.

SUMMARY

AI technology has seen rapid advances in the past decade as deep technologies have enabled vastly superior performance to prior methods. Highly accurate image classification methods have shown superhuman level performance for some tasks. AI methods also can perform tedious tasks like outlining organs or tumors with human-level accuracy efficiently. It is likely that these will see adoption into clinical practice over the next decade as the strengths and weaknesses are better understood.

A common question is whether or not deep learning is always better than traditional machine learning. It is not. Deep learning demands large data sets because the many parameters it must learn easily can result in overfitting if too few examples are provided. Traditional methods should be selected when there are few training data, although there is not an exact number for what constitutes few. Some traditional machine learning methods like decision trees also have clear and easy-to-understand models, which can be important for convincing that the decisions made make sense and also may provide valuable insight into disease.

DISCLOSURE

B.J. Erickson is a founder and stockholder in FLowSIGMA, Inc.

REFERENCES

1. PS3.1. Available at: http://dicom.nema.org/medical/dicom/current/output/html/part01.html. Accessed January 15, 2021.
2. Milletari F, Navab N, Ahmadi S-A. V-Net: Fully Convolutional Neural Networks for Volumetric Medical Image Segmentation. arXiv [cs.CV]. 2016. Available at: http://arxiv.org/abs/1606.04797. Accessed July 12, 2018.
3. Robb RA, Hanson DP, Karwoski RA, et al. Analyze: a comprehensive, operator-interactive software package for multidimensional medical image display and analysis. Comput Med Imaging Graph 1989; 13:433–54.
4. Rumelhart DE, Hinton GE, Williams RJ. Learning representations by back-propagating errors. Nature 1986;323:533–6.
5. Available at: https://papers.nips.cc/paper/2012/file/c399862d3b9d6b76c8436e924a68c45b-Paper.pdf. Accessed January 15, 2021.
6. Krizhevsky A, Sutskever I, Hinton GE. ImageNet Classification with Deep Convolutional Neural Networks. In: Pereira F, Burges C, Bottou L, Weinberger. KQ, editors.Advances in Neural Information Processing Systems 25. 2012. Available at: https://papers.nips.cc/paper/4824-imagenet-classification-with-deep-convolutional-neural-networks.pdf. Accessed July 14, 2018.
7. Santurkar S, Tsipras D, Ilyas A, et al. How Does Batch Normalization Help Optimization? arXiv [stat.ML]. 2018. Available at: http://arxiv.org/abs/1805.11604. Accessed September 3, 2019.
8. Srivastava N, Hinton GR, Krizhevsky A, et al. Dropout: A Simple Way to Prevent Neural Networks from Overfitting. J Machine Learn Res 2014;15: 1929–58.

9. Cogswell M, Ahmed F, Girshick R, et al. Reducing Overfitting in Deep Networks by Decorrelating Representations. arXiv [cs.LG]. 2015. Available at: http://arxiv.org/abs/1511.06068. Accessed November 12, 2018.

10. He K, Zhang X, Ren S, et al. Deep Residual Learning for Image Recognition. In: Bajcsy, editor. Proceedings of the IEEE Conference on computer Visions and Pattern Recognition. Los Alamitos (CA): Conference Publishing Services; 2016. p. 770–8.

11. Szegedy C, Ioffe S, Vanhoucke V, et al. Inception-v4, Inception-ResNet and the Impact of Residual Connections on Learning. arXiv [cs.CV]. 2016. Available at: http://arxiv.org/abs/1602.07261. Accessed January 18, 2017.

12. Ronneberger O, Fischer P, Brox T. U-net: convolutional networks for Biomedical image segmentation. Medical image computing and Computer-Assisted Intervention – MICCAI 2015. Cham: Springer; 2015. p. 234–41.

Basic Artificial Intelligence Techniques
Evaluation of Artificial Intelligence Performance

Jayashree Kalpathy-Cramer, PhD*, Jay B. Patel, BS,
Christopher Bridge, Dphil, Ken Chang, PhD

KEYWORDS

- Artificial Intelligence • Machine learning • Deep learning • Algorithms • Evaluation

KEY POINTS

- With the rapidly expanding use cases for AI, there is a growing need for proper evaluation of developed algorithms.
- Although the external test set is the gold standard for evaluation of model performance, algorithms ideally should be continuously evaluated prospectively and updated appropriately.
- The choice of metrics used when evaluating AI models varies depending on the application/task.
- The quality of the ground truth needs to be considered in assessing performance metrics.

Automated approaches in health care have been transformed by machine learning. Although the use of pre-engineered features combined with traditional machine learning approaches has been popular, their implementation has been limited by the need to manually extract and design features. Interest in machine learning has been catalyzed by advancements in deep learning. Breakthrough performance across various tasks within computer science spurred interest in expanding the technique to the medical domain. The need for proper evaluation of these algorithms is an active area of research. The focus of this article is on current issues, techniques, and challenges of evaluating medical artificial intelligence.

THE EXPANDING USE CASES OF ARTIFICIAL INTELLIGENCE IN HEALTH CARE

Automated approaches in health care have been fundamentally transformed by the advent of machine learning. Although the use of pre-engineered features combined with traditional machine learning approaches has been popular,[1,2] their implementation across many domains has been limited by the need to manually extract and design features. Interest in machine learning has been catalyzed in recent years by advancements in deep learning, a technique in which neural networks are used to automatically learn pertinent patterns and features directly from the input data.[3] In particular, breakthrough performance across various tasks within computer science[4–6] spurred interest in expanding the technique to the medical domain.

Recent studies have reported high performance in a variety of medical tasks in domains like cardiology,[7] ophthalmology,[8] pathology,[9] and dermatology.[10] The applications of deep learning within radiology also have been promising, with numerous algorithms developed within all subspecialties, such as neuro-,[11] musculoskeletal,[12] cardiac,[13] chest,[14] breast,[15] abdominal radiology,[16] and nuclear medicine.[17] Given that much of medicine relies on the interpretation of laboratory tests, physiologic signals, and

a Radiology, Martinos Center for Biomedical Imaging, Massachusetts General Hospital, 149 13th Street, Boston, MA 02129, USA
* Corresponding author.
E-mail address: jkalpathy-cramer@mgh.harvard.edu

Radiol Clin N Am 59 (2021) 941–954
https://doi.org/10.1016/j.rcl.2021.06.005
0033-8389/21/© 2021 Elsevier Inc. All rights reserved.

medical imaging, the use of cases for medical artificial intelligence (AI) continues to expand at a remarkable pace. The growth of medical AI studies has not come without peril, however: the need for proper evaluation of these algorithms is an active area of research, discussion, and evolution. The focus of this article is on discussing current issues, techniques, and challenges of evaluating medical AI.

GENERALIZABILITY OF ARTIFICIAL INTELLIGENCE ALGORITHMS

A machine learning study typically utilizes training, validation, internal testing, and external testing sets, all of which should be nonoverlapping. The training set is a partition of the data that is used to directly train the model. The validation set is used during training to tune hyperparameters of the model. The internal testing set is derived from the same distribution as the training and validation sets (ie, data from the same institution). The external testing set is a completely independent set of data (ie, data from a different institution). Both the internal and external testing sets are used for evaluation only after the model is fully trained.

Algorithmic performance is measured via a task-specific metric, discussed later. Algorithmic generalizability is assessed by measuring a model's performance on new, unseen data. A model with high performance on the training set is not guaranteed to be clinically useful if the model is overfit or does not generalize well. Modern neural networks are extremely large, with many millions of trainable parameters.[18] With further advancements in hardware, models continue to grow wider, deeper, and more complex. In contrast, medical data sets contain several orders of magnitude fewer data inputs. This discrepancy results in an ease of overfitting, a phenomenon known as the curse of dimensionality. Thus, perfect or near-perfect performance on the training set has no prognostic value about the generalizability of a model because a model may memorize the training data. Similarly, performance on the validation set is of little value because it is continuously being used during model training to tune model hyperparameters. This results in indirect overfitting due to leakage of information. On the other hand, the internal testing set does reveal some information about model generalizability, but it is limited in scope because the data usually are within the same distribution as the training and validation sets. Moreover, although some algorithms may perform satisfactorily on the internal testing set, they still can fail to generalize on the external testing set due to differences (minute or macro) in the data distribution. Ideally, multiple external testing sets are collected, but this can be challenging from a logistical perspective. For these reasons, the external testing set is the gold standard for evaluation of model performance.

When a model is evaluated on external testing sets, drops in performance often can be attributed to shifts in data distribution. To start, the patient populations between the training and external set could be different in terms of demographics (such as age, gender, prevalence, and race). For example, a model trained on data that have high prevalence of disease are not calibrated to a testing set with low prevalence of disease.[19] Second, the image acquisition settings may be different across different sites. For example, different mammography systems may have differing x-ray tube targets, filters, digital detector technology, and control of automatic exposures that can affect model generalizability.[20] Similarly, different magnetic resonance (MR) scanners likely have different field strengths, slice thicknesses, repetition times, and echo times.[21,22] Lastly, the neural network may have learned a confounder in the training data set that is not present in the external data set. For example, a neural network that learns that pneumonia more likely is seen on a portable chest radiograph (which more likely is used in an acute setting like the intensive care unit or emergency department) does not perform well when tested on a data set of outpatient radiographs.[19] Along the same lines, another study demonstrated that neural networks can learn to associate disease status with data set–specific laterality markers, arrows, and other forms of annotation, which is a troubling sign if trying to train an algorithm to detect disease pathology.[23] Algorithms are not explicitly trained to learn disease pathology; rather, they are optimized to correlate input data with the label of interest. Using an external testing set can elucidate these generalizability pitfalls.

Evaluation does not end with an external validation set. Just as bacteria continue to evolve with need for continual refinement of antibiotic regimens, data too evolve over time with changing technologies and patient populations. As such, the performance of algorithms needs to be continuously evaluated prospectively and updated appropriately. To facilitate this, research on algorithm development ideally is fully transparent, with clear description of methodology for ease of reproducibility by other research groups.[24] Even more preferable would be release of the source code and trained models themselves, a trend that is steadily becoming more prevalent within the literature[25–27] but challenging and potential infeasible in cases of commercial algorithms.

THE ISSUE OF BIAS IN MACHINE LEARNING

In the evaluation of an algorithm, a critical component that should be addressed is whether the algorithm is biased. Specifically, it is important to address whether there are discrepancies in performance across different subgroups, such as age, gender, and insurance status. Recent studies on deep learning algorithms for chest radiograph classification and acute kidney injury prediction have shown that there is differential performance across different subgroups.[28–30] The reasons for this discrepancy can include representation in the training set (ie, certain groups are less represented in the training set) and differences in label noise (ie, certain groups are more likely to have incorrect diagnoses).[29] In the deployment of algorithms, it is the developer's responsibility to ensure that the algorithm is ethical. That is, the use of the algorithm helps ameliorate rather than perpetuate health care disparities. Thus, assessment of algorithm fairness is a key component of algorithm evaluation. Addressing this issue, whether through the curation of fairer training sets or debiasing of algorithms, is an area of active research.[31,32]

TASKS IN MEDICAL IMAGE ANALYSIS

A majority of supervised image analysis algorithms can be categorized broadly into 4 bins: classification, detection, segmentation, and regression.[33] Classification is defined as the image-level assignment of a label from a finite set of categories. Detection involves coarsely identifying the region of the image where the label(s) is present. Segmentation involves classifying each pixel in the image to a unique label. And regression is defined as assigning each image a continuous-valued response. For example, there may only be interest if a patient's radiograph is positive for pneumonia, in which a classification algorithm should be used to differentiate normal from pathologic radiographs. If there is further interest in drawing a bounding box around the predicted pneumonia, a detection algorithm should be applied. If accurately delineating the pneumonia from healthy lung tissue is needed, a segmentation algorithm is chosen. And, finally, if assessing the severity of the pneumonia is wanted, a regression algorithm to output higher values for more severe cases is used.

TASK-SPECIFIC METRICS FOR EVALUATION OF ARTIFICIAL INTELLIGENCE MODELS

The choice of metrics used when evaluating AI models varies depending on the application/task. This section presents the most common methods used in literature for binary classification, multiclass classification, object detection, segmentation, retrieval, and regression.

Binary Classification

In binary classification, each sample has 2 possible values for its true label (positive and negative) and 2 possible values for its predicted value (also positive and negative). Each sample consequently falls into 1 of the 4 following groups, depending on the combination of its true and predicted label: (1) true positive (TP)—the sample is positive and is labeled correctly as positive by the classifier; (2) false positive (FP)—the sample is negative but is labeled incorrectly as positive by the classifier (also known as a type I error or false alarm); (3) true negative (TN)—the sample is negative and is labeled correctly as negative by the classifier; and (4) false negative (FN)—the sample is positive but is labeled incorrectly as negative by the classifier (also known as a type II error or miss). The number of samples from a test set that fall into each of these categories is denoted as N_{TP}, N_{FP}, N_{TN}, and N_{FN}, respectively; the total number of samples in the test set as N_{TOTAL}. There are several metrics that use the counts of samples in these 4 categories to summarize the performance of the model.

Accuracy

Perhaps the simplest metric is accuracy. Accuracy quantifies the proportion of samples for which the predicted label matches the true label. It, therefore, is equal to the proportion of all samples that are either TPs or TNs: $Accuracy = \frac{N_{TP}+N_{TN}}{N_{TOTAL}}$. Accuracy lies in the range 0 to 1 and is expressed commonly as a percentage. A perfect classifier has an accuracy of 1 (100%), whereas a random classifier (one that randomly chooses a class label with uniform probability) has an accuracy of 0.5 (50%) because it chooses the correct predicted label by chance half of the time.

Although simple and intuitive, accuracy commonly is considered insufficiently informative for most applications because it does not differentiate between the 2 types of errors (FPs and FNs), which commonly have very different significance in practice. Furthermore, if a test data set is highly imbalanced, a classifier may achieve a high accuracy simply by predicting the most common class label for all samples.

Sensitivity and Specificity

Sensitivity and specificity together give a more detailed view of a classifier by considering the performance on positive samples and negative samples separately.[34] Sensitivity (also referred to as the TP rate or recall) quantifies the proportion of positive samples that are labeled correctly as positive by the classifier, whereas specificity (also referred to as the TN rate) quantifies the proportion of negative samples that are labeled correctly as negative. These quantities may be expressed as follows: $Sensitivity = \frac{N_{TP}}{N_{TP}+N_{FN}}$ and $Specificity = \frac{N_{TN}}{N_{TN}+N_{FP}}$. Note that the denominators of these expressions, $(N_{TP} + N_{FN})$ and $(N_{TN} + N_{FP})$, are equal to the total number of positive and negative samples in the data set, respectively. Like accuracy, sensitivity and specificity lie in the range 0 to 1 or often are expressed as percentages. A perfect classifier has both sensitivity and specificity of 1 (or 100%), whereas a random classifier has sensitivity and specificity scores of 0.5 (50%). In practice, improving sensitivity often comes at the cost of reducing specificity and vice versa.

Because sensitivity and specificity apply, respectively, to just the positive samples and just the negative samples of a data set, they may be expected to stay approximately constant irrespective of the balance of positive and negative samples in the data set. In other words, they are properties of the classifier itself rather than its utility in the environment in which it is used. This is an important advantage if the test data set may not have a class balance that is representative of the true population. They do not capture some aspects of a classifier's performance, however, that are important when considering using a classifier for a situation with a highly imbalanced pretest probability (discussed later).

Receiver Operating Characteristics and Area Under the Receiver Operating Characteristic Metric

Many classification models do not directly output a binary classification but rather a classification score that then is compared with a threshold to give a binarized prediction. When using such models, it is possible to choose the threshold value after the model has been trained to give the desired trade-off between sensitivity and specificity for a certain application. A receiver operating characteristic (ROC)[34] aids in this process by plotting the sensitivity (TP rate) on the Y axis and the FP rate (which is equal to 1 minus

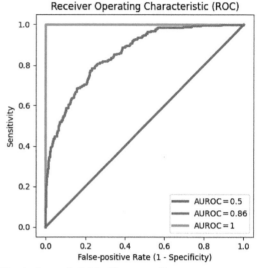

Fig. 1. Example ROCs. The green line represents a perfect classifier. The blue line represents a random classifier. The orange line represents a realistic classifier with reasonable performance for the problem.

the TN rate or, equivalently, 1 minus the specificity) on the X axis as the classification threshold is varied. By inspecting an ROC plot, it is possible to see how sensitivity and specificity jointly vary as the threshold is changed.

The area under the ROC (AUROC) summarizes the performance of the model at all possible thresholds. This important metric often is used to give a single number that captures a more complete picture of a classifier's performance than sensitivity and specificity at 1 particular threshold. This is important particularly when evaluating models that later may be used with different thresholds. The resulting metric is known as the AUROC score. It also commonly is referred to simply as the area under the score, but the authors favor the more specific term, AUROC.

Every ROC passes through the lower left corner of the axes (0, 0) corresponding to no positive predictions and the upper right corner (1, 1) corresponding to no negative predictions and increases monotonically between these 2 points. A random classifier (one that predicts random labels for each sample) has an ROC that is a straight diagonal line between the lower left and upper right corners (Fig. 1) and accordingly has an AUROC of 0.5. A perfect classifier (one for which there exists a threshold that splits the positive and negative samples perfectly) passes through the point of perfect separation of the positive and negative samples at the upper left corner of the axes (0, 1), where sensitivity and specificity are both 1. It therefore consists of a vertical line from the lower left to the upper left corner of the axes and then a horizontal line from the upper left to the upper right corner. This results in an AUROC score of 1. A good classifier has an ROC that comes close to the upper left corner of the axes and an AUROC of between 0.5 and 1.0. If a classifier is performing worse than random chance, it has an AUROC of below 0.5 and an ROC that approaches the lower right corner of the axes.

Precision and Recall

Sensitivity, specificity, and AUROC scores are the set of metrics used most commonly for binary classification performance in medical AI. As alluded to previously, however, they do not capture important aspects of a classifier's utility in imbalanced data sets. Precision (also known as positive predictive value) quantifies the proportion of the classifier's positive predictions that are in fact positive. Recall quantifies the proportion of positive samples that are labeled correctly as positive by the classifier. Specifically, the 2 metrics are defined as follows: $Precision = \frac{N_{TP}}{N_{TP}+N_{FP}}$ and $Recall = \frac{N_{TP}}{N_{TP}+N_{FN}}$. Recall is the same as sensitivity, and it is purely a matter of convention that when presented alongside precision it typically is given this alternative name.

Like sensitivity and specificity, precision and recall lie in the range 0 to 1 and alternatively may be expressed as percentages. Unlike sensitivity/recall and specificity, precision depends on the class balance in the test data set. This has 2 important implications. First, the precision of a classifier measured on a test set is not generalizable if the proportion of positive and negative samples in that test set does not match the proportion in the population in which the classifier is intended to be used. Second, the precision of a random classifier on a given data set (the baseline precision) generally is not 0.5 but rather the proportion of positive samples in that data set. This can complicate the interpretation of the precision metric.

The importance of precision as metric arises as a result of the fact that in many medical applications, the balance of positive and negative samples is highly in favor of the negative class (ie, there are many more negatives than positives).[35] In such situations, a classifier can have both high sensitivity and high specificity but low precision (ie, most of its positive predictions are incorrect), meaning that its predictions are of limited use in practice. These situations may not be identified if sensitivity and specificity alone are considered. Although it may be an unusual situation in practice in medical applications, it also is important to note that if instead the data set is heavily imbalanced in favor of the positive class a classifier may

simultaneously achieve high precision and recall even if its specificity is low (ie, it classifies most negative samples as positive). Consequently, a complete description of a classifier's performance ideally should include all 3 of these metrics (sensitivity/recall, specificity, and precision).

Describing a classifier purely by its precision and recall does not consider the number of TN samples, because N_{TN} does not appear in the definition of either of the metrics, listed previously. This may be useful in certain situations in which the number of TNs either is unimportant, difficult to determine, or even undefined (discussed later).

Precision-recall Curves and the Average Precision Metric

When working with models that output a classification score, the classification threshold can be adjusted to give the desired balance of precision and recall. The relationship between a classifier's precision and recall as the classification threshold is varied may be visualized using a precision-recall curve (PRC) (**Fig. 2**).[36] A PRC plots the precision of the classifier on the Y axis and the recall of the classifier on the X axis.

At a low classification threshold, the recall tends to 1 and the precision tends to the ratio of positives to negatives in the dataset. Therefore, on the right-hand side of the PRC, the curve tends toward the

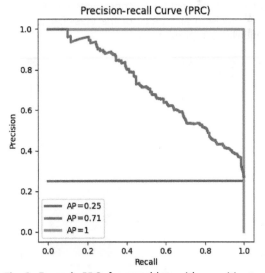

Fig. 2. Example PRCs for a problem with a positive to negative class balance of 1 to 3. The green line represents a perfect classifier. The blue line represents a random classifier with a constant precision of 0.25, reflecting the baseline class ratio. The orange line represents a realistic classifier with reasonable performance on the task.

class ratio. A random classifier has a flat PRC fixed a constant precision equal to the class ratio. A perfect classifier's PRC passes through the top-right corner of the plot, representing a precision and recall of 1. A good classifier has a high precision across a range of recall values. Unlike ROCs, PRCs do not necessarily decrease monotonically from left to right.

The area under the PRC gives a metric that quantifies the performance of the classifier over all possible thresholds. This metric may be referred to as the area under the PRC or more commonly as average precision (AP) because it measures AP of the classifier over a range of recalls. The AP score lies between 0 and 1, where a perfect classifier has an AP of 1 and a random classifier has an AP equal to the class ratio. In practice, there are several different ways to calculate the AP metric, which are not discussed.

F_1 Score

The F_1 score is a metric that combines precision and recall into a single value.[37] It is defined as the harmonic mean of precision and recall and, therefore, always lies between the 2. Specifically, it is defined as $F_1 = \frac{precision \times recall}{precision + recall} = \frac{2N_{TP}}{2N_{TP} + N_{FP} + N_{FN}}$. If a single metric to measure the performance of a classifier is required, the F_1 score often is preferred to the simple accuracy metric. Like precision and recall, the F_1 score does not consider the number of TNs. It may not be an appropriate metric when the precision and recall of the classifier are not equally as important.

Multiclass Classification

Multiclass classification problems are those in which each sample belongs to 1 of several finite, mutually exclusive classes, and the classifier predicts a single label for each sample.

Confusion Matrices

A confusion matrix (**Figs. 3–5**) is a convenient way to visualize the performance of the classifier for all classes in a single figure. A confusion matrix is a table with 1 row and 1 column for each class. Each entry in the table represents the number of cases in which a sample with the row's label was given the column's label. Often, the elements of the matrix may be shaded according to the number of cases to aid interpretation.

Elements of the confusion matrices either may contain the raw counts of the samples in the test set or, more commonly, be normalized such that each row sums to 1 in order to balance the matrix according to the proportion of samples belonging to each ground truth class. A perfect classifier has a confusion matrix with all its nonzero elements along the diagonal, meaning each sample is classified correctly by the model. A random classifier has samples uniformly distributed over all its elements.

Kappa Coefficients

The kappa coefficient (or Cohen's kappa) is a way to quantify the agreement between 2 sets of multiclass labels, giving a single number.[38] The kappa coefficient between the model's predictions and the ground truth labels, therefore, may be used

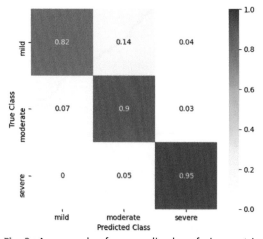

Fig. 3. An example of a normalized confusion matrix for a 3-class classification problem categorizing images into mild, moderate, and severe for an abnormality. This classifier exhibits good performance on the task, because a majority of cases are clustered in the diagonal elements of the matrix.

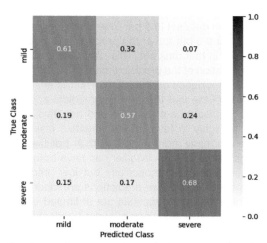

Fig. 4. Another example confusion matrix for the same classification problem. This classifier exhibits poorer performance, with more cases in the off-diagonal elements.

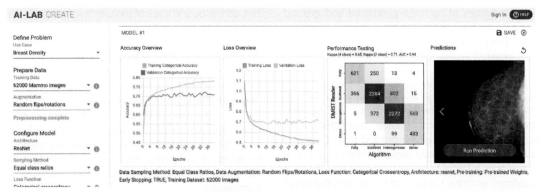

Fig. 5. Evaluation of an AI model for mammographic breast density assessment using American College of Radiology AI-LAB. After model parameters are defined, performance on training and validation sets is monitored during training. After training, performance is evaluated on the testing set by means of AUROC and Cohen's kappa. In addition, evaluation of the confusion matrix and of predictions on individual mammograms allows assessment of failure modes.

as a metric of the model's overall performance. The kappa coefficient is defined as $\kappa = \frac{P_o - P_e}{1 - P_e}$, where P_o is the proportion of samples in which the predicted label is correct (the accuracy of the model), and P_e is the probability by chance given by the formula, $P_e = \frac{1}{N^2} \sum n_{k1} n_{k2}$, where N is the number of samples and n_{k1} and n_{k2} are, respectively, the number of times label k appears in the ground truth and model predictions.

The kappa coefficient, therefore, adjusts the raw accuracy value to account for the agreement that could occur by chance. The value for kappa lies in the range -1 to 1, where a value of 1 indicates perfect agreement, a value of 0 indicates the agreement that would occur by chance, and a value below 0 indicates worse than random agreement.

Binary Segmentation

In a binary segmentation problem, each pixel (or voxel) in an image is classified as a 0 or 1. Consequently, it is possible to use the standard binary classification metrics, such as accuracy, sensitivity, specificity, and precision, to assess the binary segmentation performance within a single image. Other metrics, however, generally are preferred in practice.

Intersection over Union

The intersection over union (IoU) **(Fig. 6)** measure describes the similarity of the ground truth segmentation and the predicted segmentation in a single image. The intersection of 2 regions A and B is the area that lies within both A and B, whereas the union is the area that lies within either A or B. The IoU score between a segmented region and ground truth region is calculated as the size of

the intersection of the 2 regions divided by the size of the union of the 2 regions and lies between 0 and 1. If the predicted segmentation is perfect (ie, predicted and ground truth overlap perfectly with each other), then the IoU is 1 and if they do not overlap at all the IoU is 0. In terms of the classification results of the pixels within the image, the IoU score may be written as $IoU = \frac{N_{TP}}{N_{TP} + N_{FP} + N_{FN}}$.

One important advantage of the IoU metric over pixelwise accuracy is that it is insensitive to the size of the regions in that if the image is scaled

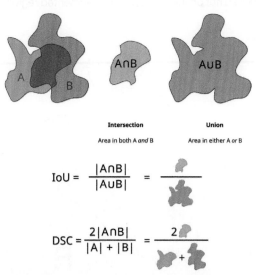

$$IoU = \frac{|A \cap B|}{|A \cup B|}$$

$$DSC = \frac{2|A \cap B|}{|A| + |B|}$$

Fig. 6. Metrics for binary segmentation. A and B represent the 2 regions to compare (ground truth and predicted). The intersection is defined as the region contained within both A and B. The union is defined as the region within either A or B (or both). The IoU and DSC metrics are defined in terms of the areas of these regions as shown in the equations.

such that sizes of both the predicted and ground truths both change, the IoU measure remains constant. The IoU metric also is referred to as the Jaccard index.[39]

Dice Similarity Coefficient

The Dice similarity coefficient (DSC, **Fig. 6**), also known as the Sørenson-Dice coefficient, describes the similarity of the ground truth segmentation and the predicted segmentation in a single image and is largely similar to the IoU metric.[40] It is defined as twice the ratio of the area of the intersection of the regions to the sum of the individual areas. It takes the value of 0 if the predicted and ground truth regions do not overlap and a value of 1 if they overlap perfectly. Like the IoU metric, it is insensitive to scale.

The DSC is mathematically equivalent to the F1 score of the classification of the pixels/voxels within a single image: $DSC = \frac{2N_{TP}}{2N_{TP}+N_{FP}+N_{FN}}$. There also is a simple mathematical relationship between DSC and IoU scores: $DSC = \frac{2IoU}{IoU+1}$ and $IoU = \frac{DSC}{2-DSC}$. As a result of this relationship, the DSC always is slightly higher than the IoU for a given segmentation, except where both are equal to 0 or 1.

Hausdorff Distance

The Hausdorff distance (HD) (**Fig. 7**) is an alternative metric used for evaluating segmentations based not on the overlap of the segmented regions but on the boundaries of the segmentations.[41] The HD from boundary A to boundary B is the furthest distance from any point on A to its closest point on B. It, therefore, represents in a sense the maximum error between the 2 boundaries. Note that the HD from boundary A to boundary B generally is not the same as the HD from boundary B to boundary A (ie, the standard HD is not symmetric, unlike DSC and IoU). For this reason, HD often is referred to as the directed HD. A related metric, the bidirectional HD, is defined as the larger of the 2 directed HD between the 2 boundaries, and, therefore, is symmetric.

The HD is a particularly useful metric when the boundaries of the segmentation are complex and/or accurate boundaries are important for the application. It is very sensitive, however, to noise and outliers in the segmentation. Therefore, the 95% HD commonly is used in practice.[42] Instead of using the maximum distance from any point on any to its closest point on B, the 95th percentile of these distance is used instead.

Information Retrieval

An information retrieval problem is one in which a query returns a set of samples, each of which may be correct (1) or incorrect (0) with respect to the query. For example, the results returned from a query to an Internet search engine or a list of similar medical images resulting from a query to an image database. In each case, the returned results may be relevant (1) or irrelevant (0) to the original query.

The information retrieval problem shares many characteristics with the binary classification problem in that each sample has a binary ground truth label. The number of TNs (ie, the number of samples that are incorrect and not returned by a query), however, either is difficult or impossible to quantify or simply irrelevant to the performance of the classifier. For example, when evaluating an Internet search engine, it is neither pertinent nor practical to consider the number of irrelevant Web pages existing on the Internet that the search engine does not return to the user. Consequently, it generally is not possible and/or not meaningful to evaluate the specificity metric of the result of a query because it depends on the number of FNs. Instead, information retrieval models are appropriately evaluated with precision, recall, AP metrics, and PRCs, as discussed previously, because they do not rely on enumeration of TN samples.

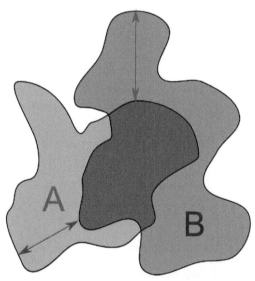

Fig. 7. The HDs between A and B (*orange line*) and between B and A (*green line*) are defined as the maximum distance from any point on the first boundary to its closest point on the second boundary.

Object Detection

Object detection models return areas of interest in an input image, typically in the form of a list of bounding boxes and their associated detection scores. Such regions may represent a tumor, lesion, fracture, or other abnormality. Taking into account all possible shapes and sizes of bounding boxes, the number of negative regions in an image is potentially infinite and not meaningful to quantify. As a result, object detection models are evaluated by considering them within the framework of information retrieval problems using precision, recall, AP metrics, and PRCs.

In order to apply these metrics, it first is necessary to first determine whether or not a particular detected bounding box is correct by referring to a set of ground truth regions. The standard method for this is to calculate the IoU of the detected bounding box and each of the ground truth boxes, as defined previously.[43]

To determine whether a given detected box is correct or not, it is compared with all ground truth boxes using the IoU score. If the IoU with any ground truth box is greater than a predetermined threshold, the detected box is considered a TP detection. Otherwise, it is considered a FP detection. Any ground truth boxes that are not detected in this way are FNs.

Equipped with a method for determining whether a given detected box is correct, it becomes possible to evaluate an object detection model using the standard precision, recall metrics. Additionally, if each detected box is associated with a score, as is the case with most modern object detection models, PRCs and the AP metric commonly are used.[43]

Mean Average Precision

The mean AP (mAP) is the mean of the AP value calculated over several different queries. In the context of object detection models, this typically is when an AP score is calculated separately for several different IoU thresholds, and the mean of these scores gives an overall mAP score for the model.[44]

Free-response Receiver Operating Characteristics

A free-response ROC (FROC) (**Fig. 8**) is a variant on the standard ROC that is used for object detection problems.[45] On the Y axis, the region-level sensitivity is plotted, that is, the proportion of positive regions that were detected as positive. Note that the sensitivity may not reach 1 if some of the positive regions are not detected at any threshold. In the place of specificity on the X axis, the number of FPs per image is used. Thus, the FROC curve gives an intuitive impression of the trade-off between the numbers of FN and FP detections as the classification threshold varies. Like a standard ROC, the closer the curve comes to the top left of the plot, the better the model.

Continuous-valued Quantification

Some AI systems produce an estimate of a continuous-valued quantity of interest for each sample. In some cases, the model may output the quantity of interest directly. In others, a quantity of interest may be derived from another type of model output. For example, the volume, diameter, or mean radiodensity may be calculated from a region segmented by a model. The authors use g_i and p_i to refer to the ground truth and predicted values, respectively, for a particular sample i in a data set of N samples.

Mean Absolute Error

The absolute error of a prediction $|p_i - g_i|$ is the difference between the prediction and the ground truth when the direction of the error is unimportant and always produces a positive number. The mean absolute error (MAE) is the mean of this quantity calculated over every sample in the test set: $MAE = \frac{1}{N}|p_i - g_i|$. The MAE gives an intuitive measurement of the average discrepancy of the predictions from the ground truth, as it is given in the units of the measurements themselves. The MAE does not indicate whether the errors are biased in a particular direction from the ground truth.

Mean Squared Error

The mean squared error (MSE) is the mean of the squared difference between the prediction and ground truth over the samples in the data set:

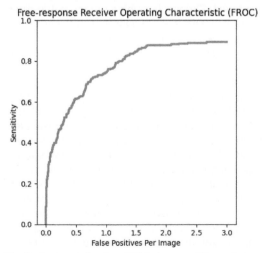

Fig. 8. An example of an FROC. As more FPs per image are allowed, model sensitivity goes up.

$MSE = \frac{1}{N}(p_i - g_i)^2$. The MSE puts more weight on cases with a large error than cases with a small error and also has other mathematical properties that make it commonly used in practice. It is not as readily interpretable, however, as MAE, and is not expressed in the same unit as the measured quantity itself (but rather in the square of that unit). Like MAE, it does not indicate whether the errors are biased in a particular direction.

Pearson Correlation Coefficient

The Pearson correlation coefficient (PCC) quantifies the strength of the relationship between 2 variables. In cases of AI models, it may be used to quantify the strength of the relationship between the ground truth and the prediction. The PCC, r_{PCC}, is calculated as follows: $r_{PCC} = \frac{\sum_{i=1}^{N}(p_i-\bar{p})(g_i-\bar{g})}{\sqrt{\sum_{i=1}^{N}(p_i-\bar{p})^2}\sqrt{\sum_{i=1}^{N}(g_i-\bar{g})^2}}$, where $\bar{p}$ and $\bar{g}$ are the means of the predictions and ground truth values over the data set, respectively. The coefficient lies in the range 1 to -1, where 1 corresponds to a perfect positive association between the 2 variables, 0 corresponds to no association, and -1 corresponds to a perfect negative association. The PCC is valid when samples of ground truth and predictions both are distributed normally. Note that the PCC measures the degree of association between the predictions and ground truth; it does not measure equality between them. In other words, the PCC does not change if the predictions are consistently higher or lower than ground truth by a constant value or are scaled with respect to the ground truth by a constant factor. Despite this important shortcoming, the PCC commonly is seen in practice due to widespread familiarity and availability in statistical software packages.

Spearman Rank Correlation Coefficient

Spearman rank is an alternative correlation coefficient that is valid when the predictions and ground truth are not distributed normally. Instead of operating on the values of the ground truth and predictions, it instead considers only their rankings in the data set. If the rank of prediction p_i in the list of all predictions is $R(p_i)$ and the rank of ground truth value g_i in the list of all ground truth values is $R(g_i)$, then the Spearman rank correlation coefficient is given by $r_{SRCC} = 1 - \frac{6\sum_{i=1}^{N}(R(p_i)-R(g_i))^2}{N(N^2-1)}$. Again, the Spearman coefficient ranges from 1 (perfect positive association) to -1 (perfect negative association). Although it is more widely applicable than the PCC, Spearman coefficient is weaker than the PCC in that only a matching ranking between the predictions and ground truth is required for a high Spearman coefficient; the actual predicted values could differ significantly from the ground truth.

Intraclass Correlation Coefficient

Intraclass correlation coefficients (ICCs) are used to measure the consistency or agreement between different raters rating the same quantity.[46] Several different ICCs are defined in literature and are appropriate in different situations. The definitions that are most applicable for measuring the agreement of an AI prediction with a ground truth are known in the taxonomy of McGraw and Wong[47] (also used by many software packages) as the 2-way, single-score, absolute agreement coefficients. Readers are referred to discussions by Koo and Li[48] and McGraw and Wong[47] for more detail on selecting appropriate coefficients and their mathematical definitions.

Like the other correlation coefficients, ICC values lie in the range 1 (perfect agreement) and are negative when the agreement between the raters is worse than random. Unlike the PCC and Spearman rank coefficients, there are ICCs defined that are measures of absolute agreement between the 2 sets of readings and reduce if, for example, their means are not equal. This makes them more appropriate choices for evaluating agreement between an AI output and a ground truth in many circumstances.

QUALITY OF GROUND TRUTH

As discussed previously, there are many different metrics to choose from, depending on the task of interest. Simply choosing a proper metric given a task of interest is not sufficient to ensure a fair and unbiased evaluation of an AI algorithm, because issues stemming directly from the ground truth (or gold standard) also can affect algorithm evaluation.

For all tasks, the absolute truth is known as the gold standard. This absolute truth, which often is unknown/unobserved, is estimated/approximated by an expert to manually generate some reference standard. For instance, the reference standard for image segmentation is the region of interest (ROI) as delineated by an expert and the reference standard for image classification is the class/category as chosen by an expert. As expected, the construction of a large database of manually generated reference standards can be an extremely time-consuming and resource-intensive task, especially with regard to image segmentation.[49]

Generating reference standard region of interest of cardiac anatomy (ventricles, atria, great vessels, and so forth) on high-resolution MR imaging can take upwards of 4 hours to 8 hours per patient.[50] As discussed previously, the absolute truth often is unknown given what information is available to the expert. For example, some pathologies may take multiple imaging modalities and clinical biomarkers to classify correctly, and the omission of a modality/biomarker leads to uncertainty in the expert's reference standard. Even in the scenario where an expert is highly certain of their reference standard, different experts often still disagree. This disagreement formally is termed inter-rater variability and intrarater variability, where inter-rater variability measures disagreement between multiple unique individuals and intrarater variability measures disagreement of a single individual over time.[51] Careful consideration must be made if a task exhibits poor inter-rater variability and/or intrarater variability, because this affects the evaluation of the proposed AI algorithm. An extreme example can be found in the Lung Image Database Consortium,[52] where 4 expert radiologists marked lung lesions on 1018 computed tomography (CT) scans. Although 2669 lesions were marked as greater than 3 mm by at least 1 expert, only 35% of those lesions had been marked by all 4 experts, showing the variance in the reference standards from the 4 different experts.[53]

Additionally, the quality of the raters themselves must be assessed. When generating reference standards for complicated and nuanced pathologies, such as the segmentation of heterogeneous high-grade gliomas, less experienced individuals (ie, undergraduate students, medical students, and new medical residents) create reference standards with higher amounts of uncertainty than specialists who have had years of dedicated training. In cases of relatively untrained individuals responsible for creating these reference standards, it is imperative to have these checked and modified as necessary by an expert to ensure a high-quality reference that is as close to the absolute truth as possible. Building off the previous point on inter-rater variability, it then is equally important to consider whether a single rater is sufficient for the task, or if the absolute truth can be approached more closely by generating a consensus label from multiple raters. Aggregation and adjudication of the assessments of a group of experts can lead to significantly more robust reference standards.[54–56] More sophisticated methods, such as those that employ expectation maximization to provide better consensus labels by estimating the quality of the rater, also may be used.[57]

So far, only reference standards that are manually generated by an expert have been discussed. In certain cases of too much data to annotate manually, it can be appropriate to use automated algorithms to generate a weak reference standard.[58] This weak reference standard generated by an algorithm should be handled as if it were generated by an untrained individual (ie, it should be checked and modified by an expert). A consensus of the outputs of many automatic algorithms also may be used, but the quality of such a reference hinges on the performance/accuracy of the algorithms.[59,60]

USER STUDIES

In certain scenarios, there may not be interest in an exact quantitative metric for evaluation purposes. Instead, it might be asked if the automatically generated segmentation is accurate enough for downstream analysis (ie, volumetric quantification or location assessment). For example, the lesion might not need to be segmented with 100% accuracy compared with the reference standard (especially in scenarios where the reference standard may differ significantly from the absolute truth). In this case, a Likert scale[61] (where a value of 1 indicates that the automatic segmentation is highly incorrect [<10%], and a value of 5 indicates that it is sufficiently correct [>90%]) can be defined and multiple raters grade the automatic outputs from the algorithm via this scale. Even if there exists minor disagreement between the raters, they all should grade similarly if the Likert scale is defined properly. This also can be more clinically useful because the algorithm is grading directly on whether the outputs are sufficient for downstream analysis.

INTERPRETABILITY

In addition to the qualitative and quantitative methods for algorithm evaluation, described previously, understanding how a model reaches its conclusion and why some samples are predicted properly whereas others are not may be of interest. This is important especially in the medical domain, where high-stakes algorithms are trained on small, homogenous cohorts of data may learn to use nonbiological and/or spurious correlations to arrive at their prediction as opposed to learning true, underlying patterns. A common critique of AI algorithms is that they are black box; in other words, these highly complex algorithms do not provide explanations for how they arrived at their predictions. A popular technique to make AI more interpretable is known as saliency maps, in which salient regions of the input medical image that are important to the model's final prediction are highlighted.[62] For instance, it is expected that a model labeling a chest radiograph for cardiomegaly makes its prediction based on the appearance of the heart; if a saliency method instead highlights other regions of the image, it may be evidence that the model has utilized spurious information for making this prediction of cardiomegaly. The clinical usability of a model is dependent not only on its raw performance but also on the soundness of its decision-making process.[23] Specifically, understanding the rationale behind predictions is important in understanding the algorithm's failure modes. Many saliency maps have been proposed in the literature and curious readers are referred to various publications on the matter.[62,63] In brief, it is important to know that these techniques still are in their infancy and there is much debate over their validity as a tool for AI interpretability. Studies have shown on both natural and medical images that most saliency methods are not sensitive to perturbations in either the data or the model parameters.[62,64] To that end, a saliency method must be evaluated rigorously and the limitations of the technique understood before using it to draw conclusions regarding AI interpretability.

SUMMARY

Many modern AI algorithms often claim to achieve or even surpass human level performance, but, as discussed in this article, it is of great importance to properly choose the metric by which an algorithm is evaluated. For instance, on a data set with a large class imbalance a very high binary classification accuracy with a largely worthless algorithm (as measured by sensitivity and specificity, which are more proper metrics for this scenario) can be obtained. In addition, proper tuning/evaluation of an algorithm on nonoverlapping validation and testing sets can help improve model generalizability, ensuring the model's utility and robustness in a clinical setting. Finally, even when the proper set of metrics is chosen along with correct usage of training, validation, and testing data sets, effective evaluation of an AI algorithm still may be marred by issues stemming directly from the ground truth (such as high inter-rater variability and/or intrarater variability). In summary, although AI holds great promise in revolutionizing image analysis across a spectrum of medical domains, such as radiology and pathology, special care must be taken with respect to algorithm evaluation in order to produce highly performant and generalizable deep-learning models.

DISCLOSURE

The authors have nothing to disclose.

REFERENCES

1. Aerts HJWL, Velazquez ER, Leijenaar RTH, et al. Decoding tumour phenotype by noninvasive imaging using a quantitative radiomics approach. Nat Commun 2014;5:4006.
2. Yun L, Syed Z, Scirica BM, et al. ECG Morphological Variability in Beat Space for Risk Stratification After Acute Coronary Syndrome. J Am Heart Assoc 2021;3:e000981.
3. LeCun Y, Bengio Y, Hinton G. Deep learning. Nature 2015;521:436.
4. Krizhevsky A, Sutskever I, Hinton GE. ImageNet Classification with Deep Convolutional Neural Networks. Commun ACM 2017;60:84–90.
5. Hinton G, Deng L, Yu D, et al. Deep Neural Networks for Acoustic Modeling in Speech Recognition: The Shared Views of Four Research Groups. IEEE Signal Process Mag 2012;29:82–97.
6. Collobert R, Weston J. A Unified Architecture for Natural Language Processing: Deep Neural Networks with Multitask Learning. in Proceedings of the 25th International Conference on Machine Learning. Association for Computing Machinery. Helsinki, Finland, July 2008. p. 160-7. https://doi.org/10.1145/1390156.1390177.
7. Hannun AY, Rajpurkar P, Haghpanahi M, et al. Cardiologist-level arrhythmia detection and classification in ambulatory electrocardiograms using a deep neural network. Nat Med 2019;25:65–9.
8. Brown J, Campbell JP, Beers A, et al. Automated Diagnosis of plus disease in retinopathy of prematurity using deep convolutional neural networks. JAMA Ophthalmol 2018;136:803–10.
9. Kather JN, Pearson AT, Halama N, et al. Deep learning can predict microsatellite instability directly from histology in gastrointestinal cancer. Nat Med 2019;25:1054–6.
10. Esteva A, Kuprel B, Novoa RA, et al. Dermatologist-level classification of skin cancer with deep neural networks. Nature 2017;542:115–8.
11. Chang K, Beers AL, Bai HX, et al. Automatic assessment of glioma burden: a deep learning algorithm for fully automated volumetric and bidimensional measurement. Neuro Oncol 2019;21:1412–22.
12. Li MD, Chang K, Bearce B, et al. Siamese neural networks for continuous disease severity evaluation and change detection in medical imaging. Npj Digit Med 2020;3:48.
13. Ouyang D, He B, Ghorbani A, et al. Video-based AI for beat-to-beat assessment of cardiac function. Nature 2020;580:252–6.

14. Irvin J, Rajpurkar P, Ko M, et al. CheXpert: {A} Large Chest Radiograph Dataset with Uncertainty Labels and Expert Comparison. CoRR abs/1901.0, (2019).

15. Yala A, Lehman C, Schuster T, et al. A Deep Learning Mammography-based Model for Improved Breast Cancer Risk Prediction. Radiology 2019;292:60–6.

16. Lu JT, Brooks R, Hahn S, et al. DeepAAA: clinically applicable and generalizable detection of abdominal aortic aneurysm using deep learning. (2019).

17. Chen KT, Gong E, de Carvalho Macruz FB, et al. Ultra–Low-Dose 18F-Florbetaben Amyloid PET Imaging Using Deep Learning with Multi-Contrast MRI Inputs. Radiology 2018;290:649–56.

18. Huang Y, Cheng Y, Bapna A, et al. GPipe: Efficient Training of Giant Neural Networks using Pipeline Parallelism. In: Wallach H, et al, editors. Advances in neural information processing systems. Curran Associates, Inc.; 2019. p. 32.

19. Zech JR, Badgeley MA, Liu M, et al. Variable generalization performance of a deep learning model to detect pneumonia in chest radiographs: A cross-sectional study. PLoS Med 2018. https://doi.org/10.1371/journal.pmed.1002683a.

20. Chang K, Beers AL, Brink L, et al. Multi-Institutional Assessment and Crowdsourcing Evaluation of Deep Learning for Automated Classification of Breast Density. J Am Coll Radiol 2020. https://doi.org/10.1016/j.jacr.2020.05.015.

21. Albadawy EA, Saha A, Mazurowski MA. Deep learning for segmentation of brain tumors: Impact of cross-institutional training and testing: Impact. Med Phys 2018. https://doi.org/10.1002/mp.12752.

22. Mårtensson G, Ferreira D, Granberg T, et al. The reliability of a deep learning model in clinical out-of-distribution MRI data: A multicohort study. Med Image Anal 2020;66:101714.

23. DeGrave AJ, Janizek JD, Lee S-I. AI for radiographic COVID-19 detection selects shortcuts over signal. medRxiv 2020. https://doi.org/10.1101/2020.09.13.20193565.

24. Haibe-Kains B, Adam GA, Hosny A, et al. Transparency and reproducibility in artificial intelligence. Nature 2020;586:E14–6.

25. Gibson E, Li W, Sudre C, et al. NiftyNet: a deep-learning platform for medical imaging. Comput Methods Programs Biomed 2018;158:113–22.

26. Isensee F, Jaeger PF, Kohl SAA, et al. a self-configuring method for deep learning-based biomedical image segmentation. Nat Methods 2021;18:203–11.

27. Beers A, Brown J, Chang K, et al. DeepNeuro: an open-source deep learning toolbox for neuroimaging. Neuroinformatics 2020. https://doi.org/10.1007/s12021-020-09477-5.

28. Larrazabal AJ, Nieto N, Peterson V, et al. Gender imbalance in medical imaging datasets produces biased classifiers for computer-aided diagnosis. Proc Natl Acad Sci 2020;117:12592–4.

29. Seyyed-Kalantari L, Liu G, McDermott M, et al. CheXclusion: Fairness gaps in deep chest X-ray classifiers 2020;26:232–43.

30. Tomašev N, Glorot X, Rae JW, et al. A clinically applicable approach to continuous prediction of future acute kidney injury. Nature 2019;572:116–9.

31. van Amsterdam WAC, Verhoeff JJC, de Jong PA, et al. Eliminating biasing signals in lung cancer images for prognosis predictions with deep learning. Npj Digit Med 2019;2:122.

32. Amini A, Soleimany AP, Schwarting W, et al. Uncovering and Mitigating Algorithmic Bias through Learned Latent Structure. In Proceedings of the 2019 AAAI/ACM Conference on AI, Ethics, and Society. Association for Computing Machinery. Honolulu, HI, January 2019. p. 289–95. doi:10.1145/3306618.3314243.

33. Mendoza F, Lu R. Basics of Image Analysis. Food Eng Ser 2015;9–56. https://doi.org/10.1007/978-1-4939-2836-1_2.

34. Fawcett T. An introduction to ROC analysis. Pattern Recognit Lett 2006;27:861–74.

35. Saito T, Rehmsmeier M. The Precision-Recall Plot Is More Informative than the ROC Plot When Evaluating Binary Classifiers on Imbalanced Datasets. PLoS One 2015;10:e0118432.

36. He H, Garcia EA. Learning from Imbalanced Data. IEEE Trans Knowl Data Eng 2009;21:1263–84.

37. Chinchor, N. MUC-4 Evaluation Metrics. in Proceedings of the 4th Conference on Message Understanding. Association for Computational Linguistics. McLean, VA, June 1992. p. 22–9. doi:10.3115/1072064.1072067.

38. McHugh ML. Interrater reliability: the kappa statistic. Biochem Med 2012;22:276–82.

39. Jaccard P. The Distribution of the Flora in the Alpine Zone. New Phytol 1912;11:37–50.

40. Dice LR. Measures of the Amount of Ecologic Association Between Species. Ecology 1945;26:297–302.

41. Huttenlocher, D. P., Rucklidge, W. J. & Klanderman, G. A. Comparing images using the Hausdorff distance under translation. in Proceedings 1992 IEEE Computer Society Conference on Computer Vision and Pattern Recognition. Champaign, IL, June 1992. 654–6. doi: 10.1109/CVPR.1992.223209.

42. Taha AA, Hanbury A. Metrics for evaluating 3D medical image segmentation: analysis, selection, and tool. BMC Med Imaging 2015;15:29.

43. Everingham M, Van Gool L, Williams CKI, et al. The Pascal Visual Object Classes (VOC) Challenge. Int J Comput Vis 2010;88:303–38.

44. Lin, T.-Y. et al. Microsoft COCO: Common Objects in Context. in ECCV (European Conference on Computer Vision). Zürich, Switzerland, September 2014.

45. Bandos AI, Rockette HE, Song T, et al. Area under the free-response ROC curve (FROC) and a related summary index. Biometrics 2009;65:247–56.

46. Shrout PE, Fleiss JL. Intraclass correlations: uses in assessing rater reliability. Psychol Bull 1979;86: 420–8.

47. McGraw KO, Wong SP. Forming inferences about some intraclass correlation coefficients. Psychol Methods 1996;1:30–46.

48. Koo TK, Li MY. A Guideline of Selecting and Reporting Intraclass Correlation Coefficients for Reliability Research. J Chiropr Med 2016;15:155–63.

49. Despotović I, Goossens B, Philips W. MRI Segmentation of the Human Brain: Challenges, Methods, and Applications. Comput Math Methods Med 2015;2015:450341.

50. Pace DF, Dalca AV, Geva T, et al. Interactive Whole-Heart Segmentation in Congenital Heart Disease. Med Image Comput Comput Assist Interv 2015; 9351:80–8.

51. Prevedello LM, Halabi SS, Shih G, et al. Challenges Related to Artificial Intelligence Research in Medical Imaging and the Importance of Image Analysis Competitions. Radiol Artif Intell 2019;1:e180031.

52. Armato SG 3rd, McNitt-Gray MF, Reeves AP, et al. The Lung Image Database Consortium (LIDC): an evaluation of radiologist variability in the identification of lung nodules on CT scans. Acad Radiol 2007;14:1409–21.

53. Armato SG 3rd, McLennan G, Bidaut L, et al. The Lung Image Database Consortium (LIDC) and Image Database Resource Initiative (IDRI): a completed reference database of lung nodules on CT scans. Med Phys 2011;38:915–31.

54. Taylor-Phillips S, Jenkinson D, Stinton C, et al. Double Reading in Breast Cancer Screening: Cohort Evaluation in the CO-OPS Trial. Radiology 2018; 287:749–57.

55. Barnett ML, Boddupalli D, Nundy S, et al. Comparative Accuracy of Diagnosis by Collective Intelligence of Multiple Physicians vs Individual Physicians. JAMA Netw Open 2019;2:e190096.

56. Krause J, Gulshan V, Rahimy E, et al. Grader Variability and the Importance of Reference Standards for Evaluating Machine Learning Models for Diabetic Retinopathy. Ophthalmology 2018;125:1264–72.

57. Jordan MI, Jacobs RA. Hierarchical mixtures of experts and the EM algorithm. in Proceedings of 1993 International Conference on Neural Networks (IJCNN-93-Nagoya, Japan), October 1993. p. 1339–44. vol.2. doi: 10.1109/IJCNN.1993.716791.

58. Ratner A, Bach SH, Ehrenberg H, et al. Snorkel: Rapid Training Data Creation with Weak Supervision. Proc VLDB Endow 2017;11:269–82.

59. Rolnick D, Veit A, Belongie S, et al. Deep Learning is Robust to Massive Label Noise. 2018.

60. Wang X, Peng Y, Lu L, et al. ChestX-Ray8: Hospital-Scale Chest X-Ray Database and Benchmarks on Weakly-Supervised Classification and Localization of Common Thorax Diseases. 2017 IEEE Conference on Computer Vision and Pattern Recognition (CVPR). Honolulu, HI, July 21-26, 2017. p. 3462–71. doi: 10.1109/CVPR.2017.369.

61. Likert R. A technique for the measurement of attitudes. Arch Psychol 1932;22(140):55.

62. Adebayo J, Gilmer J, Muelly M, et al. Sanity Checks for Saliency Maps. 2020.

63. Reyes M, Meier R, Pereira S, et al. On the Interpretability of Artificial Intelligence in Radiology: Challenges and Opportunities. Radiol Artif Intell 2020;2: e190043.

64. Arun N, Gaw N, Singh P, et al. Assessing the (Un) Trustworthiness of Saliency Maps for Localizing Abnormalities in Medical Imaging. (2020).

Optimization of Radiology Workflow with Artificial Intelligence

Erik Ranschaert, MD, PhD[a,b,*], Laurens Topff, MD[c], Oleg Pianykh, PhD[d]

KEYWORDS

• Artificial intelligence • Machine learning • Workflow • Operational efficiency • Radiology

KEY POINTS

- Artificial intelligence (AI) can be used not only for diagnostic purposes but also for a variety of operational tasks in the radiology workflow.
- Machine learning algorithms can guide workflow optimization by identifying the key factors responsible for workflow outcomes.
- Although operational AI tools demonstrate remarkable potential for improving radiology workflow, more work needs to be done to make them widely available.

INTRODUCTION

Over the past few years, artificial intelligence (AI) has made a significant advance in the medical world, particularly due to developments in the field of machine learning (ML) and deep learning (DL), coupled with tremendous increases in computational processing power. This has led to the development of new tools enabling computerized image analysis, mainly for tasks of classification and detection of abnormalities.[1] Combining these tools with radiomics (providing quantitative image data not perceptible to the human eye) and data from the electronic medical record (EMR) makes it possible to evaluate patients' response to therapy, paving the way to personalized treatments.[2]

The potential applications of AI in radiology, however, go well beyond image analysis for diagnostic and prognostic purposes. It is becoming increasingly clear that AI algorithms also can be used for a variety of nondiagnostic tasks to provide support in all levels of the radiology workflow for purposes, such as scheduling, prioritizing, quality, safety, and operational efficiency.[1,3] Radiology business intelligence and management tools, providing real-time dashboarding and performing workflow analysis, also can be guided by ML.[2,4] Time to image, modality utilization, and report turnaround time (RTAT) are just a few of the metrics that already are utilized. As health care progresses from volume to value, such intelligent enterprise view of the radiology department will be useful to maintain the highest-quality services at the lowest cost.

Although the technology is present and already reported in multiple health care institutions, clinical implementation of AI tools in its broadest sense still is in its early phase and remains rather limited. One of the major reasons is because integration often is hampered by a lack of infrastructure, processes, and tools.[5] Complex radiology information technology (IT) environments pose unique challenges in implementing AI-based solutions.[6] Moreover, AI tools cannot work on their own and need to be properly integrated and maintained. To do so, serious work is needed to ensure the readiness

a Elisabeth-Tweesteden Hospital, Hilvarenbeekseweg 60, 5022 GC Tilburg, The Netherlands; b Ghent University, C. Heymanslaan 10, 9000 Gent, Belgium; c Netherlands Cancer Institute, Plesmanlaan 121, 1066 CX, Amsterdam, The Netherlands; d Department of Radiology, Harvard Medical School, Massachusetts General Hospital, 25 New Chardon Street, Suite 470, Boston, MA 02114, USA
* Corresponding author. Elisabeth-Tweesteden Hospital, Hilvarenbeekseweg 60, 5022 GC Tilburg, The Netherlands.
E-mail address: erik.ranschaert@ugent.be

Radiol Clin N Am 59 (2021) 955–966
https://doi.org/10.1016/j.rcl.2021.06.006

and suitability of the existing informatics infrastructure in the radiology department and in the hospital.

Another reason for the slow-moving implementation of AI in clinical practice can be found in tight policies and regulations, governing the use of AI in clinical environments. AI-based applications for "diagnosis, prevention, monitoring, treatment, or alleviation of disease" belong to the category of Software as a Medical Device (SaMD), as defined by the International Medical Device Regulators Forum (IMDRF).[7] This means that they must meet more stringent requirements and thus also have to go through a longer trajectory before they can be marketed and used effectively in the clinical setting.[8,9] The IMDRF also has outlined quality management system principles to systematically evaluate for SaMD applications in terms of their functionalities and performance.[7] Because nondiagnostic AI tools for workflow improvement are not considered as SaMD, there is no regulatory obligation to prove their robustness and validity. It is expected that many of such operational tools will be implemented in the more immediate future.[3]

Financial gains play another important role in determining the applicability of operational AI. With a few exceptions, insurance reimbursements are not currently available in most countries for the use or purchase of AI software.[10] Consequently, the return on investment (ROI) must be evaluated by the demonstration of quality and/or efficiency improvement. For diagnostic-type AI, quality improvement could be achieved by reducing errors or increasing diagnostic accuracy, which by assumption not only could be of clinical benefit but also reduce downstream costs in liability insurance.[11] Demonstrating the ROI for tools that improve efficiency, however, is easier than for tools that improve quality. Reduction of study read times by using diagnostic AI-based software, for example, can be translated directly into person-hours and subsequent cost savings. So, for nondiagnostic applications that in general are more focused on workflow improvement and efficiency, the cost-saving effect is easier to calculate, which also facilitates their implementation. Most of these tools probably will not be sold separately but as an (optional) feature of the vendor's modality, picture archiving and communication system (PACS), EMR, or speech recognition system, which also facilitates their integration in the existing radiology IT environment.

In this article the authors take a closer look at the types of nondiagnostic AI solutions, which are focused on the automation of operational tasks, such as the evaluation of appropriateness of imaging, patient scheduling, selection of examination protocols, improvement of radiologists' workflow, and more, to ultimately improve the radiology workflow and patient services (**Fig. 1**).

ORDER ENTRY SUPPORT

Ordering a patient examination is the first step in the diagnostic imaging chain. It is about not only identifying the right imaging modality to help the patient but also about ensuring the safe execution of the imaging examination or procedure.[3] Over the past few decades, medical imaging utilization has been increasing rapidly. In the United States alone, the number of imaging examinations increased by 26% between 1998 and 2010, mainly due to more advanced types of services, such as computed tomography (CT) and MR imaging.[12] Similarly, a 2018 report by a UK workforce reported a 54% increase in demand for CT examinations and 48% for MR imaging examinations over the previous 5 years, confirming this trend.[13] Due to this relentless increase in workload for radiologists and the associated growing health care costs, continuing with adding more work is not a feasible option. As a result, it is necessary to find solutions to manage this growth while maintaining quality standards of patient care.[14,15]

In the 2 recent decades, in the pre-AI era, several clinical decision support (CDS) systems have been created with the intention of providing referrers with the best possible guidance when ordering imaging examinations, in the belief that this will reduce inappropriate utilization of low-value, high-cost imaging.[16] The Select module of the American College of Radiology (ACR) and the iGuide from the European Society of Radiology (ESR) provide recommendations based on appropriateness criteria and referral guidelines, as defined by dedicated experts and committees.[17,18] ACR Select works with a database comprising more than 3000 clinical scenarios and 15,000 criteria. These CDS modules can be incorporated into computerized ordering and EHR systems to guide providers when ordering medical imaging scans.[17,19] They calculate an appropriateness score for the requested imaging imagination, based on the clinical information and abnormal prior tests as selected from an examination-specific menu of choices. The benefits of these CDS systems have been documented throughout the literature and are promoted by the ACR and the ESR.[17] A recent trial[20] demonstrated that CDS systems can reduce targeted (ie, likely inappropriate) imaging orders by a statistically

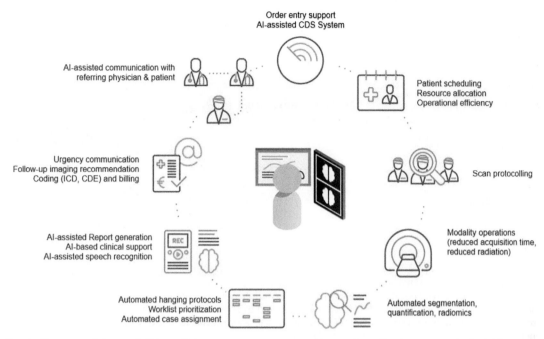

Fig. 1. The potential use of AI in radiology encompasses an amalgam of applications, several of which are not interpretative but aimed at automation of operational tasks, such as the evaluation of appropriateness of imaging, patient scheduling, selection of examination protocols, improvement of radiologists' reporting workflow. and much more.

significant 6%, allowing reducing imaging-associated costs. The potential of using ML for creating CDS-based order entry support systems nowadays is considered as an important area of research.[16,17] Pre-AI CDS systems mostly are developed as rule-based (also known as if-then systems), operating by applying a set of relevant predefined rules and then providing a recommendation. A weakness of such systems is that they become difficult to operate (and even more difficult to maintain) when the number of rules is large or when separate rules contradict each other. In addition, they are able to account for only a limited amount of clinical data as presented in a selection menu, making them impractical for more complex clinical situations.[19] To address these problems, more adaptive data-driven systems can be developed to operate on large data sets through data mining the most appropriate imaging tests by analyzing notes and other EMR features. By integrating ML, the existing shortcomings of CDS systems could be overcome, either by teaching the system much more complex rules or by letting it discover some optimal rules on its own. Such AI-based CDS systems could perform automated screening for renal insufficiency when placing orders for contrast-enhanced studies. Another example is screening for duplicate examination orders within a predetermined timeframe.[16] As was

shown by Hassanpour and colleagues,[21] it is possible to develop ML classifiers to analyze narrative radiology reports and to identify high utilizers of imaging services with 94% accuracy. In the future, it should be possible to create a complete digital representation of a patient, a so-called digital twin, allowing a CDS system to make recommendations based on a more holistic approach.[1,17,22] By combining this in-depth knowledge with adaptive decision-making in complex and uncertain environments, AI-based frameworks will have great value for optimizing radiology examination ordering, reducing overuse of imaging, and erroneous ordering and protocolling of scans.[1,23]

SCHEDULING AND RESOURCE ALLOCATION

Scheduling and any resource allocation in general represent another recent and interesting development in radiology AI. They also can be viewed as an important direction in health care operations analysis, a relatively new field, aiming at optimizing health care delivery. For years, the clinical aspects of health care were prioritized, looking into better practices and more informative models.[23] Many health care failures, however—delayed or unavailable services, incorrect decisions, and overloaded workflows—have purely operational

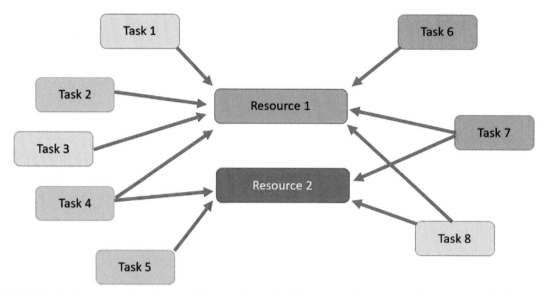

Fig. 2. Standard resource allocation problem—such as scheduling outpatient examinations on several radiology scanners. There are different task types to be scheduled, and different resources; some tasks may be done on any resource and some only on certain resources. The goal is to assign tasks to resources to minimize specific cost function, such as resource idling and patient wait time.

causes and can have a dramatic impact on the overall quality and safety of patient care.[24,25]

In this regard, resource allocation represents one of the most important and classic problems of workflow optimization (**Fig. 2**). Each hospital process can be seen as a series of tasks assigned to different resources: for example, specific patient examinations must be scheduled for a particular MRI scanner, depending on the type of examination. Each task can have its own complexity (such as examination duration time or scanning protocol) and each resource its own cost (such as scanner time or negative impact of scanner delays). As a result, for any workflow in question, its resource utilization cost function can be set—for instance, total idle time for all MR imaging scanners in a given outpatient facility. The goal of resource allocation is to compute optimal task-to-resource assignments (schedules), to minimize this predefined cost.

For a single resource or task type (such as scheduling the same MR imaging examination on the same scanner), the problem looks rather trivial and often can be resolved by a human. This virtually never is the case with real-life scheduling, however, where multiple intertwined resources, scheduling constraints, and workflow disruptions make simple solutions impossible. As a result, real operational problems call for more exhaustive, algorithmic solvers.

Therefore, many pre-ML scheduling solvers already have been attempted for decades,

including linear programming,[26–28] genetic programming,[29] and branch-and-bound, simulated annealing[30,31] as well as more ad hoc algorithms.[32] They were followed by simulation models—discrete event simulations (DESs), in particular—capable of modeling virtually any operational environment.[28,33–36] The entire premise of pre-ML algorithms (such as DES), however, was based on the ability to fully understand the existing environment, and to rewrite it as a logical computer model (**Fig. 3**).

Although attractive from the interpretability point of view, this workflow model approach ran into a major obstacle: current health care environments could be too complex to interpret. The emergency department (ED) chart in **Fig. 4** illustrates this better than anything: it shows the real ED workflow map, which was reconstructed from the actual ED data by a process mining algorithm.[25] When the authors did this for 1 project, it took several weeks to explain it to the emergency physicians, who spent years working in this environment. The main complexity comes from the fact that real health care environments are probabilistic: in a couple minutes, a patient who enters such an environment may end up in any of its branches, with a great degree of probabilistic uncertainty. This probabilistic mess undermines the ability to package the problem into a nice clean flowchart model (such as DES) or define exact relationships among the model parameters (such as required by pre-ML solvers). Therefore, the only way to model

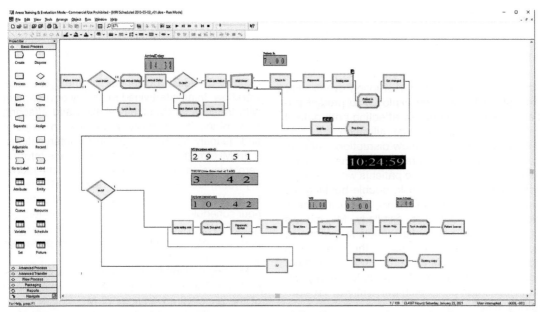

Fig. 3. DES model built to simulate MR imaging scanner workflow (Mass General Hospital, Arena software). Each model block can be defined with its own properties, such as processing time or task queueing logic. When the model is executed, it creates new patient entities entering the workflow (*top left corner*), runs them through the model, and outputs simulation metrics. Changing model parameters can be used to tune the model (manual analogy to ML model training), and to answer what if questions.

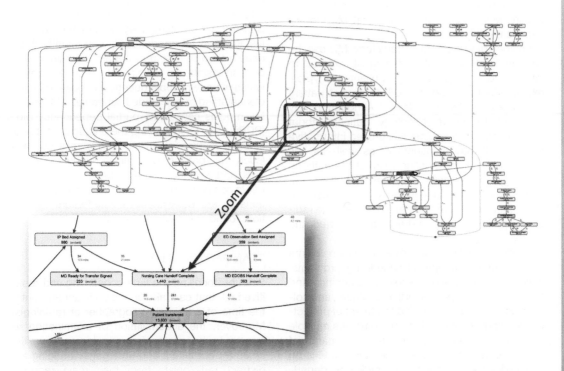

Fig. 4. Process mining algorithm, applied to reconstruct the real workflow in an ED. Note the overall flow complexity and interconnectivity of different steps. (*Courtesy of* Oleg Pianykh, Medical Analytics Group, Mass General Hospital.)

this environment is to make the model learn all these complexities on its own, by fitting the model coefficients into the actual workflow data. And this is precisely what ML models are capable of.

First, ML models prove efficient in predicting scheduling and workflow-disrupting events. For example, ML has been explored to predict patient no-shows, negatively affecting both patient care and radiology resource utilization.[19,37,38] As a result, predicting no-show disruptions with ML can be used for taking practical actions: appointment reminder calls to the patients with the highest predicted no-show risk, double-booking the slots with predicted no-shows, and using these slots for other activities. Similarly, ML models predicting patient risks (implants, adverse contrast reaction, and so forth) could help schedule these patients better and ensure safer scans. Thus, using ML to correctly classify examinations can provide an efficient way for optimizing scheduling.[39]

Second, ML demonstrated good potential in many shared resource problems, when the same resource must be used by multiple concurrent workflows. Waiting rooms in multimodality outpatient centers, recovery rooms in interventional radiology, scanners used by different radiology departments, and more frequently can be shared by radiology and other hospital services and require well-planned scheduling that ML models can create.[40,41]

Another development in radiology ML can be seen in increasing patient-facing AI, created to inform and engage radiology patients. A typical example includes models built to predict patient wait times and facility delays.[42] Although initially designed to inform radiology patients about possible delays, these models proved informative for the radiology management as well—as has been learned, implementing them at the authors' radiology department.[43] The authors believe that more work will be done in this direction, particularly with using ML models to closely engage radiology patients and address their scheduling needs.[44]

Finally, predicting radiology examination volume offers another example of scheduling problems, aimed at improving radiology planning and finance. For example, the article by Zhang and colleagues[45] provides a detailed treatment of predicting radiology volume in ED and compares multiple ML models as well as identifies the cyclic nature of the model and its features. The study of Guitron and colleagues[46] shows how radiology department volume can be projected accurately a few weeks ahead, even during the uncertain times of pandemic volume drops.

OPERATIONAL EFFICIENCY

The role AI can play in allocating optimal resources immediately points to another important and currently developing direction: identification and removal of hidden bottlenecks in the operational workflow. In an intertwined radiology environment with traffic jams constantly shifting and affecting each other, it is virtually impossible to pinpoint and quantify the best direction for interventions. If an MR imaging outpatient facility runs into severe delays, then should the capacity of the recovery room be increased? Or extra MR imaging technologists be added? Or more patients per hour schedule? Or more MR imaging scanners acquired? When only a couple of possible interventions can be afforded and chosen, their projected gains have to be known.

ML-driven workflow optimization solves this problem. This becomes possible because of one of the principal advantages of ML modeling—its built-in ability to detect the best (most predictive) features. This functionality was completely missing in pre-ML models, where one working with unfeasibly exhaustive "what if" model tweaking was possible. Running ML optimal feature selection algorithms—from feature importance to more in-depth feature subset selection—can pinpoint the most critical workflow parameters efficiently and, therefore, suggest the best ways of fixing the problems they are pointing to.[47] For instance, an ML model easily can identify that a certain time of day, or a certain modality queue, is responsible for significant reporting delays, which, if known, subsequently can point to insufficient staffing or overloaded schedule.[48] Moreover, ML models can create partial dependency plots (PDPs) (Fig. 5), identifying the unique contribution of each feature into the main process outcome (such as patient wait time, workflow delay, queueing problem, or no-show).[19] In this way, PDPs can be used to answer many "what if" questions as well but without manual feature exploration, found in pre-ML approaches.

SCAN PROTOCOLLING

Scan protocolling is a time-consuming and repetitive task that can take up a significant amount of the time of a trained radiographer or radiologist. Moreover, the accumulation of examination requests to be protocoled can increase waiting times for outpatient and emergency imaging and distract radiologists from their main reporting work. Therefore, efficient and streamlined preparation of radiology examinations may present several administrative and operational challenges.

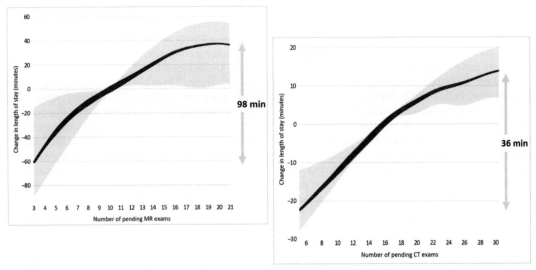

Fig. 5. Using PDP from an ML model to study the impact of CT (*left*) and MR (*right*) imaging scheduling on emergency patient length of stay (vertical axis, in minutes). Note that ML model was used to isolate each feature and identify its individual impact. (*Courtesy of* Steven Guitron, Medical Analytics Group, Mass General Hospital.)

Proper protocolling of scans is inevitably linked to specific medical information. In addition, protocols often can be suboptimal, depending on the expertise or personal preferences of the protocolling radiologist. Although automated CDS systems using ML techniques are growing in popularity, few investigators so far have studied their applicability for protocolling.[1] To build systems for automated protocol selection, different natural language processing (NLP) techniques can be used, to extract and to process relevant clinical text data from the field of clinical information as well as from prior study reports.[1] Besides clinical information and history, other features, such as patient demographics (age and sex) and ordering service or referring physician, can be used.

Trivedi and colleagues[49] have successfully demonstrated that NLP can be used for free-text analysis of the clinical indication for a study, to automatically determine the need for IV contrast in musculoskeletal MR imaging, with an accuracy of 80%. In another study, Lee[50] showed that DL-based convolutional neural networks can be utilized clinically to select a tumor versus routine protocol for musculoskeletal MR imaging, with an accuracy of 94%. More recently Kalra and colleagues[51] were able to train an NLP-based classification algorithm for CT and MR imaging protocol assignment, able to provide 69% of protocols in automation mode with 95% accuracy. The administrative scheduling process in the radiology department can be enhanced significantly by implementation of these semiautomated or automated protocolling algorithms. This could

free up radiologists for more important, high-level activities.

Currently, in most radiology departments, choosing the most appropriate scanning protocol sometimes is complicated by the limited information provided on the application form, where other relevant information from the patient record might not always be (timely) available. In the future, when it is possible to automatically analyze and include more in-depth information from the EMR, it will be possible to facilitate this process, which also will contribute to choosing the best scanning protocol. In addition, this should help identify any superfluous or redundant scans, which also will give a requesting physician or radiologist the opportunity to propose a more appropriate solution. With the increasing sophistication of NLP and ML applications, it also is possible to perform efficient safety screening of patients before scheduling a scan, identifying any contraindications when planning a contrast-enhanced study.[1,23]

Finally, combining ML optimal features selection and interpretable models with scan protocolling and NLP can lead to another interesting direction: auto-discovering interpretable protocolling rules from the historical protocolling data. This rule-discovering ML can create even better decision support systems, thus enhancing knowledge of critical decision-making factors.

WORKLIST OPTIMIZATION

In most institutions, radiologists report examinations in their chronologic order, with exceptions for emergency and hospitalized patients, who are given higher priority. This idea of prioritization corresponds nicely to the fact that many of the first clinically available AI applications for radiology have been developed to detect acute imaging findings and, therefore, can be used to prioritize cases in the radiologist's reading worklist. By detecting critical conditions and alerting the radiologist, these tools potentially can reduce the time to diagnosis and treatment and improve patient outcomes. This becomes relevant especially when there is a significant backlog of unreported examinations. Because prioritization tools are assistive and do not provide a final diagnosis, a limited number of false positive alerts can be tolerated.

This approach makes worklist integration one of the preferred ways to implement the currently available single-task AI applications in the radiologist workflow. Some examples of use cases are the detection and prioritization of intracranial hemorrhage on head CT,[52–55] pulmonary embolism on CT,[56] and pneumothorax on chest radiography.[57,58] Baltruschat and colleagues[58] demonstrated in a simulation environment that AI-based worklist prioritization can reduce the RTAT for critical findings on chest radiographs while not exceeding the maximum RTAT for nonprioritized examinations, to account for possible false-negative AI predictions.

A study from O'Neill and colleagues[53] showed that the method of implementing critical AI results in the radiologist's workflow is important to having a positive impact on wait time, defined as the interval between image acquisition and viewing of the images by the radiologist. They investigated the implementation of an AI tool for the detection of intracranial hemorrhage in nonenhanced head CTs. There was no significant impact on examination wait time when the critical notifications were solely displayed in a pop-up widget or with a worklist flag. Only by reprioritizing the positive examinations to the top of the worklist, a significant reduction in wait time was achieved.

Radiology departments and practices that handle high volumes of examinations, especially when managing multiple imaging facilities, might benefit from more advanced workflow orchestration tools to increase operational efficiency, maximize quality, and improve service levels. Case assignments in the radiologists' worklists can be automated, ensuring an evenly distributed workload and complexity among radiologists. In a multireader practice, Wong and colleagues[59] used analytics-driven worklists based on individual radiologists' interpretation times for musculoskeletal MR imaging studies to reduce the overall group interpretation times for such examinations. This

was done by redistributing examinations based on the calculated relative interpretation times of individual radiologists. Radiologists with relatively faster interpretation times for certain examinations would be assigned more of those examinations and vice versa. There are many more factors, however, than the radiologist's reading speed that need to be taken into account. AI has the potential to optimize workflow management software by using all available data, for example, a radiologist's schedule and availability, reporting history, behavioral patterns, subspecialty expertise, and so forth.

Another possible way in which AI applications can optimize the reading workflow is to label examinations that are normal or completely unchanged from a prior examination. If such classification could be achieved with a high sensitivity, then this could reduce interpretation time significantly. In the future, normal examinations may not even require the interpretation of a radiologist.

HANGING PROTOCOLS

Hanging protocols determine how imaging series are displayed in a PACS viewer when an examination is opened. They also control which relevant prior examinations are loaded for comparison. Ideally, the user does not need to make any manual adjustments in the viewing layout before being able to start with image interpretation. Therefore, hanging protocols can contribute significantly to an efficient reading workflow.

The configuration of hanging protocols in most PACS viewers is based on rules using Digital Imaging and Communications in Medicine (DICOM) metadata. This can be time-intensive, especially in centers where there is a lot of variation in modality vendors, imaging from external sources, and individual user preferences. ML and DL techniques have the potential to automate semantic labeling of radiology examinations. Effective AI solutions are not restricted to using DICOM metadata, which often can be inconsistent or incomplete but also can analyze pixel data to identify anatomic region, pulse sequences, and scan parameters.[60,61] Intelligent systems also can learn personal preferences for hanging protocols based on the users' past adjustments.

REPORT GENERATION

Automated speech recognition (ASR) software nowadays is assisting most radiologists in generating radiology reports. The impact of ASR systems on report error rates and productivity in radiology departments, however, still seems to be variable. A systematic literature review by Hammana and colleagues[62] shows that by using ASR the percentage of reports with at least 1 error still varies between 4.8% and 89%, whereas the RTAT can be improved by 35% to 99%. Although recent information about ongoing research is scarce, it is expected that the accuracy of ASR will be improved significantly by AI algorithms and that new features will be added to streamline image interpretation and reporting, with a positive effect on the radiology workflow.[3]

The report generation falls toward the end of the workflow, making it very sensitive to errors from preceding steps and requiring thorough quality management.[3,63] The algorithm's output can be presented in different ways, one of them being a DICOM Structured Report (DICOM SR).[64] By using a DICOM SR output, the algorithm's results can be integrated automatically in the reports. Examples of such AI-based results that can be automatically integrated within the radiology report include calculated organ-specific dose estimates, volume calculations of detected pulmonary lesions, or dual-energy x-ray absorptiometry scores obtained from routine CT scans.[1,65] Automation of reporting of more complex examinations, such as oncological CT scans containing a multitude of quantifiable findings, is more challenging due to the risk for information overload.[66] To make these solutions efficient, integration of prior examinations and reports needs to be performed, to avoid missing important prior findings, and to evaluate the size or treatment response of a specific abnormality. Despite increasing efforts to improve data exchange, supporting the workflow by automatically displaying crucial information from prior examinations when measuring specific lesions on cross-sectional examinations remains a challenge.[12]

FINAL CONSIDERATIONS

As this review demonstrates, operational AI solutions begin to enter many areas of radiology workflow management, demonstrating significant practical potential. They help investigate, monitor, and forecast operational environments with dozens of intertwined variables, thus greatly surpassing simple human estimates and pre-ML algorithms. Moreover, ML models can help understand the hidden dependencies between various workflow parameters, and their exact contribution into the main efficiency metrics, which can be used to identify the real problems behind the observed numbers. Nevertheless, significant work needs to be done to make operational AI solutions widespread and robustly implemented.[3]

In the authors' opinion, the radiologist's non-diagnostic workflow also can benefit greatly from AI, for example, by improving scan protocolling, worklist orchestration, and hanging protocols. Intelligent tools need to be developed that focus on an optimal user experience. One of the main practical obstacles to this work lies in the current lack of integration between various IT systems and data sources in the radiology department and hospital. Therefore, transitioning radiology data flows from the currently siloed to an all-inclusive integration will greatly benefit not only the operational AI but also diagnostic AI applications.

CLINICS CARE POINTS

- Operational AI solutions are developed to improve healthcare delivery and management, and they are beginning to make inroads into many areas of radiology.
- AI and machine learning models can efficiently solve challenging operational problems with complex, multi-variable workflows.
- Radiology workflow management can benefit greatly from AI, for example, by improving scan protocolling, worklist orchestration, hanging protocols, and user experience.
- Significant work remains to be done to make operational AI solutions widely adopted and robustly implemented.
- Transitioning radiology data flows from the currently siloed to an all-inclusive integration will greatly benefit not only the operational AI but also diagnostic AI applications.

DISCLOSURE STATEMENT

No disclosures.

REFERENCES

1. Letourneau-Guillon L, Camirand D, Guilbert F, et al. Artificial Intelligence Applications for Workflow, Process Optimization and Predictive Analytics. Neuroimaging Clin N Am 2020;30(4):e1–15.
2. Petersilge CA. The Enterprise Imaging Value Proposition. J Digit Imaging 2020;33(1):37–48.
3. Kapoor N, Lacson R, Khorasani R. Workflow Applications of Artificial Intelligence in Radiology and an Overview of Available Tools. J Am Coll Radiol 2020;17(11):1363–70.

4. Cook TS, Nagy P. Business Intelligence for the Radiologist: Making Your Data Work for You. J Am Coll Radiol 2014;11(12):1238–40.

5. Gauriau R, Bridge C, Chen L, et al. Using DICOM Metadata for Radiological Image Series Categorization: a Feasibility Study on Large Clinical Brain MRI Datasets. J Digit Imaging 2020;33(3):747–62.

6. Sohn JH, Chillakuru YR, Lee S, et al. An Open-Source, Vender Agnostic Hardware and Software Pipeline for Integration of Artificial Intelligence in Radiology Workflow. J Digit Imaging 2020;33(4):1041–6.

7. Larson DB, Harvey H, Rubin DL, et al. Regulatory Frameworks for Development and Evaluation of Artificial Intelligence–Based Diagnostic Imaging Algorithms: Summary and Recommendations. J Am Coll Radiol 2020;18(3):413–24. https://doi.org/10.1016/j.jacr.2020.09.060.

8. Mehrizi MHR, van Ooijen P, Homan M. Applications of artificial intelligence (AI) in diagnostic radiology: a technography study. Eur Radiol 2020;1–7. https://doi.org/10.1007/s00330-020-07230-9.

9. Kruskal JB, Larson DB. Strategies for Radiology to Thrive in the Value Era. Radiology 2018;289(1):3–7.

10. Nicola GN. Has AI Reimbursement in Healthcare Entered a New Era?. 2020. Blog ACR Data Science Institute. Available at: https://www.acrdsi.org/DSIBlog/2020/10/17/14/56/Has-AI-Reimbursement-in-Healthcare-Entered-a-New-Era. Accessed January 17, 2021.

11. Tadavarthi Y, Vey B, Krupinski E, et al. The State of Radiology AI: Considerations for Purchase Decisions and Current Market Offerings. Radiol Artif Intell 2020;2(6):e200004.

12. Wichmann JL, Willemink MJ, Cecco CND. Artificial Intelligence and Machine Learning in Radiology: Current State and Considerations for Routine Clinical Implementation. Invest Radiol 2020;55(9). https://doi.org/10.1097/RLI.0000000000000673.

13. Clinical radiology UK workforce Census report 2018. The Royal College of Radiologists; 2019. p. 53. Available at: https://www.rcr.ac.uk/system/files/publication/field_publication_files/clinical-radiology-uk-workforce-census-report-2018.pdf. Accessed January 17, 2021.

14. Huang S-C, Pareek A, Seyyedi S, et al. Fusion of medical imaging and electronic health records using deep learning: a systematic review and implementation guidelines. Npj Digital Med 2020;3(1):136.

15. McDonald RJ, Schwartz KM, Eckel LJ, et al. The Effects of Changes in Utilization and Technological Advancements of Cross-Sectional Imaging on Radiologist Workload. Acad Radiol 2015;22(9):1191–8.

16. Makeeva V, Gichoya J, Hawkins CM, et al. The Application of Machine Learning to Quality Improvement Through the Lens of the Radiology Value Network. J Am Coll Radiol 2019;16(9):1254–8.

17. Bizzo BC, Almeida RR, Michalski MH, et al. Artificial Intelligence and Clinical Decision Support for Radiologists and Referring Providers. J Am Coll Radiol 2019;16(9):1351–6.

18. ESR)communications@myesr.org ES of R. Methodology for ESR iGuide content. Insights Imaging 2019;10(1):32.

19. Glover M, Daye D, Khalilzadeh O, et al. Socioeconomic and Demographic Predictors of Missed Opportunities to Provide Advanced Imaging Services. J Am Coll Radiol 2017;14(11). https://doi.org/10.1016/j.jacr.2017.05.015.

20. Doyle J, Abraham S, Feeney L, et al. Clinical decision support for high-cost imaging: A randomized clinical trial. Plos One 2019;14(3):e0213373.

21. Hassanpour S, Langlotz CP. Predicting High Imaging Utilization Based on Initial Radiology Reports: A Feasibility Study of Machine Learning. Acad Radiol 2016;23(1):84–9.

22. Morey JM, Haney NM, Kim W. Artificial Intelligence in Medical Imaging, Opportunities, Applications and Risks. undefined 2019;129–43. https://doi.org/10.1007/978-3-319-94878-2_11.

23. Choy G, Khalilzadeh O, Michalski M, et al. Current Applications and Future Impact of Machine Learning in Radiology. Radiology 2018;288(2):318–28.

24. Lakhani P, Prater AB, Hutson RK, et al. Machine Learning in Radiology: Applications Beyond Image Interpretation. J Am Coll Radiol 2018;15(2):350–9.

25. Rosenthal D, Pianykh O. Efficient radiology, how to optimize radiology operations. undefined 2020;33–60.

26. Gass SI. In: Books D, editor. Linear programming: Methods and applications. New York: Dover Publications; 2010.

27. Yılmaz AO, Baykal N. A novel approach to optimize workflow in grid-based teleradiology applications. Comput Methods Programs Biomed 2016;123:159–69.

28. Granja C, Almada-Lobo B, Janela F, et al. An optimization based on simulation approach to the patient admission scheduling problem using a linear programing algorithm. J Biomed Inform 2014;52:427–37.

29. O'Neill M, Langdon RPB, McPhee NF, et al. A Field Guide to Genetic Programming. Genet Program Evol M 2009;10(2):229–30.

30. Cohen O, Rosen MS. Algorithm comparison for schedule optimization in MR fingerprinting. Magn Reson Imaging 2017;41:15–21.

31. Azadeh A, Farahani MH, Torabzadeh S, et al. Scheduling prioritized patients in emergency department laboratories. Comput Methods Programs Biomed 2014;117(2):61–70.

32. Vermeulen IB, Bohte SM, Elkhuizen SG, et al. Adaptive resource allocation for efficient patient scheduling. Artif Intell Med 2009;46(1):67–80.

33. Tellis R, Starobinets O, Prokle M, et al. Identifying Areas for Operational Improvement and Growth in IR Workflow Using Workflow Modeling, Simulation, and Optimization Techniques. J Digit Imaging 2020;1–10. https://doi.org/10.1007/s10278-020-00397-z.

34. Patrick J, Puterman ML. Improving resource utilization for diagnostic services through flexible inpatient scheduling: A method for improving resource utilization. J Oper Res Soc 2007;58(2):235–45.

35. Idigo F, Idigo V, Agwu K, et al. Workflow estimation of a radiology department using modelling and simulation. Int J Adv Operations Manag 2020;12(2):122–41.

36. Lu L, Li J, Gisler P. Improving Financial Performance by Modeling and Analysis of Radiology Procedure Scheduling at a Large Community Hospital. J Med Syst 2011;35(3):299–307.

37. H S FS. Using machine learning for no show prediction in the scheduling of clinical exams. Int J Radiol Radiat Ther 2020;7(1):34.

38. Harvey HB, Liu C, Ai J, et al. Predicting No-Shows in Radiology Using Regression Modeling of Data Available in the Electronic Medical Record. J Am Coll Radiol 2017;14(10):1303–9.

39. Patil MA, Patil RB, Krishnamoorthy P, et al. A Machine Learning Framework for Auto Classification of Imaging System Exams in Hospital Setting for Utilization Optimization. 2016 38th Annu Int Conf IEEE Eng Med Biol Soc Embc 2016;2016:2423–6.

40. Fairley M, Scheinker D, Brandeau ML. Improving the efficiency of the operating room environment with an optimization and machine learning model. Health Care Manag Sci 2019;22(4):756–67.

41. Bellini V, Guzzon M, Bigliardi B, et al. Artificial Intelligence: A New Tool in Operating Room Management. Role of Machine Learning Models in Operating Room Optimization. J Med Syst 2020;44(1):20.

42. Pianykh OS, Rosenthal DI. Can We Predict Patient Wait Time? J Am Coll Radiol 2015;12(10):1058–66.

43. Curtis C, Liu C, Bollerman TJ, et al. Machine Learning for Predicting Patient Wait Times and Appointment Delays. J Am Coll Radiol 2018;15(9):1310–6.

44. Towbin AJ, O'Connor T, Perry LA, et al. Using informatics to engage patients. Pediatr Radiol 2020;50(11):1514–24.

45. Zhang Y, Luo L, Zhang F, et al. Emergency patient flow forecasting in the radiology department. Health Inform J 2020;26(4):2362–74.

46. Guitron S, Pianykh OS, Succi MD, et al. COVID-19: Recovery Models for Radiology Departments. J Am Coll Radiol 2020;17(11):1460–8.

47. Pianykh OS, Guitron S, Parke D, et al. Improving healthcare operations management with machine learning. Nat Mach Intell 2020;2(5):266–73.

48. Crowley C, Guitron S, Son J, et al. Modeling workflows: Identifying the most predictive features in healthcare operational processes. Plos One 2020;15(6):e0233810.

49. Trivedi H, Mesterhazy J, Laguna B, et al. Automatic Determination of the Need for Intravenous Contrast in Musculoskeletal MRI Examinations Using IBM Watson's Natural Language Processing Algorithm. J Digit Imaging 2018;31(2):245–51.

50. Lee YH. Efficiency Improvement in a Busy Radiology Practice: Determination of Musculoskeletal Magnetic Resonance Imaging Protocol Using Deep-Learning Convolutional Neural Networks. J Digit Imaging 2018;31(5):604–10.

51. Kalra A, Chakraborty A, Fine B, et al. Machine Learning for Automation of Radiology Protocols for Quality and Efficiency Improvement. J Am Coll Radiol 2020;17(9):1149–58.

52. Ginat DT. Analysis of head CT scans flagged by deep learning software for acute intracranial hemorrhage. Neuroradiology 2020;62(3):335–40.

53. O'Neill TJ, Xi Y, Stehel E, et al. Active Reprioritization of the Reading Worklist Using Artificial Intelligence Has a Beneficial Effect on the Turnaround Time for Interpretation of Head CTs with Intracranial Hemorrhage. Radiol Artif Intell 2020;e200024. https://doi.org/10.1148/ryai.2020200024.

54. Arbabshirani MR, Fornwalt BK, Mongelluzzo GJ, et al. Advanced machine learning in action: identification of intracranial hemorrhage on computed tomography scans of the head with clinical workflow integration. Npj Digital Med 2018;1(1):9.

55. Titano JJ, Badgeley M, Schefflein J, et al. Automated deep-neural-network surveillance of cranial images for acute neurologic events. Nat Med 2018;24(9):1337–41.

56. Weikert T, Winkel DJ, Bremerich J, et al. Automated detection of pulmonary embolism in CT pulmonary angiograms using an AI-powered algorithm. Eur Radiol 2020;30(12):6545–53.

57. Annarumma M, Withey SJ, Bakewell RJ, et al. Automated Triaging of Adult Chest Radiographs with Deep Artificial Neural Networks. Radiology 2019;291(1):180921.

58. Baltruschat I, Steinmeister L, Nickisch H, et al. Smart chest X-ray worklist prioritization using artificial intelligence: a clinical workflow simulation. Eur Radiol 2020;1–9. https://doi.org/10.1007/s00330-020-07480-7.

59. Wong TT, Kazam JK, Rasiej MJ. Effect of Analytics-Driven Worklists on Musculoskeletal MRI Interpretation Times in an Academic Setting. Am J Roentgenol 2019;212(5):1091–5.

60. Yi PH, Kim TK, Wei J, et al. Automated semantic labeling of pediatric musculoskeletal radiographs using deep learning. Pediatr Radiol 2019;49(8):1066–70.

61. Pizarro R, Assemlal H-E, Nigris DD, et al. Using Deep Learning Algorithms to Automatically Identify the Brain MRI Contrast: Implications for Managing Large Databases. Neuroinformatics 2019;17(1):115–30.

62. Hammana I, Lepanto L, Poder T, et al. Speech Recognition in the Radiology Department: A Systematic Review. Health Inf Manag J 2015;44(2):4–10.

63. Hosny A, Parmar C, Quackenbush J, et al. Artificial intelligence in radiology. Nat Rev Cancer 2018; 18(8):500–10.

64. Dikici E, Bigelow M, Prevedello LM, et al. Integrating AI into radiology workflow: levels of research, production, and feedback maturity. J Med Imaging 2020;7(01):1.

65. Tajmir SH, Alkasab TK. Toward Augmented Radiologists Changes in Radiology Education in the Era of Machine Learning and Artificial Intelligence. Acad Radiol 2018;25(6):747–50.

66. Rubin J, Sanghavi D, Zhao C, et al. Large Scale Automated Reading of Frontal and Lateral Chest X-Rays using Dual Convolutional Neural Networks. Arxiv 2018. Available at: https://arxiv.org/abs/1804.07839. Accessed January 17, 2021.

Upstream Machine Learning in Radiology

Christopher M. Sandino, PhD[a], Elizabeth K. Cole, MS[a], Cagan Alkan, MS[a], Akshay S. Chaudhari, PhD[b,c], Andreas M. Loening, MD, PhD[c], Dongwoon Hyun, PhD[c,1], Jeremy Dahl, PhD[c,1], Abdullah-Al-Zubaer Imran, PhD[c], Adam S. Wang, PhD[c], Shreyas S. Vasanawala, MD, PhD[c,*]

KEYWORDS

• Deep learning • Artificial intelligence • Medical imaging • Image reconstruction

KEY POINTS

- This article reviews multiple applications of artificial intelligence (AI) in which it has been used to vastly improve upstream components of the medical imaging pipeline.
- All medical imaging examinations can be accelerated by using AI to help manage examination schedules and imaging protocols.
- In ultrasound, AI has been used to form high-quality images with enhanced robustness to speckle noise.
- In computed tomography, AI-based image reconstruction approaches have been used to reconstruct high-quality images from low-dose acquisitions.
- In MR imaging, AI has been used to design optimal data sampling schemes, and reconstruction approaches to accelerate scan time.

INTRODUCTION

Machine learning (ML) approaches have many applications in radiology. Over the last several years, much attention has been garnered by applications focused on assisted interpretation of medical images. However, a significant component of radiology encompasses the generation of medical images before interpretation, the upstream component. These elements include modality selection for an examination, hardware design, protocol selection for an examination, data acquisition, image reconstruction, and image processing. Here, the authors give the reader insight into these aspects of upstream artificial intelligence (AI), conveying the breadth of the emerging field, some of the techniques, and the potential impact of the applications.

DISCUSSION

The standard radiology workflow can undergo 7 steps: (1) conversion of a patient's clinical question into a radiology examination order, usually performed by a nonradiologist physician; (2) conversion of an examination order into an examination protocol, usually performed by a radiologist or radiology technologist based on institution-specific guidelines; (3) scheduling of an examination onto a specific scanner, usually performed by a radiology scheduler or technologist; (4) adaption of a protocol to a specific device, usually performed by a radiology technologist; (5) acquisition and reconstruction of acquired imaging data into images, usually performed automatically with software algorithms directly on the imaging hardware; (6) image processing, to retrospectively improve

[a] Department of Electrical Engineering, Stanford University, 350 Serra Mall, Stanford, CA 94305, USA;
[b] Department of Biomedical Data Science, 1201 Welch Road, Stanford, CA 94305, USA; [c] Department of Radiology, Stanford University, 1201 Welch Road, Stanford, CA 94305, USA
[1] Present address: 3155 Porter Drive, Palo Alto, CA 94304.
* Corresponding author.
E-mail address: admin_vasanawala@stanford.edu

Radiol Clin N Am 59 (2021) 967–985
https://doi.org/10.1016/j.rcl.2021.07.009

image quality and produce multiplanar reformations and quantitative parameter maps, typically performed directly on the imaging hardware; and (7) evaluation of images to render a diagnosis related to the patient's clinical question, usually performed by a radiologist (Fig. 1). Applications and research areas for AI algorithms in radiology have typically focused on the final 2 steps in the radiology workflow.[1] Several AI techniques exist to perform automated classification, detection, or segmentation of medical images, many of which are even approved for clinical use by the Food and Drug Administration. Furthermore, the acquisition of raw data for generating diagnostic quality images is also being used for reducing scan time or radiation dosage of medical images, or retrospectively improving resolution or signal-to-noise ratio (SNR) of images.

Despite a dearth of research studies, there exist substantial challenges for all steps in the "preimage acquisition" workflow (steps 1–4) that may be alleviated using data-driven benefits that AI techniques can offer. For example, a patient's initial examination order may not always be correctly defined by a radiology specialist, which can lead to delays in insurance authorizations and the schedule of the correct examination. Next, conversion of an order to a protocol is commonly performed by radiology fellows at many academic institutions, whereas many private practice organizations may not have such a luxury. Furthermore, with "protocol creep" of new protocols being aggregated in an unorganized manner, choosing the appropriate protocol for the patient becomes a more challenging task.[2] The scheduling of patients to different scanners also requires

considerations for complex cases that may require a radiologist present. Following successful protocoling and scheduling, tuning the scanner parameters to cater to the specific examination order needs and patient requirements (such as image resolution, coils, and breath holds for MR imaging, dose optimization and contrast needs for computed tomography [CT], and so on) can directly affect image quality, and consequently, downstream utility for eventual image interpretation.

Errors can occur during any part of the radiology preimage-acquisition workflow and can lead to delayed diagnoses, or, in the worst case, missed diagnoses. Each of these 4 steps is repetitive, but because of the innate variability between patients, these tasks have not lent themselves to automated techniques. Using manual techniques to complete such tasks is prone to user error, leads to delays in the workflow, and is an inefficient use of human capital particularly when these tasks require radiologist oversight. The application of premage-acquisition AI can lead to potential gains in efficiency and patient care. There are several factors that make these tasks ripe for automation with AI techniques. First, all the tasks are already performed on computer systems, entailing that all inputs to and output of the tasks are already digitized and recorded and can be retrospectively extracted. Second, as large volumes (hundreds to thousands) of most examination types are performed every year, even at a single academic center, large institution-specific data sets needed to train AI algorithms are already available. Finally, a stepped pathway for incorporating these algorithms into the radiology workflow

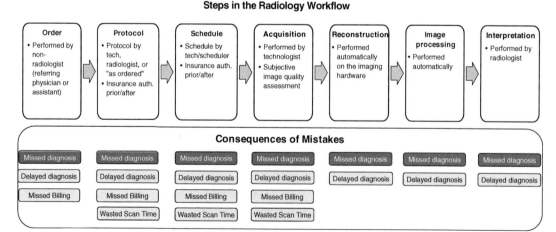

Fig. 1. The radiology workflow starting from the ordering of an examination and ending with a radiologist interpretation of the acquired imaging. Errors during each of the 7 stages of this workflow can lead to delays or the rendering of an incorrect final diagnosis decision.

can be achievable. Initial versions of the ML algorithms can suggest or preselect choices for use as a clinical decision support system with continued human oversight. Following this, continual-learning strategies can be used to improve such algorithms to have higher reliability than humans for eventual transition to full automation.

Recent advances in natural language processing (NLP) have been used to perform automated assignment for CT and MR imaging protocols using procedure names, modality, section, indications, and patient history as inputs to guide a clinical decision support model.[3] Similar NLP systems have also been previously used to use unstructured data for performing automated protocoling for musculoskeletal MR imaging examinations[4,5] as well as brain MR imaging examinations.[6] Newer AI techniques for NLP that use the Bidirectional Encoder Representations from Transformers model[7] have also been used in the context of automated protocoling.[8] Advances in multimodality data integration present an exciting opportunity to improve the upstream workflow by further combining data from a patient's medical record, along with AI models that rely on conventional computer vision and NLP techniques.[9]

Although the techniques and applications of upstream AI are broad, the authors later discuss some representative examples across various commonly used medical imaging modalities.

Improved Image Formation in Ultrasound

In ultrasound image reconstruction, raw echo data are received by an array of transducer sensors. These "channel data" are processed to produce an image of the underlying anatomy and function.

Traditional ultrasound image reconstruction can include various noise artifacts that degrade signal and image quality. Rather than attempting to correct these using already-reconstructed images, upstream ultrasound research uses the raw channel data to address the artifacts at their source. AI has found a wide range of early uses in upstream ultrasound, a few of which are highlight here.

A major source of ultrasound image degradation is reverberation clutter.[10] Clutter arises from shallow reverberations that are incorrectly superimposed on echoes from deeper tissue, resulting in decorrelated channel data. This decorrelation manifests in ordinary B-mode images as a dense haze and also degrades the ability to perform Doppler and other advanced imaging techniques. Several non-AI techniques have been proposed to remove clutter from channel data directly, improving channel data correlations and B-mode image contrast, albeit at great computational cost.[11–13] Recently, AI has been used to achieve the same goal using a data-driven approach.[14,15] In the authors' work, they used matched simulations of ultrasound sensor data with reverberation clutter (input) and without reverberation clutter (output) to train a convolutional neural network (CNN).[15] **Fig. 2** demonstrates how the CNN removes high-frequency clutter from simulated channel data. In **Fig. 3**, the CNN removes clutter from in vivo channel data, resulting in B-mode images with improved structure visualization and contrast. The CNN restores correlations in the raw channel data and thus enables subsequent advanced imaging techniques, such as sound speed estimation and phase aberration correction.

Another major noise source in ultrasound images is a pervasive grainy texture called speckle.

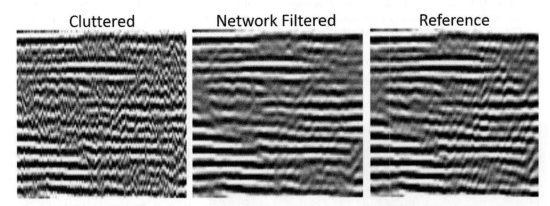

Fig. 2. Simulated channel data comparing cluttered, CNN-filtered, and reference uncluttered images. Reverberation clutter, which appears as a high-frequency noise across the channels, is removed by the CNN while preserving the structure of reflections from true targets. (*Data from* Brickson LL, Hyun D, Jakovljevic M, Dahl JJ. Reverberation Noise Suppression in Ultrasound Channel Signals Using a 3D Fully Convolutional Neural Network. IEEE Trans Med Imaging. 2021;PP.)

Original   **Network Filtered**

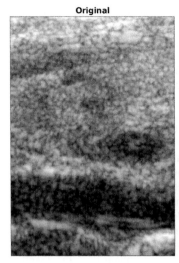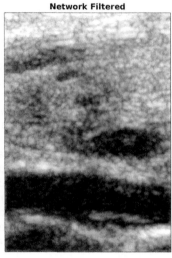

Fig. 3. B-mode images of a longitudinal cross-section of a carotid artery and thyroid. The CNN-filtered image visualizes several hypoechoic and anechoic targets that were originally obscured by clutter. (*Data from* Brickson LL, Hyun D, Jakovljevic M, Dahl JJ. Reverberation Noise Suppression in Ultrasound Channel Signals Using a 3D Fully Convolutional Neural Network. IEEE Trans Med Imaging. 2021;PP.)

Speckle is an unavoidable artifact arising from the finite resolution of ultrasound imaging systems. Although speckle can be useful for certain applications, it is largely treated as an undesirable noise that degrades B-mode images of the underlying tissue echogenicity. Rather than filtering speckle from already-reconstructed B-mode images, the authors trained a CNN to estimate the tissue echogenicity directly from raw channel data using simulations of ultrasound speckle and known ground-truth echogenicity.[16] In simulations, the trained CNN accurately and precisely estimated the true echogenicity. In phantom and in vivo experiments, where the ground-truth echogenicity is unknown, the CNN outperformed traditional signal processing and image processing speckle reduction techniques according to standard image quality metrics, such as contrast, contrast-to-noise ratio, and SNR. **Fig. 4** shows an in vivo example of a liver lesion acquired using a clinical scanner. This CNN has been further demonstrated in real time on a prototype scanner.[17]

Another emerging application in ultrasound is contrast-enhanced imaging, including with targeted contrast agents, to detect the presence of disease. Contrast-enhanced images are presented alongside ordinary B-mode images to highlight any disease-bound contrast agents in the field of view. A key challenge in contrast-enhanced imaging, particularly molecular imaging, is to detect echoes from contrast agents while suppressing echoes from background tissue. Current state-of-the-art imaging identifies molecular signals retrospectively after a strong destructive ultrasound pulse eliminates them from the field of view and thus cannot be used for real-time imaging. The authors recently used CNNs to nondestructively emulate the performance of destructive imaging, enabling real-time molecular imaging for early cancer detection.[18] Rather than treating B-mode and contrast-enhanced modes as separate images, the CNN combines raw data from both to improve the final molecular image. As shown in **Fig. 5**, the trained CNN (panel D) was able to mimic the performance of the state-of-the-art destructive approach (panel C), enabling high-quality real-time ultrasound molecular imaging.

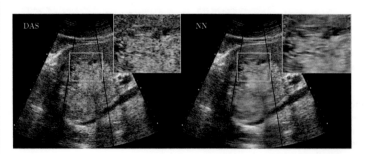

Fig. 4. CNN-based ultrasound speckle reduction and detail preservation. (*left*) A traditional B-mode image of a complex focal liver lesion. (*right*) The CNN output when provided with the same raw data. (*Data from* Hyun D, Brickson LL, Looby KT, Dahl JJ. Beamforming and Speckle Reduction Using Neural Networks. *IEEE Trans Ultrason Ferroelectr Freq Control.* 2019;66(5):898-910.)

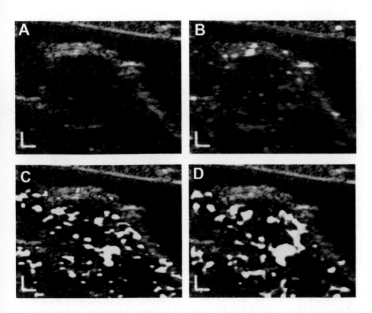

Fig. 5. Ultrasound molecular imaging of a breast cancer tumor in a transgenic mouse. (*A*) B-mode image, with the tumor in the center. (*B*) Contrast-enhanced image overlaid on the B-mode image. (*C*) Destructive state-of-the-art molecular image. (*D*) Output of the trained CNN using only nondestructive input data. The nondestructive CNN closely matched the destructive image, showing the potential for AI-enabled real-time molecular imaging.

In addition to these, AI has found numerous other upstream ultrasound applications, including adaptive beamforming,[19] ultrasound localization microscopy,[20] surgical guidance,[21] vector flow Doppler imaging,[22,23] as well as many others.[24] The range and variety of applications highlight the extraordinary adaptability of AI techniques to ultrasound signal and image processing.

Computed Tomography Dose Optimization

More than 75 million CT scans are performed annually in the United States, with the number expected to continue increasing.[25] Despite clear clinical value, ionizing radiation dose has been a major concern for CT. In addition, there are significant variations in radiation dose and image quality across institutions, protocols, scanners, and patients. Although CT has evolved from the manual adjustment of dose control parameters, such as tube current, to automatic tube current modulation, CT dose optimization still has major challenges in achieving the most efficient use of radiation dose for each patient and clinical task.[26,27] An overview of existing technologies for controlling dose and image quality is shown in **Fig. 6**.

Reconstructed CT images contain quantum noise when the ALARA (as low as reasonably achievable) principle is followed to reduce radiation exposure. As a result, important details in the image could be hidden by the noise, leading to degradation in the diagnostic value of CT. It is therefore crucial to assess the quality of reconstructed CT images at reduced dose. Dose and

image noise have a complex dependency on patient size (ranging from pediatrics to obese adults), patient anatomy, CT acquisition, and reconstruction. As can be seen in **Fig. 7**, CT images at lower doses relative to the routine dose induce higher noise. Unfortunately, there is no consistent image quality assessment measure that has been established to objectively quantify images from different imaging protocols, vendors, sites, and so forth.[28] Having such capabilities would help balance image quality and radiation dose. At every step of the CT scan, from system design to acquisition to reconstruction, efforts could then be made to lower radiation dose.[29] As a result, the quality of the acquired CT images could be varied and assessed to guide dose reduction. In addition, effective dose to the patient needs to account for the different radiosensitivity of different organs (for example, using the International Commission on Radiological Protection tissue weights).[30] Therefore, an accurate, reliable, and region-focused assessment of dose and image quality is extremely important.

In an effort to combat increased noise in low-dose settings, CT image reconstruction has been going through a paradigm shift, from conventional filtered backprojection (FBP) to model-based iterative reconstruction (MBIR), and now to deep learning (DL) image reconstruction.[31] FBP, although fast and computationally efficient, incurs higher noise and streak artifacts at low dose. Toward improving image quality at low dose, iterative reconstruction has emerged that preserves diagnostic information, although low-contrast detail remains a challenge and can impact detectability of

System Design	Acquisition	Reconstruction
Scanner Geometry	Tube Voltage	Method (FBP/MBIR/DLIR)
View Sampling	Tube Current Modulation	Kernel / Parameters
Anti-Scatter Grid	Filtration	Post-Processing
Detector Efficiency	Bowtie	
Detector Electronic Noise	Collimation	
	Pitch	

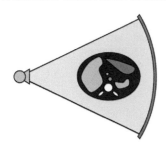
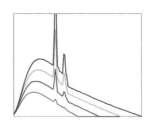
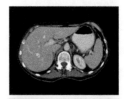
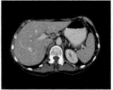

Fig. 6. Various technologies for controlling CT dose and image quality are listed under the categories of system design, acquisition, and reconstruction. Subfigures show (*left to right*): overall scanner geometry, x-ray spectra from different tube voltages, and 2 reconstructions with different kernels showing sharper image but higher noise (*top*) and lower noise but smoother image (*bottom*).

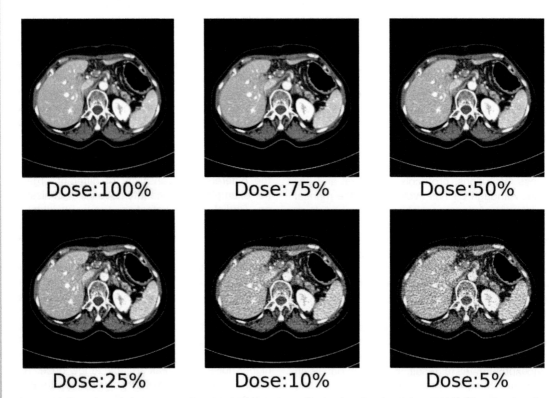

Fig. 7. CT slice of an abdomen scan showing higher noise at lower dose levels. Mayo patient CT projection data library[93] provides routine (100%) dose and low (25%) dose after inserting noise in the projection data. The additional 4 dose levels are synthesized from these two, assuming only quantum noise.

subtle pathologic conditions. With the advent of machine learning and DL, in particular, high diagnostic quality is created with reduced noise at low dose, with the additional benefit of faster reconstruction than iterative reconstruction,[32] for example, (1) generating standard-dose images from low-dose images in DL-based CT denoising[33]; (2) through incorporating deep CNN in the complex iterative reconstruction process, less noisy images can be obtained at low dose[34]; (3) improved image quality of dual-energy CT, particularly for large patients, low-energy virtual monoenergetic images, and material decomposition[35]; (4) reduction of metal artifacts through DL techniques.[36,37] DL-based image reconstruction enables significantly lower image noise and higher image quality (IQ score and better CNR [contrast to noise ratio]) over FBP and MBIR, which can be traded off for dose reduction.[38] However, dose reduction needs to be balanced against an acceptable level of diagnostic accuracy. Therefore, not only phantom data but also patient data are needed to understand the impacts of dose reduction on image quality (using objective metrics) as well as the task-specific diagnostic performance (such as detecting liver lesions).[39]

Conventionally, medical images are assessed subjectively requiring manual labor, long times, and observer variations, which is impractical for use in a clinical workflow. It is therefore desirable to perform fast, automatic, and objective image quality assessment. Objective assessment can be of 2 types: reference-based and non-reference-based. Several reference-based image assessment metrics have been widely used in medical imaging. For example, PSNR, MSE, CNR, SSIM, and RMSE are often used. However, these metrics rely on the availability of high-quality reference images. Because the goal is to acquire CT scans at reduced dose, one cannot assume to have access to high-quality (and high-dose) images of the same patient.[40] Therefore, nonreference assessments are preferred so that any CT image can be quantified without requiring the corresponding reference images at high dose. In addition to the established image quality assessment metrics, a few nonreference assessment methods are also available, such as a blind/referenceless image spatial quality evaluator based on natural scene statistics that operates in the spatial domain.[41] A growing body of research has recently emerged focusing on no-reference and automated image quality assessment using DL. For example, Patwari and colleagues[42] used a regression CNN to learn mapping noisy CT images to GSSIM scores, as an assessment of the reconstructed image quality. Kim and

colleagues[43] proposed a no-reference image quality assessment framework via 2-stage training: regression into objective error map and subjective score. Another DL-based nonreference assessment has recently been proposed leveraging self-supervised prediction of noise levels.[44]

In summary, reduction of CT dose directly impacts image quality. Preserving image quality at low dose has been an active area of research. DL-based methods have achieved some promising results in CT image reconstruction, denoising, artifact reduction, and image quality assessment. However, to bring dose optimization to CT acquisition, prediction of the expected dose and image quality must be real time, patient specific, organ specific, and task specific. This problem is a complex and challenging one for which DL algorithms are likely to excel.

Optimized Data Acquisition in MR Imaging via Deep Learning

In MR imaging, data are acquired in the Fourier domain, or k-space, which represents spatial and temporal frequency information in the object being imaged. Sampling of k-space is necessarily finite. Therefore, optimizing sampling patterns and designing k-space readout trajectories that enable collecting the most informative k-space samples for image reconstruction can improve the resulting diagnostic information in images. Besides improved image quality, the design of optimized sampling trajectories can lead to shortened data acquisition for improved efficiency. Recently, several DL methods have been proposed for learning k-space sampling patterns jointly with image reconstruction algorithmic parameters. These methods have shown improved reconstructed image quality compared with reconstructions obtained with predetermined trajectories, such as variable density sampling. DL methods for data sampling can be separated into 2 categories: active and nonactive (fixed) strategies. These 2 strategies differ primarily in whether the learned sampling schemes are fixed or not at inference time.

Given a target k-space undersampling or acceleration factor, the nonactive (fixed) strategies produce undersampling masks or sampling trajectories using a set of fully sampled images. After the training procedure is completed, the learned sampling pattern is *fixed,* and new scans can be acquired using the learned trajectory (Fig. 8A, B). Image reconstruction can then be performed using the reconstruction network learned as a part of the training process. Several studies[45,46] focus on the Cartesian sampling case and model binary sampling masks

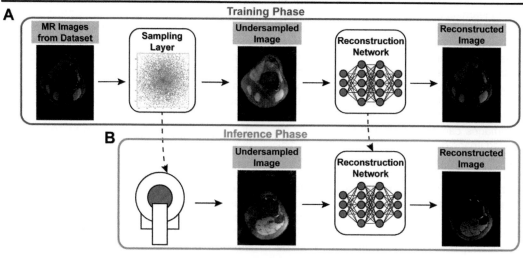

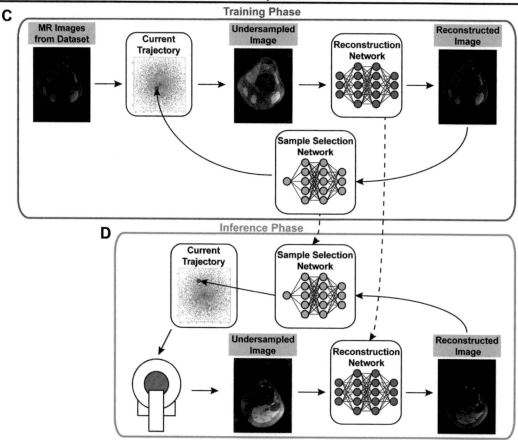

Fig. 8. Nonactive and active data strategies for DL-based data sampling methods. Nonactive (fixed) strategies optimize sampling trajectories and reconstruction networks at training time (*A*). At inference time (*B*), the sampling trajectory is fixed, and the corresponding gradient waveforms are programmed in the scanner for acquisition. The optimized reconstruction network is then used for reconstructing images from undersampled measurements. Active strategies (*C*, *D*) use an additional neural network that suggests the next sample to collect using the reconstruction obtained from existing samples. The process is repeated until a desired metric or uncertainty threshold is met. Because of their sequential nature, active strategies require an additional mechanism that generates gradient waveforms on the fly for acquiring the samples proposed by the sample selection network.

probabilistically. These methods can be applied to either 2-dimensional (2D) or 3-dimensional (3D) Cartesian sampling to determine the optimal set of phase encodes. As an extension to more general parameterized, or non-Cartesian, k-space trajectories,[47] one can directly optimize for k-space coordinates by restricting the optimization to a set of separable variables, such as horizontal and vertical directions in the 2D plane. The framework presented in Weiss and colleagues[48] additionally incorporates gradient system constraints into the learning process. This enables finding the optimal gradient waveforms in a data-driven manner.

Active acquisition strategies,[49–52] on the other hand, attempt to predict in real time the next k-space samples to be acquired using information from existing samples from the same acquisition, that is, the same patient/scan (see **Fig. 8**C, D). These methods use an additional neural network that suggests the next sample to collect by measuring the reconstruction quality or uncertainty during the acquisition. Active techniques therefore have the benefit of obtaining subject-specific data acquisition strategies. In other words, active sampling strategies *tailor* the sampling pattern to new scans and patients.

In general, the nonactive acquisitions are easier to implement in scanner hardware. However, such acquisitions can be suboptimal on new types of data or scans. For example, a sampling pattern that is optimal for brain imaging might not be the best trajectory for abdominal imaging. On the other hand, active acquisitions could adapt to new kinds of data at the expense of added complexity in determining and generating gradient waveforms on the fly.

Optimization of data sampling using DL is an active area of research, and many open questions exist for further investigation. The effects of imaging nonidealities, such as off-resonance, relaxation effects, and motion, on the optimized sampling pattern have not yet been fully investigated. In addition, the findings on DL-based data sampling approaches in MR literature typically rely on retrospective studies and simulations. Their applicability to prospective studies and clinical settings should be investigated to understand the full potential and applicability of learned sampling patterns.

Image Reconstruction in MR Imaging: Supervised Deep Learning

To reconstruct rapidly acquired k-space data into high-quality images, advanced image reconstruction methods are necessary. Previously, parallel imaging and compressed sensing (PI-CS) methods[53,54] have been used to iteratively reconstruct highly undersampled data, thus enabling rapid MR imaging scans. However, because of their iterative nature, PI-CS methods suffer from impractically long reconstruction times, which limit their clinical applicability. More recently, DL-based reconstruction approaches have demonstrated much faster reconstruction times, and in some cases, better image quality than PI-CS methods. These approaches are based on machine learning models, which must first be trained to learn the process of reconstructing raw data into images.

The most common way of training a model to reconstruct MR images is through supervised learning. In the case of reconstruction, the inputs are undersampled k-space data, which the model uses to output a reconstructed image. Supervision here is enabled by using fully sampled k-space data, which may have either been directly acquired through a lengthy scan or synthesized from undersampled data via more conventional image reconstruction techniques. The model itself is learned by updating the model parameters such that the difference between the model output and the fully sampled ground truth is minimized. This process, known as stochastic gradient descent, is done repeatedly for each example in the training data set until the model has fully converged (**Fig. 9**).

Choosing the type of model to use for reconstruction tasks remains an active area of research. Similar to image classification approaches, the most common type of model used to learn MR image reconstruction is a deep CNN.[55–57] CNNs consist of convolutions, cascaded with nonlinear activation functions, which are able to extract features from images at various hierarchical levels of detail and use them for reconstruction (**Fig. 10**A). As in any other application of DL, deeper networks (ie, more cascades) are capable of learning better, more accurate reconstruction models. However, deeper networks also consist of more learnable parameters and are therefore more likely to overfit to the training data set. In other words, if not provided with enough training data to support the number of network parameters, the network will begin to memorize the data, degrading performance on data that were not seen during training.

Recently, it has been demonstrated that deep CNN methods benefit from incorporating additional information about the MR imaging acquisition as an aid for image reconstruction. This is done by interleaving shallow CNNs with projections of a simulated MR imaging scanning model (see **Fig. 10**B).[58–60] This interleaved model, known as an unrolled neural network (UNN), is treated as

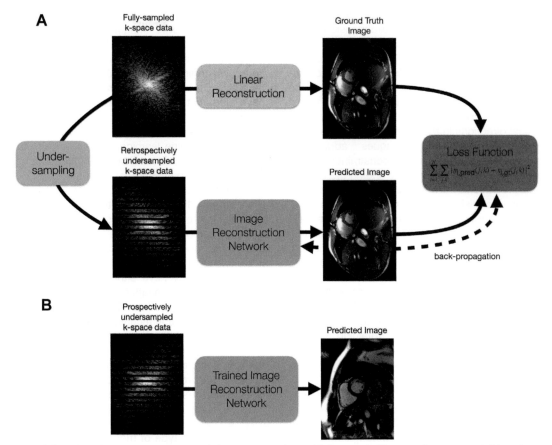

Fig. 9. (A) MR imaging reconstruction model training pipeline. If fully sampled k-space data are available, a linear reconstruction is performed to generate the high-quality, ground-truth image. The fully sampled k-space data are then retrospectively undersampled by throwing away k-space lines, simulating how the scanner would undersample data in a true, accelerated acquisition. This undersampled data are given to the network for reconstruction. The network is then trained to output a predicted image, which is enforced to be "close" to the ground-truth image via a loss function. A simple mean-squared error loss is shown here. The model parameters are then iteratively updated by a stochastic gradient descent algorithm, which intends to minimize the loss function, thereby minimizing the difference between the predicted image and the ground-truth image. (B) Once the model is fully trained, it can be used to "infer" or reconstruct images from prospectively undersampled data in an efficient manner.

one deep model and trained end-to-end in the same way as a conventional CNN. By incorporating additional acquisition information, the network is never allowed to produce images that are relatively inconsistent with the raw k-space data. As a result, UNN reconstruction methods reduce the overfitting problem and allow for better generalizability to unseen data. Initial proof-of-concept studies have demonstrated that UNNs outperform conventional reconstruction methods across a wide variety of clinical applications, such as 2D cardiac cine MR imaging scans,[61] for example (Fig. 11). However, further research is necessary to demonstrate their robustness and effectiveness across large clinical populations.

Besides undersampled MR imaging reconstruction that uses raw k-space data, an additional class of techniques performs image-to-image translations (for example, low resolution to high resolution, low SNR to high SNR) in order to overcome the challenge that raw k-space data are not always archived from clinical MR imaging scans. Such techniques have previously been used to transform low-resolution images into higher-resolution images, under the constraints of maintaining segmentation, quantitative parameter mapping, and diagnostic accuracy.[62–64] These methods have been demonstrated across varying anatomies, including neuro, cardiac, and musculoskeletal MR imaging.[65–68] DL-based approaches

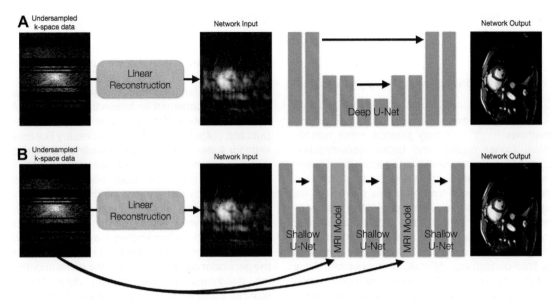

Fig. 10. (*A*) An example of a deep CNN for MR imaging reconstruction. There are many degrees of freedom in designing CNNs. One popular architecture is called a U-Net, which repeatedly applies convolutions and down-sampling layers to extract both low-resolution and high-resolution features. (*B*) UNN instead apply shallow CNNs (again U-Nets are shown) cascaded with simulated MR imaging model projections, which ensure that the output of each CNN does not deviate from the raw, undersampled k-space data. These projections also make use of Fourier transforms and coil sensitivity information to convert intermediate network outputs back to the original multichannel k-space domain where the projection is performed.

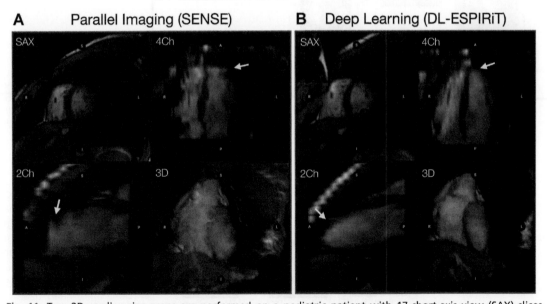

Fig. 11. Two 2D cardiac cine scans are performed on a pediatric patient with 17 short-axis view (SAX) slices covering the heart and scan parameters: TE = 1.4 milliseconds, TR = 3.3 milliseconds, matrix size = 200 × 180. Reformats are shown to visualize 4-chamber (4Ch), 2-chamber (2Ch) views along with a 3D rendering. (*A*) The first scan is performed with 2× undersampling and reconstructed using a standard parallel imaging technique. (*B*) The second scan is performed with 12× undersampling and reconstructed using a DL approach. With DL-powered acceleration, the scan time is shortened from 6 breath-holds down to a single breath-hold. This has important implications not only for patient comfort but also for the accuracy of volumetric assessments from these images, because the inevitable variations between breath-holds are significantly reduced in the DL images (*arrows*).

have also been used to alleviate the constraints of long scan times for accelerating quantitative MR imaging[69–71] scans.

MR Image Reconstruction: Unsupervised Deep Learning

As described above, supervised DL reconstruction methods[56,58,59,72–78] may provide more robustness, higher quality, and faster reconstruction speed than conventional image reconstruction approaches. However, the need for fully sampled data for supervised training poses a problem for applications, such as dynamic contrast enhancement (DCE), 3D cardiac cine, 4-dimensional flow, low-dose contrast agent imaging, and real-time imaging, where collecting fully sampled data sets is time-consuming, difficult, or impossible. As a result, supervised DL-based methods often cannot be used in these applications. There are 2 main possible ways to address this problem. First, PI-CS reconstructions can be used as ground truth for DL frameworks.[75] However, reconstructions of the DL model are unlikely to surpass PI-

CS reconstruction methods with respect to image quality. Another way is to reformulate DL training in a way that only leverages undersampled data sets for training, otherwise known as unsupervised learning.[79–86]

In unsupervised learning, the goal is to train a network to reconstruct an image that is consistent with a distribution of images. Therefore, paired inputs and outputs are no longer necessary like they were for supervised learning. This can be achieved using generative adversarial networks (GAN),[87] which, in the past, have been used to learn and model complex distributions of images.[88,89] GAN training involves jointly training 2 networks: a generator network whose goal is to reconstruct an image from undersampled k-space data, and a discriminator whose goal is to discern whether the generator output came from the same underlying distribution as the training data. During training, these 2 networks are pitted against each other such that the generator continuously learns to reconstruct higher-quality images, whereas the discriminator becomes better at discerning outputs from the generator.

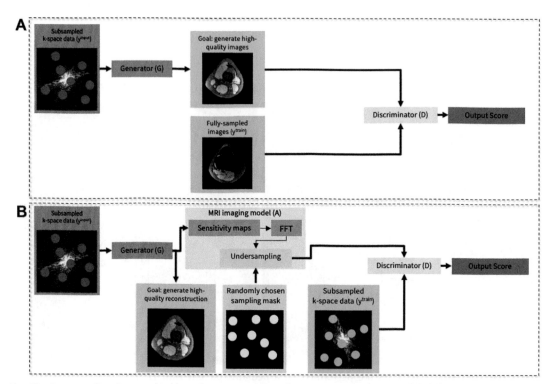

Fig. 12. A conventional supervised learning system (*A*) and an unsupervised system (*B*). (*A*) Framework overview in a supervised setting with a conditional GAN when fully sampled data sets are available. (*B*) Framework overview in an unsupervised setting. The input to the generator network is an undersampled complex-valued k-space data and the output is a reconstructed 2D complex-valued image. Next, a sensing matrix comprising coil sensitivity maps, an FFT, and a randomized undersampling mask (drawn independently from the input k-space measurements) is applied to the generated image to simulate the imaging process. The discriminator takes simulated and observed measurements as inputs and tries to differentiate between them.

GAN can be used to train MR imaging reconstruction models in an unsupervised fashion in 2 situations. If fully sampled data are available, the generator can be trained to output images that match the distribution of a training data set comprising fully sampled images[90] (**Fig. 12A**). If only undersampled data are available, a slightly different framework, known as AmbientGAN,[91] can be used (see **Fig. 12B**). In AmbientGAN, the generator output is converted back to k-space and is undersampled through simulation. Then, the discriminator is tasked with determining if the undersampled output is consistent with the undersampled training data distribution. This approach has been demonstrated to be effective for unsupervised DL reconstruction, when the undersampling is sufficiently varied throughout the training data set.[92]

As shown in **Fig. 13**, the unsupervised method achieves superior SSIM, PSNR, and NRMSE on a knee data set compared with compressed sensing reconstruction. However, the supervised GAN is superior in comparison to the proposed unsupervised GAN, which is expected because the supervised GAN has access to fully sampled data, giving the network a stronger prior. Of note, the superior performance of the unsupervised GAN compared with compressed sensing is negligible for lower accelerations but becomes more significant at accelerations of 4 to 6 (**Fig. 14**), highlighting the potential of achieving imaging speedups greater than can be obtained conventionally. Representative results from a DCE data set are shown in **Fig. 15**. The generator greatly improves input image quality by recovering sharpness and adding more structure to input images. In addition, the proposed method produces a sharper reconstruction compared with CS. In the first row, the anatomic right kidney of the unsupervised GAN is visibly much sharper than input and CS.

The main advantage of this method over existing DL reconstruction methods is eliminating the need for fully sampled data. Another benefit is that other additional data sets are not needed to use as ground truth, as in some other works on semisupervised training.[90] In addition, the method produces better-quality reconstruction compared with baseline compressed sensing methods.

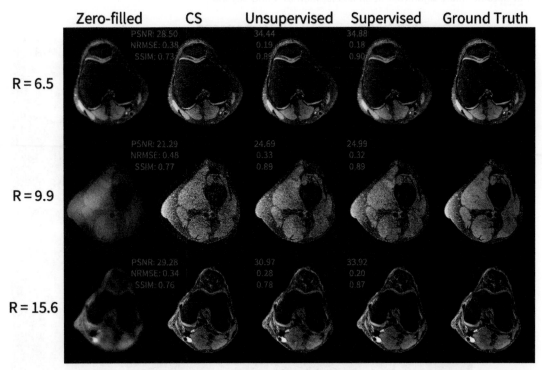

Fig. 13. Knee application representative results, showing, from left to right, the input undersampled complex image to the generator, the output of the unsupervised generator, the output of the supervised generator, and the fully sampled image. The acceleration factors of the input image are 6.5, 9.9, and 15.6, from top to bottom. The quantitative metrics that are plotted next to the images are for the slice that is shown. In all rows, the unsupervised GAN has superior PSNR, NRMSE, and SSIM compared with CS. In the first row, the unsupervised GAN has metrics that are notably worse than the supervised GAN. In the middle row and last rows, the unsupervised GAN has metrics that come close to the performance of the supervised GAN.

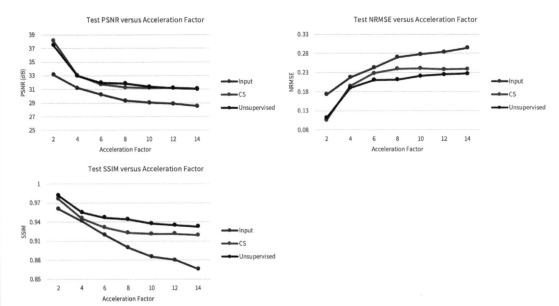

Fig. 14. The results of the reconstruction performance on the set of knee scans of the unsupervised GAN as a function of the acceleration factor of the training data sets. The y-axis represents PSNR, NRMSE, or SSIM, depending on the plot. The x-axis represents the acceleration factor of the data sets. The gap between PSNR of CS and the unsupervised model is negligible over the range of accelerations. The gap between NRMSE of CS and the unsupervised model is negligible at first, for low accelerations, but becomes more significant at an acceleration of 6 and beyond. The gap between SSIM of CS and the unsupervised model is negligible at first, for an acceleration of 2, but becomes more significant at an acceleration of 4 and beyond.

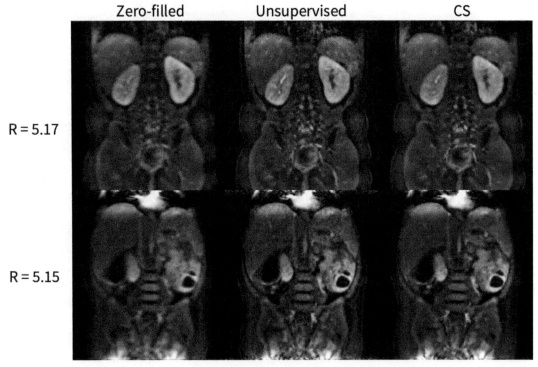

Fig. 15. 2D DCE application representative results, where the left slice is the magnitude of one input undersampled complex image to the generator; the middle slice is the output of the generator, and the right slice is a compressed sensing L1-wavelet regularization. The generator greatly improves the input image quality by recovering sharpness and adding more structure to the input images. In addition, the proposed method produces a sharper reconstruction compared with CS. In the first row, the kidneys of the unsupervised GAN are visibly much sharper than that of the input and CS.

One significant challenge in the implementation of unsupervised methods is ensuring adequate clinical validation. In supervised methods, a ground-truth image can be obtained for comparison. In that circumstance, comparison can be by quantitative image quality metrics, such as SNR. However, an open question in the field is whether conventional image quality metrics are adequate to ensure diagnostic performance. Thus, clinical assessment by expert radiologists is critical. The challenge of clinical validation in unsupervised methods is often harder, because the big applications are for cases whereby a gold standard is impossible to obtain, such as high spatiotemporal resolution DCE or perfusion MR imaging. In this case, validation would require comparison against either another modality, such as CT, or by assessing clinical outcomes.

SUMMARY

The field of upstream AI for medical imaging is broad, covering the steps in the medical imaging process from selection of an imaging modality to image processing. Potential benefits include a more streamlined clinical practice, faster and more accurate examination scheduling and protocoling, faster examinations, and improved image quality. In this article, the authors highlighted only a few representative applications, giving the reader insight into directions in this rapidly evolving field.

CLINICS CARE POINTS

- As of today, there has been little research on validating upstream artificial intelligence approaches in large clinical cohorts for deep learning-based image reconstruction approaches.

- Although these methods demonstrate great potential for accelerating clinical workflows in radiology, further studies are necessary to understand and determine the robustness of such approaches across a variety of patient populations.

- Future studies should validate upstream artificial intelligence approaches based not only on standard image quality metrics but also on quantitative measurements, which serve as clinical endpoints to ensure that the algorithms are truly improving the standard of care.

DISCLOSURE

Dr J. Dahl receives technical and in-kind support from Siemens Healthcare and serves as a technical advisor to Cephasonics Ultrasound and Vortex Imaging, Inc. Dr A.S. Chaudhari has provided consulting services to Skope MR, Subtle Medical, Culvert Engineering, Edge Analytics, Image Analysis Group, ICM, and Chondrometrics GmbH; and is a shareholder in Subtle Medical, LVIS Corp, and Brain Key; and received research support from GE Healthcare and Philips. Dr D. Hyun has a consulting relationship with Exo Imaging, Inc. Dr A.A.Z. Imran receives research support from GE Healthcare. Dr A.S. Wang receives research support from GE Healthcare, Siemens Healthineers, and Varex Imaging. Elizabeth Cole receives support from GE Healthcare. Drs A.M. Loening, S.S. Vasanawala, and A.S. Chaudhari receive research support from GE Healthcare. Dr S.S. Vasanawala has a consulting relationship with Arterys and HeartVista. This research was supported by NIBIB grants R01 EB013661, R01 EB015506, P41 EB015891, R01 EB002524, R01 EB009690, R01 EB026136, and R01 EB027100, by NIAMS grant R01 AR063643, by NCI grant R01-CA218204, by NICHD grant R01-HD086252, by a seed grant from the Stanford Cancer Institute, and an NCI-designated Comprehensive Cancer Center.

REFERENCES

1. Chaudhari AS, Sandino CM, Cole EK, et al. Prospective deployment of deep learning in MRI: a framework for important considerations, challenges, and recommendations for best practices. J Magn Reson Imaging 2020;54(2):357–71.

2. Sachs PB, Hunt K, Mansoubi F, et al. CT and MR protocol standardization across a large health system: providing a consistent radiologist, patient, and referring provider experience. J Digit Imaging 2017;30(1):11–6.

3. Kalra A, Chakraborty A, Fine B, et al. Machine learning for automation of radiology protocols for quality and efficiency improvement. J Am Coll Radiol 2020;17(9):1149–58.

4. Lee YH. Efficiency improvement in a busy radiology practice: determination of musculoskeletal magnetic resonance imaging protocol using deep-learning convolutional neural networks. J Digit Imaging 2018;31(5):604–10.

5. Trivedi H, Mesterhazy J, Laguna B, et al. Automatic determination of the need for intravenous contrast in musculoskeletal MRI examinations using IBM Watson's Natural Language Processing Algorithm. J Digit Imaging 2018;31(2):245–51.

6. Brown AD, Marotta TR. Using machine learning for sequence-level automated MRI protocol selection in neuroradiology. J Am Med Inform Assoc 2018; 25(5):568–71.

7. Devlin J, Chang MW, Lee K, Toutanova K. BERT: Pre-training of deep bidirectional transformers for language understanding. Paper presented at: Proceedings of the 2019 Conference of the North American Chapter of the Association for Computational Linguistics: Human Language Technologies2019; Minneapolis, Minnesota, June 2-7, 2019.

8. Lau W, Aaltonen L, Gunn M, Yetisgen-Yildiz M. Automatic Assignment of Radiology Examination Protocols Using Pre-trained Language Models with Knowledge Distillation. ArXiv. 2020;abs/2009.00694.

9. Huang SC, Pareek A, Seyyedi S, et al. Fusion of medical imaging and electronic health records using deep learning: a systematic review and implementation guidelines. NPJ Digit Med 2020;3:136.

10. Pinton GF, Trahey GE, Dahl JJ. Sources of image degradation in fundamental and harmonic ultrasound imaging using nonlinear, full-wave simulations. IEEE Trans Ultrason Ferroelectr Freq Control 2011;58(4):754–65.

11. Byram B, Dei K, Tierney J, et al. A model and regularization scheme for ultrasonic beamforming clutter reduction. IEEE Trans Ultrason Ferroelectr Freq Control 2015;62(11):1913–27.

12. Shin J, Huang L. Spatial prediction filtering of acoustic clutter and random noise in medical ultrasound imaging. IEEE Trans Med Imaging 2017;36(2): 396–406.

13. Jennings J, Jakovljevic M, Biondi E, Dahl J, Biondi B. Estimating signal and structured noise in ultrasound data using prediction-error filters. Paper presented at: 2019 SPIE Medical Imaging2019; San Diego, California, February 16-21, 2019.

14. Luchies AC, Byram BC. Deep neural networks for ultrasound beamforming. IEEE Trans Med Imaging 2018;37(9):2010–21.

15. Brickson LL, Hyun D, Jakovljevic M, et al. Reverberation noise suppression in ultrasound channel signals using a 3D fully convolutional neural network. IEEE Trans Med Imaging 2021;40(4):1184–95.

16. Hyun D, Brickson LL, Looby KT, et al. Beamforming and speckle reduction using neural networks. IEEE Trans Ultrason Ferroelectr Freq Control 2019;66(5): 898–910.

17. Hyun D, Li L, Steinberg I, Jakovljevic M, Klap T, Dahl JJ. An Open Source GPU-Based Beamformer for Real-Time Ultrasound Imaging and Applications. Paper presented at: 2019 IEEE International Ultrasonics Symposium (IUS) 2019; Glasgow, United Kingdom, October 6-9, 2019.

18. Hyun D, Abou-Elkacem L, Bam R, et al. Nondestructive detection of targeted microbubbles using dual-mode data and deep learning for real-time ultrasound molecular imaging. IEEE Trans Med Imaging 2020;39(10):3079–88.

19. Luijten B, Cohen R, de Bruijn FJ, et al. Adaptive ultrasound beamforming using deep learning. IEEE Trans Med Imaging 2020;39(12):3967–78.

20. van Sloun RJ, Solomon O, Bruce M, et al. Super-resolution ultrasound localization microscopy through deep learning. IEEE Trans Med Imaging 2020; 40(3):829–39.

21. Nair AA, Washington KN, Tran TD, et al. Deep learning to obtain simultaneous image and segmentation outputs from a single input of raw ultrasound channel data. IEEE Trans Ultrason Ferroelectr Freq Control 2020;67(12):2493–509.

22. Stanziola A, Robins T, Riemer K, M. T. A Deep Learning Approach to Synthetic Aperture Vector Flow Imaging. Paper presented at: 2018 IEEE International Ultrasonics Symposium (IUS)2018; Kobe, Japan, October 22-25, 2018.

23. Li Y, Hyun D, Dahl JJ. Vector Flow Velocity Estimation from Beamsummed Data Using Deep Neural Networks. Paper presented at: 2019 IEEE International Ultrasonics Symposium (IUS)2019; Glasgow, United Kingdom, October 6-9, 2019.

24. van Sloun RJ, Cohen R, Eldar YC. Deep learning in ultrasound imaging. Proc IEEE 2020;108(1):11–29.

25. Over 75 million CT scans are performed each year and growing despite radiation concerns. 2018. Available at: https://idataresearch.com/over-75-million-ct-scans-are-performed-each-year-and-growing-despite-radiation-concerns. Accessed January 4, 2021.

26. Larson DB, Boland GW. Imaging quality control in the era of artificial intelligence. J Am Coll Radiol 2019;16(9 Pt B):1259–66.

27. Lell MM, Kachelriess M. Recent and upcoming technological developments in computed tomography: high speed, low dose, deep learning, multienergy. Invest Radiol 2020;55(1):8–19.

28. Meineke A, Rubbert C, Sawicki LM, et al. Potential of a machine-learning model for dose optimization in CT quality assurance. Eur Radiol 2019;29(7):3705–13.

29. McCollough CH, Bruesewitz MR, Kofler JM Jr. CT dose reduction and dose management tools: overview of available options. Radiographics 2006; 26(2):503–12.

30. ICRP. The 2007 Recommendations of the International Commission on Radiological Protection. 2007.

31. Willemink MJ, Noel PB. The evolution of image reconstruction for CT-from filtered back projection to artificial intelligence. Eur Radiol 2019;29(5):2185–95.

32. Eberhard M, Alkadhi H. Machine learning and deep neural networks: applications in patient and scan preparation, contrast medium, and radiation dose optimization. J Thorac Imaging 2020;35(Suppl 1):S17–20.

33. Tian C, Fei L, Zheng W, et al. Deep learning on image denoising: an overview. Neural Netw 2020; 131:251–75.

34. Kambadakone A. Artificial intelligence and CT image reconstruction: potential of a new era in radiation dose reduction. J Am Coll Radiol 2020;17(5):649–51.

35. Liu SZ, Cao Q, Tivnan M, et al. Model-based dual-energy tomographic image reconstruction of objects containing known metal components. Phys Med Biol 2020;65(24):245046.

36. Katsura M, Sato J, Akahane M, et al. Current and novel techniques for metal artifact reduction at CT: practical guide for radiologists. Radiographics 2018;38(2):450–61.

37. Zhang Y, Yu H. Convolutional neural network based metal artifact reduction in x-ray computed tomography. IEEE Trans Med Imaging 2018;37(6):1370–81.

38. Akagi M, Nakamura Y, Higaki T, et al. Deep learning reconstruction improves image quality of abdominal ultra-high-resolution CT. Eur Radiol 2019;29(11):6163–71.

39. Greffier J, Hamard A, Pereira F, et al. Image quality and dose reduction opportunity of deep learning image reconstruction algorithm for CT: a phantom study. Eur Radiol 2020;30(7):3951–9.

40. Kaza RK, Platt JF, Goodsitt MM, et al. Emerging techniques for dose optimization in abdominal CT. Radiographics 2014;34(1):4–17.

41. Mittal A, Moorthy AK, Bovik AC. No-reference image quality assessment in the spatial domain. IEEE Trans Image Process 2012;21(12):4695–708.

42. Patwari M, Gutjahr R, Raupach R, Maier A. Measuring CT reconstruction quality with deep convolutional neural networks. In: Knoll F, Maier A, Rueckert D, et al, editors. Machine Learning for Medical Image Reconstruction. Cham: Springer International Publishing; 2019. p. 113- 24.

43. Kim J, Nguyen AD, Lee S. Deep CNN-based blind image quality predictor. IEEE Trans Neural Netw Learn Syst 2019;30(1):11–24.

44. Imran AAZ, Pal D, Patel B, et al. SSIQA: Multi-Task learning for non-reference CT image quality assessment with self-supervised noise level prediction. 2021 IEEE 18th International Symposium on Biomedical Imaging (ISBI). Nice, France, April 13-16, 2021, p. 1962-5. doi:10.1109/ISBI48211.2021.9434044.

45. Bahadir CD, Dalca AV, Sabuncu MR. Learning-Based Optimization of the Under-Sampling Pattern in MRI. Paper presented at: International Conference on Information Processing in Medical Imaging2019; Hong Kong, China, June 2-7, 2019.

46. Huijben IAM, Veeling BS, van Sloun RJ. Learning Sampling and Model-Based Signal Recovery for Compressed Sensing MRI. Paper presented at: 2020 IEEE International Conference on Acoustics, Speech and Signal Processing (ICASSP)2020; Barcelona, Spain, May 4-8, 2020.

47. Aggarwal HK, Jacob M. J-MoDL: joint model-based deep learning for optimized sampling and reconstruction. IEEE J Selected Top Signal Process 2020;14(6):1151–62.

48. Weiss T, Senouf O, Vedula S, Michailovich O, Zibulevsky M, Bronstein A. PILOT: Physics-Informed Learned Optimal Trajectories for Accelerated MRI. ArXiv. 2019;abs/1909.05773.

49. Bakker T, Hoof HV, Welling M. Experimental design for MRI by greedy policy search. ArXiv. 2020;abs/2010.16262.

50. Jin K, Unser M, Yi K. Self-Supervised Deep Active Accelerated MRI. ArXiv. 2019;abs/1901.04547.

51. Pineda L, Basu S, Romero A, Calandra R, Drozdzal M. Active MR k-space Sampling with Reinforcement Learning. Paper presented at: Medical Image Computing and Computer-Assisted Intervention 2020; Lima, Peru, October 4-8, 2020.

52. Zhang Z, Romero A, Muckley M, Vincent P, Yang L, Drozdzal M. Reducing Uncertainty in Undersampled MRI Reconstruction With Active Acquisition. Paper presented at: 2019 IEEE/CVF Conference on Computer Vision and Pattern Recognition (CVPR) 2019; Long Beach, CA, June 16-20, 2019.

53. Lustig M, Donoho D, Pauly JM. Sparse MRI: the application of compressed sensing for rapid MR imaging. Magn Reson Med 2007;58(6):1182–95.

54. Vasanawala SS, Alley MT, Hargreaves BA, et al. Improved pediatric MR imaging with compressed sensing. Radiology 2010;256(2):607–16.

55. Jin KH, McCann MT, Froustey E, et al. Deep convolutional neural network for inverse problems in imaging. IEEE Trans Image Process 2017;26(9):4509–22.

56. Mardani M, Gong E, Cheng JY, et al. Deep generative adversarial neural networks for compressive sensing MRI. IEEE Trans Med Imaging 2019;38(1):167–79.

57. Lee D, Yoo J, Tak S, et al. Deep residual learning for accelerated MRI using magnitude and phase networks. IEEE Trans Biomed Eng 2018;65(9):1985–95.

58. Hammernik K, Klatzer T, Kobler E, et al. Learning a variational network for reconstruction of accelerated MRI data. Magn Reson Med 2018;79(6):3055–71.

59. Aggarwal HK, Mani MP, Jacob M. MoDL: model-based deep learning architecture for inverse problems. IEEE Trans Med Imaging 2019;38(2):394–405.

60. Sandino CM, Cheng JY, Chen F, et al. Compressed sensing: from research to clinical practice with deep neural networks. IEEE Signal Process Mag 2020;37(1):111–27.

61. Sandino CM, Lai P, Vasanawala SS, et al. Accelerating cardiac cine MRI using a deep learning-based ESPIRiT reconstruction. Magn Reson Med 2021;85(1):152–67.

62. Chaudhari AS, Stevens KJ, Wood JP, et al. Utility of deep learning super-resolution in the context of osteoarthritis MRI biomarkers. J Magn Reson Imaging 2020;51(3):768–79.

63. Chaudhari AS, Fang Z, Hyung Lee J, Gold GE, Hargreaves BA. Deep Learning Super-Resolution

Enables Rapid Simultaneous Morphological and Quantitative Magnetic Resonance Imaging. Paper presented at: Machine Learning for Medical Image Reconstruction 2018; Granada, Spain, September 16, 2018.

64. Chaudhari AS, Grissom MJ, Fang Z, et al. Diagnostic accuracy of quantitative multi-contrast 5-minute knee MRI using prospective artificial intelligence image quality enhancement. AJR Am J Roentgenol 2020;216(6):1614–25.

65. Tian Q, Bilgic B, Fan Q, et al. Improving in vivo human cerebral cortical surface reconstruction using data-driven super-resolution. Cereb Cortex 2021; 31(1):463–82.

66. Chen Y, Xie Y, Zhou Z, Shi F, Christodoulou A, Li D. Brain MRI super resolution using 3D deep densely connected neural networks. Paper presented at: 2018 IEEE 15th International Symposium on Biomedical Imaging (ISBI 2018)2018; Washington, DC, April 4-7, 2018.

67. Oktay O, Bai W, Lee M, et al. Multi-input Cardiac Image Super-Resolution Using Convolutional Neural Networks. Paper presented at: International Conference on Medical Image Computing and Computer-Assisted Intervention2016; Athens, Greece, October 17-21, 2016.

68. Chaudhari AS, Fang Z, Kogan F, et al. Super-resolution musculoskeletal MRI using deep learning. Magn Reson Med 2018;80(5):2139–54.

69. Cai C, Wang C, Zeng Y, et al. Single-shot T2 mapping using overlapping-echo detachment planar imaging and a deep convolutional neural network. Magn Reson Med 2018;80(5):2202–14.

70. Bollmann S, Rasmussen KGB, Kristensen M, et al. DeepQSM - using deep learning to solve the dipole inversion for quantitative susceptibility mapping. Neuroimage 2019;195:373–83.

71. Gibbons EK, Hodgson KK, Chaudhari AS, et al. Simultaneous NODDI and GFA parameter map generation from subsampled q-space imaging using deep learning. Magn Reson Med 2019;81(4): 2399–411.

72. Chen F, Taviani V, Malkiel I, et al. Variable-density single-shot fast spin-echo MRI with deep learning reconstruction by using variational networks. Radiology 2018;289(2):366–73.

73. Yang G, Yu S, Dong H, et al. DAGAN: deep de-aliasing generative adversarial networks for fast compressed sensing MRI reconstruction. IEEE Trans Med Imaging 2018;37(6):1310–21.

74. Diamond S, Sitzmann V, Heide F, Wetzstein G. Unrolled Optimization with Deep Priors. ArXiv. 2017; abs/1705.08041.

75. Cheng JY, Chen F, Alley M, Pauly J, Vasanawala S. Highly Scalable Image Reconstruction using Deep Neural Networks with Bandpass Filtering. ArXiv. 2018;abs/1805.03300.

76. Souza R, Lebel RM, Frayne R. A Hybrid, Dual Domain, Cascade of Convolutional Neural Networks for Magnetic Resonance Image Reconstruction. Proceedings of the 2nd International Conference on Medical Imaging with Deep Learning; 2019; London, England, July 8-10, 2019.

77. Eo T, Jun Y, Kim T, et al. KIKI-net: cross-domain convolutional neural networks for reconstructing undersampled magnetic resonance images. Magn Reson Med 2018;80(5):2188–201.

78. Cole E, Cheng JY, Pauly J, Vasanawala S. Analysis of Complex-Valued Convolutional Neural Networks for MRI Reconstruction. ArXiv. 2020;abs/2004.01738.

79. Tamir JI, Yu S, Lustig M. Unsupervised Deep Basis Pursuit: Learning inverse problems without ground-truth data. Paper presented at: International Society for Magnetic Resonance in Medicine 27th Annual Meeting & Exhibition 2019; Montreal, Quebec, Canada, May 11-16, 2019.

80. Zhussip M, Soltanayev S, Chun S. Training Deep Learning Based Image Denoisers From Undersampled Measurements Without Ground Truth and Without Image Prior. Paper presented at: 2019 IEEE/CVF Conference on Computer Vision and Pattern Recognition (CVPR) 2019; Long Beach, CA, June 16-20, 2019.

81. Lehtinen J, Munkberg J, Hasselgren J, et al. Noise2Noise: Learning Image Restoration without Clean Data. Proceedings of the 35th International Conference on Machine Learning. Stockholm, Sweden, July 10-15, 2018.

82. Soltanayev S, Chun SY. Training deep learning based denoisers without ground truth data. 32nd Conference on Neural Information Processing Systems (NeurIPS); 2018; Montreal, Canada, December 2-8, 2018.

83. Yaman B, Hosseini SAH, Moeller S, Ellermann J, Ugurbil K, AkÁakaya M. Self-Supervised Physics-Based Deep Learning MRI Reconstruction Without Fully-Sampled Data. Paper presented at: 2020 IEEE 17th International Symposium on Biomedical Imaging (ISBI) 2020; Iowa City, IA, USA, April 3-7, 2020.

84. Chen F, Cheng JY, Pauly JM, Vasanawala SS. Semi-Supervised Learning for Reconstructing Under-Sampled MR Scans. Paper presented at: International Society for Magnetic Resonance in Medicine 27th Annual Meeting & Exhibition2019; Montreal, Quebec, Canada, May 11-16, 2019.

85. Wu Z, Xiong Y, Yu S, Lin D. Unsupervised Feature Learning via Non-Parametric Instance-level Discrimination. Paper presented at: 2018 IEEE/CVF Conference on Computer Vision and Pattern Recognition2018; Salt Lake City, UT, USA, June 18-22, 2018.

86. Sim B, Oh G, Ye JC. Optimal Transport Structure of CycleGAN for Unsupervised Learning for Inverse

Problems. Paper presented at: 2020 IEEE International Conference on Acoustics, Speech and Signal Processing (ICASSP) 2020; Barcelona, Spain, May 4-8, 2020.

87. Goodfellow IJ, Pouget-Abadie J, Mirza M, et al. Generative Adversarial Nets. 28th Conference on Neural Information Processing Systems; 2014; Montreal, Canada, December 8-13, 2014.

88. Zhu JY, Krähenbühl P, Shechtman E, Efros AA. Generative Visual Manipulation on the Natural Image Manifold. Paper presented at: Computer Vision – ECCV 20162016; Amsterdam, The Netherlands, October 11-14, 2016.

89. Radford A, Metz L, Chintala S. Unsupervised Representation Learning with Deep Convolutional Generative Adversarial Networks. 4th International Conference on Learning Representations; 2016; San Juan, Puerto Rico, May 2-4, 2016.

90. Lei K, Mardani M, Pauly J, et al. Wasserstein GANs for MR imaging: from paired to unpaired training. IEEE Trans Med Imaging 2021;40(1):105–15.

91. Bora A, Price E, Dimakis A. AmbientGAN: Generative models from lossy measurements. Paper presented at: 6th International Conference on Learning Representations2018; Vancouver, Canada, April 30-May 3, 2018.

92. Cole EK, Pauly J, Vasanawala S, Ong F. Unsupervised MRI Reconstruction with Generative Adversarial Networks. ArXiv. 2020;abs/2008.13065.

93. Chen B, Duan X, Yu Z, et al. Technical note: development and validation of an open data format for CT projection data. Med Phys 2015;42(12):6964–72.

Clinical Artificial Intelligence Applications in Radiology: Chest and Abdomen

Sungwon Lee, MD, PhD, Ronald M. Summers, MD, PhD*

KEYWORDS

- Deep learning • Artificial intelligence • Radiology • Chest • Thorax • Abdomen • Pelvic

KEY POINTS

- Organ segmentation, chest radiograph classification, and lung and liver nodule detections are some of the popular artificial intelligence (AI) tasks in the chest and abdominal radiology due to the wide availability of public datasets.
- AI algorithms have achieved performance comparable to humans in less time for several organ segmentation tasks, and some lesion detection, and classification tasks.
- The complexity of organs and diseases in the chest and abdomen and the imbalance in the availability of public datasets are some of the challenges.

INTRODUCTION

How wonderful would it be if an automated assistant would go through our daily chest radiographs and sort out the ones that need our immediate attention; or maybe pick out the diagnostic errors in our computed tomography (CT) reports that could be as high as 5%[1] before we hit that confirm button. Compared with other body parts, chest and abdominal images have a larger field of view, multiple freely moving organs, and greater variability in shape and size. This is one of the reasons why the chest and abdominal images have been latecomers to the field of artificial intelligence (AI).[2] However, with the growing number of public datasets and increases in computational power, the number of published articles has vastly accelerated in the past few years, especially with the outbreak of the Coronavirus Disease 2019 (COVID-19).

For the clinical application of AI, the sophisticated task of interpreting a radiologic image is broken down into separate simplified tasks: measuring an organ or lesion (segmentation), detecting the region of abnormality from the whole image (detection), providing a diagnosis for the detected lesion (classification), and predicting the pathology or prognosis from an image. This review briefly introduces the current AI-derived published articles on the chest and abdominal radiology, accordingly.

Depending on the nature of the task, some algorithms perform better than others. Radiomics, a technique for extracting a large number of quantitative features, is used to link meaningful features to diagnose diseases or predict prognosis.[3] Most segmentation tasks work best with deep learning (DL) algorithms such as convoluted neural networks, especially U-Net[4] and its variants. With DL, the algorithm does not need predefined features, and unsupervised feature learning is

Funding: Not applicable.
Conflicts of interest: Author R.M. Summers receives royalties from iCAD, ScanMed, Philips, Translation Holdings, and Ping An. His laboratory received research support from Ping An and NVIDIA.
Imaging Biomarkers and Computer-Aided Diagnosis Laboratory, Department of Radiology and Imaging Sciences, National Institutes of Health Clinical Center, Building 10, Room 1C224D, 10 Center Drive, Bethesda, MD 20892-1182, USA
* Corresponding author.
E-mail address: rms@nih.gov

radiologic.theclinics.com

possible. However, to do so, it requires a large amount of data and the performance is unstable with insufficient datasets. Radiomics has the advantage of being able to incorporate human knowledge into the algorithm and also has explainability because we know exactly what predefined features have brought the algorithm to its conclusion. However, the feature extraction in radiomics may be affected by factors such as image resolution, low signal-to-noise ratio, and other artifacts.[5] Algorithms for detection are many and include DenseNet,[6] AlexNet,[7] ResNet,[8] and MaskRCNN.[9] Classification algorithms include AlexNet, ResNet, VGG16,[10] GoogLeNet (Inception-v3),[11] and Unet-like architectures. Generative adversarial networks (GAN) have also been used to create saliency maps.[12]

CHEST IMAGING APPLICATIONS
Organ Segmentation

An image segmentation task is a process of partitioning an image into multiple segments, and in radiologic images, it is used to outline the borders of an organ or lesion of interest. Although segmentation is not a task a radiologist would do daily, image segmentation provides us with the volume, shape, and densities of an organ or lesion of interest. This can then be used to quantify the severity or diagnose diseases such as cardiomegaly,[13] chronic obstructive pulmonary disease (COPD),[14] acute respiratory distress syndrome (ARDS),[15] and aortic aneurysm.[16] Image segmentation is also an important building block in improving other AI-derived tasks such as lesion detection[17] and classification.[18]

Organ segmentation was one of the first areas to be explored by AI, and now DL-derived segmentation algorithms have outperformed traditional segmentation algorithms that had rules for segmentation hard-coded into the software.[19] Currently, fully automated segmentation is possible in areas such as the lung fields[20] and heart shadow[21] of chest radiographs and lung lobes[22] and airways[23] in CT scans exceeding Dice similarity coefficients (DSCs) of 0.93 to 0.98. These automated organ segmentation techniques may assist us in situations such as calculating cardiothoracic ratio (correlation coefficient with reference 0.96),[24] detecting malpositioned feeding tubes (area under the curve [AUC] 0.82–0.87)[25] and endotracheal tubes (AUC 0.81)[26] and generating clavicle and rib-free chest radiograph images[27] (Fig. 1) to improve lung mass detection rate (increase receiver operating characteristic curve 10%).[28] Multiorgan segmentation on chest CT scans[29] show equally good results, suggesting

potential use on thoracic radiotherapy planning. However, it should be noted that many of the ground truth lung field segmentation in the chest radiograph datasets[30,31] do not include the retrocardiac and posterior base of the lung lobes. Also, the segmentation performances are still lower in organs with high variances in shapes, such as the esophagus (DSC 0.75)[29] and right middle lobe, or diseased lung (Intersection over Union of the right middle lobe was 0.89 in the COVID-19 dataset).[32]

Lesion Detection

Lesion detection is a task of computing the location information of an abnormal lesion in an image, which traditionally involved long processing pipelines.[33] With DL approaches, many of these steps can be avoided, and recently multitask algorithms have achieved lesion detection and segmentation simultaneously in pneumothorax (DSC 0.88),[34] lung nodules (DSC 0.80, 0.82),[35] and rib fractures (DSC 0.72).[36] Although these performances are not fit for clinical use alone, they can be applied to enhance the performance of radiologists in detecting lung nodules[37] and rib fractures[36] in CT.

Classification

Disease diagnosis in chest radiograph
Classification is a task of predicting a category for a presented example, and one of the perfect applications for this is the task of predicting the diagnosis in chest radiograph images. This task can be done as a binary task in which the categories may be normal versus abnormal (AUC 0.98),[38,39] normal versus pneumonia (AUC 0.99),[40] pneumothorax versus nonpneumothorax (accuracy 87.3%),[41] and pulmonary tuberculosis versus nontuberculosis (AUC 0.75).[42] A more realistic setting would be to solve this as a multiclass task in which the chest radiograph categories may be critical, urgent, nonurgent, and normal (sensitivities 65%, 76%, 48%, and 71%)[43] or 4 different diseases (AUCs 0.95 for pneumothorax, 0.72 for nodule or mass, 0.91 for opacity, and 0.86 for fracture)[44] or 8 different diseases (average per-class AUC approximately 0.7),[45] or 14 different diseases (average per-class AUC 0.83).[46] The performances for the multiclass algorithms were lower than binary models and were generally good for emphysema, cardiomegaly, and pneumothorax, and poor for infiltration, pneumonia, and mass. However, multiclass algorithms have proven to reduce report time in a simulation study (from 11.2 to 2.7 days for radiographs with critical imaging findings)[43] and improve performance of radiology residents in the emergency department

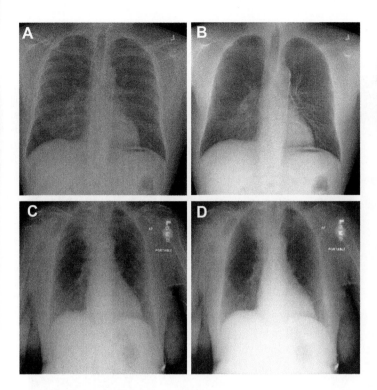

Fig. 1. Example of real and the corresponding bone-suppressed chest radiographs obtained from a Cycle-GAN model. (*A, C*) Standard chest radiographs. (*B, D*) The corresponding bone-suppressed images. (*From* Liang J, Tang Y-X, Tang Y-B, Xiao J, Summers R. *Bone suppression on chest radiographs with adversarial learning.* Vol 11314: SPIE; 2020.)

when used as a second reader (sensitivity improved from 66% to 73%).[47] Although perhaps with more limited use, DL-based automatic lung nodule detection algorithms improved nodule detection performances by physicians[48,49] or show performance superior to that of human readers.[50]

To consider the AI-derived prediction as a second reader, it is also important to understand "how" the algorithm came up with such prediction and radiologic imaging saliency maps[51] are the most common explanation method. Recently, Tang and colleagues[12] used a deep disentangled generative model to generate a patient-specific "normal" chest radiograph image from an abnormal radiograph and obtained residue maps and saliency maps from them (**Fig. 2**).

Lung nodule detection and classification in computed tomography

Low-dose chest CT is now the recommended method for lung cancer screening.[52] However, detecting and classifying pulmonary nodules is a time-consuming task and also prone to interobserver and intraobserver variability.[53] AI-derived algorithms have now gone beyond the old computer-aided detection systems and can suggest a possible diagnosis for the automatically detected lung nodules.[54] With DL-derived methods, the nodule classifications do not have

to be limited to the hand-crafted features of the nodule, such as size, density, and growth. DL algorithms can be trained to give a probability of malignancy score with excellent performance in predicting cancerous and noncancerous nodules (sensitivity 94.8%,[55] AUCs more than 0.9[56]), surpassing the performance of the Lung CT Screening Reporting and Data System (Lung-RADS) in predicting deaths from lung cancer.[56] Algorithms detecting and classifying nodules into 4[37,57] or 6[58] types (solid, nonsolid, part-solid, calcified, perifissural, and spiculated nodules) have shown performances comparable to human observers, and sometimes better if no previous CT imaging are available.[54] One thing we should keep in mind is that these algorithms were trained on carefully prepared nodule-only data, whereas the real-world data is mixed with nodule and non-nodule diseases. Also, because of the black-box nature of the DL algorithms, it may be difficult to explain why it has come up with such a conclusion or in which step (detection, segmentation, classification) it went wrong.

Classification of diffuse lung disease in computed tomography

Diffuse lung disease includes a group of heterogeneous diseases with considerably different prognoses and treatment.[59] As many of these diseases have similar appearances on CT and tend to have

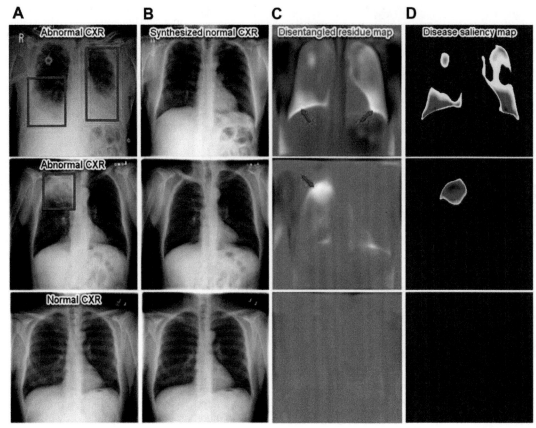

Fig. 2. Example of synthesized patient-specific normal chest radiograph generated from a deep disentangled generative model. (*A*) Original chest radiograph with abnormalities annotated by radiologists (*pink boxes*). (*B*) Synthesized normal radiograph generated from the original image. (*C, D*) Residual map and saliency map to delineate the potential diseased areas. (*From* Tang Y, Tang Y, Zhu Y, Xiao J, Summers RM. A disentangled generative model for disease decomposition in chest X-rays via normal image synthesis. *Med Image Anal.* 2021;67:101839.)

much disagreement between readers,[60,61] quantitative tools in CT scans are being used to assist in the diagnosis and disease severity assessment of diseases such as emphysema, cystic fibrosis, asthma, idiopathic pulmonary fibrosis, and hypersensitivity pneumonitis.[62] These quantitative tools have been applied with DL-derived algorithms or texture analysis to automatically assess the extent of systemic sclerosis-related interstitial lung disease (ILD),[63] emphysema,[64] and COPD[65] to show good correlation with pulmonary function tests. DL models have also been used to classify lung parenchyma into regional patterns (ground-glass opacity, consolidation, reticular opacity, emphysema, and honeycombing)[66] or classify lung CT scans according to idiopathic pulmonary fibrosis guidelines achieving human-level accuracy.[67] Although with relatively low performance, ILD classifying models that allow the whole lung as input

have been reported[68,69] and should be encouraged.

Predicting prognosis

With the emerging field of radiomics[70] and DL, we can now automatically extract large numbers of features from a lesion of interest and use them to predict pathology, prognosis, and mortality. Risk scores can be obtained from images to predict mortality in chest radiographs (mortality rates were 53.0% and 33.9% for high-risk score groups)[71] and CT (C index 0.72 in smoker group).[72] Radiomics can also find certain features that may have a better response with adjuvant chemotherapy,[73] differentiate squamous cell carcinoma from adenocarcinoma (AUC 0.89),[74] or predict epidermal growth factor receptor genotyping in lung adenocarcinoma CT (AUC 0.8).[75] Studies can be designed to predict the time to progression and overall survival in a baseline CT (hazard ratio 2.8, 2.4)[76] or time-series CT (hazard ratio 6.2 in overall survival).[77]

Artificial Intelligence on Coronavirus Disease 2019

In 2020 the world was hit by COVID-19, and up to the point of writing this review, more than 500 DL papers using COVID-19 images have been published.[78] Before the diagnostic test kit was available around the world, many studies were focused on screening COVID-19 in chest radiographs[79] and CT.[80] Although many of them had a good performance, radiologic images have less advantage in diagnosing COVID-19 infection because more than half of the symptomatic patients have a normal chest CT.[81] We are now looking toward using DL to ease the hospital resource allocation in the pandemic. One of those tasks is automatically assessing the severity of patients with COVID-19 by classifying them into severity scores.[82] DL and quantitative analysis can help discriminate between patients with and without COVID-19 (AUC 0.88 for external data),[83] evaluate disease progression,[84,85] predict patients who develop ARDS,[86] predict oxygen therapy, intubation,[87] hospitalized days,[88] or mortality.[89,90] We hope AI will continue to support us with decisions such as when to image patients for extrapulmonary manisfestations[91] and how to incorporate information about underlying diseases or patient demographics in treating COVID, especially now that vaccines and treatment therapies are starting to be used.

ABDOMINAL IMAGING APPLICATIONS
Organ Segmentation

Fully automated organ segmentation in the abdominal and pelvic regions must deal with problems such as high anatomic variability, indistinctive boundaries with neighboring structures, and mobility of the patient and organs.[92] This explains why the segmentation Dice scores are approximately 0.95 for the spleen,[93] visceral and subcutaneous adipose tissue,[94] muscle,[95] and vertebrae[96]; approximately 0.9 and higher for the liver,[97] kidneys,[98] prostate,[99] bladder, and rectum[99,100]; approximately 0.8 and higher for the esophagus,[101] pancreas,[102,103] and uterus[104]; and less than 0.8 for the stomach,[105] colon,[105] and small bowel.[106] There are multiorgan segmentation models that segment several organs at once with equally good accuracies.[107,108] The segmentation task is now turning toward more detailed substructures, such as hepatic vessels,[109]

Couinaud liver segments,[110] biliary tree anatomy,[111] and prostate zonal anatomy.[112]

Clinicians have been using manual or semiautomated measurements of organs for various medical decisions, and now fully automated segmentation algorithms may assist them in surgical[113,114] or radiotherapy planning,[115] or diagnose organomegaly in the spleen[93] and prostate.[116] There are several commercially available liver segmentation software packages and solutions that even have picture archiving and communication system (PACS) interfaces.[117] Measurements from these automated segmentations may be used as biomarkers to assess diseases such as sarcopenia,[95] liver steatosis,[118] liver fibrosis,[119] or cardiovascular events and mortality.[120]

Lesion Detection

Automatically detecting and segmenting a certain tumor or disease has been a popular topic, especially in organs with good organ segmentation. The performances are better for tumors of the liver (DSC 0.83, **Fig. 3**),[121] kidney (DSC 0.87),[122] prostate (detection sensitivity 86%, DSC 0.87),[123] rectum (DSC 0.9),[124] and uterine fibroids (DSC 0.9).[125] Performances are poorer for pancreas tumors (DSC 0.71),[126] cervical tumors (DSC 0.82),[127] and small-sized tumors (detection sensitivity 10% vs 85%, DSC 0.14 vs 0.68 for liver tumor smaller than 1 cm vs larger than 2 cm).[128] A few preliminary studies have focused on segmenting the active and necrotic parts of liver tumors.[129,130] This would potentially be helpful in assessing the accurate tumor burden.

Other nontumoral disease entities such as colonic polyps,[131] abdominal calcified plaque,[132,133] hemoperitoneum,[134] pneumoperitoneum,[135] and urinary stones[136] have been targeted for detection and segmentation and have shown promising results. However, more work needs to be done on detecting "universal lesions" on the whole abdomen. For instance, detecting metastatic lymph nodes[137] or multiple diseases (average sensitivity 69.2%,[138] 86.1%)[139] in the entire abdomen and pelvic CT.

Classification

Disease diagnosis

DL-based diagnosis is outperforming the human-made measurements, such as the hepatorenal index method in liver steatosis[140] or PI-RADS (prostate imaging–reporting and data system) in prostate cancer.[141] With the help of U-Net,[4] radiomics, and ensemble DL algorithms, disease diagnosis can be approached as a binary or multiclass classification problem.[142–144] The task of classifying

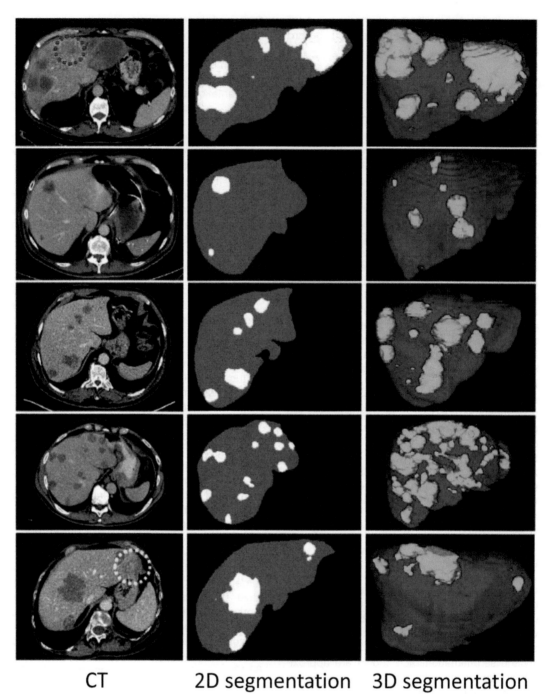

CT   2D segmentation   3D segmentation

Fig. 3. Example of 2-dimensional and 3-dimensional liver tumor segmentation generated from a coarse liver segmentation network followed by an edge-enhanced network. The yellow/red dashed circles indicate some cases in which the tumor boundaries are blurry on the original image. (*From* Tang Y, Tang Y, Zhu Y, Xiao J, Summers RM. E2Net: An Edge Enhanced Network for Accurate Liver and Tumor Segmentation on CT Scans. Paper presented at: International Conference on Medical Image Computing and Computer-Assisted Intervention2020.)

abdominal tumors into 2 types or multiple types has achieved variable results. Examples include benign or malignant classification in liver tumors on ultrasound (AUC 0.94),[145] pancreas tumors on CT (sensitivity 97%),[146] adrenal tumors on CT (AUC 0.8),[147] kidney tumors on CT (accuracy 77.3%),[148] prostate tumors on magnetic resonance (MR) images (AUC 0.79),[149] ovary tumors on MR (AUC 0.86),[150] cervical tumors on MR (accuracy 0.9%),[151] 6 liver tumor types on MR (sensitivity 82.9%),[152] and PI-RADS classification on MR (moderate agreement with expert radiologists).[153] The interpretation of these performances can sometimes be confusing, because the imaging modality, tumor types, gold-standard methods, and dataset populations vary between studies. Some of the studies show that they achieve similar[153] or better performances[150] than radiologists in predicting pathology-proven diagnosis, but many of the studies lack comparisons with both radiologists' evaluation and traditional methods.[154]

Sometimes radiologists are challenged with difficult differential diagnoses that have crucial consequences. This is a good situation to use AI-derived algorithms. Some studies have achieved interesting results in differentiating ambiguous lesions, such as fat-poor renal angiomyolipoma from renal cell carcinoma in CT (AUC 0.96),[155] hepatocellular carcinoma (HCC) from intrahepatic cholangiocarcinoma in CT (AUC 0.72),[156] stromal benign prostatic hyperplasia from transitional zone prostate cancer (AUC 0.9),[157] and benign borderline ovarian tumors from malignant ovarian tumors (AUC 0.89).[150] AI algorithms can also lend a hand in stressful tasks such as detecting vessel invasion of pancreatic cancer in CT (AUC 0.85, comparable performance to senior radiologist),[158] or early-stage cervical cancer in MR (AUC 0.9),[159] detecting extraprostatic extension of prostate cancer (AUC 0.88),[160] detecting local recurrence of rectal cancer anastomosis in MR (AUC 0.86),[161] and detecting HCC in patients with cirrhosis (AUC 0.7).[162] They can even be tried on tasks in which radiologists feel less confident, such as differentiating HCC in noncontrast MR,[163] classifying small hypoattenuating hepatic nodules in colorectal carcinoma CT (AUC 0.84, lower than radiologist),[164] and diagnosing appendicitis in acute abdominal pain CT (accuracy more than 90%).[165]

Disease grading
The classification does not have to be limited to traditional labels. Transfer learning radiomics models can be used to classify liver fibrosis in grayscale and elastogram ultrasounds that perform better than prior liver stiffness

measurements.[166] Contrast-enhanced CT scans can be used as inputs to classify grades of liver steatosis (AUC of 0.67, 0.85, and 0.97 for predicting MR proton density fat fraction thresholds of 5%, 10%, and 15%)[118] or liver fibrosis (AUC of 0.96, 0.97, and 0.95 for significant fibrosis, advanced fibrosis, and cirrhosis).[119]

Texture analysis and DL-derived classification algorithms use features beyond the human vision, allowing creative classification tasks, such as predicting estimated glomerular filtration rate (correlation coefficient of 0.74)[167] or interstitial fibrosis and tubular atrophy grades (F1 84%)[168] from ultrasound images, distinguishing aldosterone-producing and cortisol-producing functional adrenocortical adenomas in CT (AUC 0.88),[169] classifying dysplasia grades of intraductal papillary mucinous neoplasia in MR (AUC 0.78),[170] differentiating renal cell carcinoma subtypes in MR (accuracy 81.2%),[171] or grading pancreatic neuroendocrine neoplasm histology types in CT (AUC 0.81).[172] Radiomic features have even shown better results than PI-RADS in diagnosing prostate cancer (AUC 0.96 vs 0.88).[141]

Predicting prognosis
The whole point of classifying any disease into stages or categories is to predict the prognosis and plan a treatment strategy. Radiomics features coupled with machine learning approaches are now used to bypass this hand-crafted staging and directly predict clinical outcome, or predict certain gene expression,[173] and even discover new image biomarkers for well-known diseases.[174] Radiomics features extracted from pretreatment radiologic images have been shown to improve the detection of early recurrence, or predict treatment response or overall survival in HCC,[175,176] liver metastasis,[177] prostate cancer,[178] and many more malignancies.[179,180] Models can predict future events of gastro-esophageal variceal bleeding,[181] hepatic encephalopathy[182] in liver cirrhotic CT, or predict intraoperative blood loss in pernicious placenta previa MR (accuracy 75.6%).[183]

CHALLENGES OF ARTIFICIAL INTELLIGENCE APPLICATION AND FUTURE WORKS

There are more than a dozen different kinds of organs in the chest and abdomen, many of which are constantly moving, and each of them can have multiple diseases. This makes it challenging for many AI tasks, including registration, detection, and classification. Currently, most studies are focused on a certain organ, a single phase or sequence, and a specific disease condition, on a carefully collected dataset.[149] However, the real-world task needs more than 1 diagnosis on more than 1 organ, and more research needs to be done on multitask algorithms with a universal approach. Also, the real-world dataset may have a much lower disease prevalence and a broader spectrum of diseases.[184] Thus, more research needs to be done on larger imaging datasets with external validation on data from multiple institutions. The availability of large radiologic datasets is currently a bottleneck for AI research, contributed by many factors including institutional review board approvals, patient privacy and anonymity, the complexities of working with DICOM (digital imaging and communications in medicine) files and their size, and the cost of assembling and maintaining a database.[185] Despite all the efforts to minimize training data,[186] it is still true that where there is no data there is no study. This is proven by how the AI methods thrive on fields with large public datasets (chest radiograph frontal view,[45] lung nodule CT,[187] and liver tumor CT[188]) and are scarce in fields such as chest radiograph lateral view, bowels, and pelvic organs.

For the same reason described previously, one must be careful when interpreting the results of the chest and abdominal AI studies. The accuracies depend greatly on the dataset, the complexity of the task, how the gold standard was chosen, image modality, scanner types, and protocol.[19,189,190] The results need to be presented as case-control studies in which the AI results could be statistically compared with human experts, conventionally used measurements, or results of other AI methods.

Currently, the accuracies of these single-task AI algorithms are approximately 80%, and depending on the nature of the task, this may be clinically helpful in the emergency department,[47] improve inter-reader agreements,[191] or monitor disease progression.[47,192] To be of more practical value, the algorithms should be ready to incorporate additional information, such as the chief complaint, medical history, and laboratory results, and be able to interact with human corrections, preferably on PACS, ultrasound, and intervention machines. Future AI studies should not dwell on mimicking human radiologists. They should be targeted to outperform the human eye by training on clinical and pathology-proven gold standards.

In conclusion, the chest and abdominal AI studies are latecomers but have advanced immensely in the past few years, in some fields more than others, probably due to the imbalance of dataset availability. Organ segmentation, chest radiograph diagnosis, detection, and classification of lung and liver tumors have relatively better performance.

CLINICS CARE POINTS

- Organ segmentation tools will be able to assist in surgical or radiotherapy planning and diagnose diseases such as organomegaly, sarcopenia, and diffuse liver and lung diseases.

- Currently, the accuracies of single-task classification algorithms are approximately 80%, but this may still be clinically helpful in the emergency department, improve inter-reader agreements, or monitor disease progression.

- Caution is needed in interpreting the accuracies of AI as the studies greatly depend on the data they were trained on.

- More clinical validation is needed for AI to be of help to radiologists and clinicians.

ACKNOWLEDGMENTS

This research was supported by the Intramural Research Program of the National Institutes of Health Clinical Center.

REFERENCES

1. Itri JN, Tappouni RR, McEachern RO, et al. Fundamentals of diagnostic error in imaging. Radiographics. 2018;38(6):1845–65.
2. Summers RM. Progress in fully automated abdominal CT interpretation. AJR Am J Roentgenol 2016; 207(1):67–79.
3. Gillies RJ, Kinahan PE, Hricak H. Radiomics: images are more than pictures, they are data. Radiology 2016;278(2):563–77.
4. Ronneberger O, Fischer P, Brox T. U-net: Convolutional networks for biomedical image segmentation. Paper presented at: International Conference on Medical image computing and computer-assisted intervention. Munich, Germany, October 5-9, 2015. p. 234-41.
5. Wang Y, Yue W, Li X, et al. Comparison study of radiomics and deep learning-based methods for thyroid nodules classification using ultrasound images. IEEE Access. 2020;8:52010–7.
6. Huang G, Liu Z, Van Der Maaten L, Weinberger KQ. Densely connected convolutional networks. Paper presented at: Proceedings of the IEEE conference on computer vision and pattern recognition. Honolulu, HI, July 21-26, 2017. p. 4700-8.
7. Krizhevsky A, Sutskever I, Hinton GE. Imagenet classification with deep convolutional neural

networks. Adv Neural Inf Process Syst 2012;25: 1097–105.

8. Li D, He K, Sun J, Zhou K. A geodesic-preserving method for image warping. Paper presented at: Proceedings of the IEEE Conference on Computer Vision and Pattern Recognition. Boston, MA, June 7-12, 2015. p. 213-21.

9. He K, Gkioxari G, Dollár P, Girshick R. Mask r-cnn. Paper presented at: Proceedings of the IEEE international conference on computer vision. Honolulu, HI, July 21-26, 2017. p. 2961-9.

10. Simonyan K, Zisserman A. Very deep convolutional networks for large-scale image recognition. arXiv preprint arXiv:14091556. 2014.

11. Szegedy C, Liu W, Jia Y, et al. Going deeper with convolutions. Paper presented at: Proceedings of the IEEE conference on computer vision and pattern recognition. Boston, MA, June 7-12, 2015. p. 1-9.

12. Tang Y, Tang Y, Zhu Y, et al. A disentangled generative model for disease decomposition in chest X-rays via normal image synthesis. Med Image Anal 2021;67:101839.

13. Sogancioglu E, Murphy K, Calli E, et al. Cardiomegaly detection on chest radiographs: segmentation versus classification. IEEE Access. 2020;8:94631–42.

14. Fischer AM, Varga-Szemes A, Martin SS, et al. Artificial intelligence-based fully automated per lobe segmentation and emphysema-quantification based on chest computed tomography compared with global initiative for chronic obstructive lung disease severity of smokers. J Thorac Imaging 2020;35:S28–34.

15. Nishiyama A, Kawata N, Yokota H, et al. A predictive factor for patients with acute respiratory distress syndrome: CT lung volumetry of the well-aerated region as an automated method. Eur J Radiol 2020;122:108748.

16. Cao L, Shi R, Ge Y, et al. Fully automatic segmentation of type B aortic dissection from CTA images enabled by deep learning. Eur J Radiol 2019;121: 108713.

17. Rahman T, Khandakar A, Kadir MA, et al. Reliable tuberculosis detection using chest x-ray with deep learning, segmentation and visualization. IEEE Access. 2020;8:191586–601.

18. Liu H, Wang L, Nan Y, et al. Segmentation-based deep fusion network for thoracic disease classification in chest X-ray images. Comput Med Imaging Graphics. 2019;75:66–73.

19. Auffermann WF, Gozansky EK, Tridandapani S. Artificial intelligence in cardiothoracic radiology. AJR Am J Roentgenol 2019;212(5):997–1001.

20. Portela RDS, Pereira JRG, Costa MGF, Filho CFFC. Lung region segmentation in chest x-ray images using deep convolutional neural networks. Paper presented at: 2020 42nd Annual International Conference of the IEEE Engineering in Medicine &

Biology Society (EMBC). Virtual, July 20-24, 2020. p. 1246-9.

21. Gómez O, Mesejo P, Ibáñez O, et al. Deep architectures for high-resolution multi-organ chest X-ray image segmentation. Neural Comput Appl 2020;32(20):15949–63.

22. Park J, Yun J, Kim N, et al. Fully automated lung lobe segmentation in volumetric chest CT with 3D U-Net: validation with intra- and extra-datasets. J Digit Imaging 2020;33(1):221–30.

23. Nadeem SA, Hoffman EA, Sieren JC, et al. A CT-based automated algorithm for airway segmentation using freeze-and-grow propagation and deep learning. IEEE Trans Med Imaging 2020;1.

24. Li Z, Hou Z, Chen C, et al. Automatic cardiothoracic ratio calculation with deep learning. IEEE Access. 2019;7:37749–56.

25. Singh V, Danda V, Gorniak R, et al. Assessment of critical feeding tube malpositions on radiographs using deep learning. J Digit Imaging 2019;32(4): 651–5.

26. Lakhani P. Deep convolutional neural networks for endotracheal tube position and X-ray image classification: challenges and opportunities. J Digit Imaging 2017;30(4):460–8.

27. Liang J, Tang Y-X, Tang Y-B, Xiao J, Summers R. Bone suppression on chest radiographs with adversarial learning. 11314: SPIE. Houston, TX, February 15-20, 2020.

28. Baltruschat IM, Steinmeister L, Ittrich H, et al. When does bone suppression and lung field segmentation improve chest x-ray disease classification? Paper presented at: 2019 IEEE 16th International Symposium on Biomedical Imaging (ISBI 2019). Venice, Italy, April 8-11, 2019. p. 1362-6.

29. Dong X, Lei Y, Wang T, et al. Automatic multiorgan segmentation in thorax CT images using U-net-GAN. Med Phys 2019;46(5):2157–68.

30. Shiraishi J, Katsuragawa S, Ikezoe J, et al. Development of a digital image database for chest radiographs with and without a lung nodule: receiver operating characteristic analysis of radiologists' detection of pulmonary nodules. AJR Am J Roentgenol 2000;174(1):71–4.

31. Candemir S, Jaeger S, Palaniappan K, et al. Lung segmentation in chest radiographs using anatomical atlases with nonrigid registration. IEEE Trans Med Imaging 2014;33(2):577–90.

32. Xie W, Jacobs C, Charbonnier JP, et al. Relational modeling for robust and efficient pulmonary lobe segmentation in CT scans. IEEE Trans Med Imaging 2020;39(8):2664–75.

33. Sahiner B, Pezeshk A, Hadjiiski LM, et al. Deep learning in medical imaging and radiation therapy. Med Phys 2019;46(1):e1–36.

34. Wang X, Yang S, Lan J, et al. Automatic segmentation of pneumothorax in chest radiographs based

on a two-stage deep learning method. IEEE Trans Cogn Developmental Syst 2020;1.

35. Wang S, Zhou M, Liu Z, et al. Central focused convolutional neural networks: developing a data-driven model for lung nodule segmentation. Med Image Anal 2017;40:172–83.

36. Jin L, Yang J, Kuang K, et al. Deep-learning-assisted detection and segmentation of rib fractures from CT scans: development and validation of FracNet. EBioMedicine. 2020;62: 103106.

37. Liu K, Li Q, Ma J, et al. Evaluating a fully automated pulmonary nodule detection approach and its impact on radiologist performance. Radiol Artif Intelligence. 2019;1(3):e180084.

38. Dunnmon JA, Yi D, Langlotz CP, et al. Assessment of convolutional neural networks for automated classification of chest radiographs. Radiology 2019;290(2):537–44.

39. Tang Y-X, Tang Y-B, Peng Y, et al. Automated abnormality classification of chest radiographs using deep convolutional neural networks. NPJ Digit Med 2020;3(1):70.

40. Narayanan BN, Davuluru VSP, Hardie R. Two-stage deep learning architecture for pneumonia detection and its diagnosis in chest radiographs, 11318. SPIE. Houston, TX, February 15-20, 2020.

41. Park S, Lee SM, Kim N, et al. Application of deep learning-based computer-aided detection system: detecting pneumothorax on chest radiograph after biopsy. Eur Radiol 2019;29(10):5341–8.

42. Harris M, Qi A, Jeagal L, et al. A systematic review of the diagnostic accuracy of artificial intelligence-based computer programs to analyze chest x-rays for pulmonary tuberculosis. PLoS One. 2019;14(9): e0221339.

43. Annarumma M, Withey SJ, Bakewell RJ, et al. Automated triaging of adult chest radiographs with deep artificial neural networks. Radiology 2019; 291(1):196–202.

44. Majkowska A, Mittal S, Steiner DF, et al. Chest radiograph interpretation with deep learning models: assessment with radiologist-adjudicated reference standards and population-adjusted evaluation. Radiology 2020;294(2):421–31.

45. Wang X, Peng Y, Lu L, Lu Z, Bagheri M, Summers RM. Chestx-ray8: hospital-scale chest x-ray database and benchmarks on weakly-supervised classification and localization of common thorax diseases. Paper presented at: Proceedings of the IEEE conference on computer vision and pattern recognition. Honolulu, HI, July 21-26, 2017. p. 2097-106.

46. Wang H, Wang S, Qin Z, et al. Triple attention learning for classification of 14 thoracic diseases using chest radiography. Med Image Anal 2021; 67:101846.

47. Hwang EJ, Nam JG, Lim WH, et al. Deep learning for chest radiograph diagnosis in the emergency department. Radiology 2019;293(3):573–80.

48. Nam JG, Park S, Hwang EJ, et al. Development and validation of deep learning-based automatic detection algorithm for malignant pulmonary nodules on chest radiographs. Radiology 2019; 290(1):218–28.

49. Sim Y, Chung MJ, Kotter E, et al. Deep convolutional neural network-based software improves radiologist detection of malignant lung nodules on chest radiographs. Radiology 2020;294(1): 199–209.

50. Cha MJ, Chung MJ, Lee JH, et al. Performance of deep learning model in detecting operable lung cancer with chest radiographs. J Thorac Imaging 2019;34(2):86–91.

51. Adebayo J, Gilmer J, Muelly M, et al. Sanity checks for saliency maps. Adv Neural Inf Process Syst 2018;31:9505–15.

52. Oudkerk M, Devaraj A, Vliegenthart R, et al. European position statement on lung cancer screening. Lancet Oncol 2017;18(12):e754–66.

53. van Riel SJ, Sánchez CI, Bankier AA, et al. Observer variability for classification of pulmonary nodules on low-dose CT images and its effect on nodule management. Radiology 2015;277(3): 863–71.

54. Ardila D, Kiraly AP, Bharadwaj S, et al. End-to-end lung cancer screening with three-dimensional deep learning on low-dose chest computed tomography. Nat Med 2019;25(6):954–61.

55. Agnes SA, Anitha J. Appraisal of deep-learning techniques on computer-aided lung cancer diagnosis with computed tomography screening. J Med Phys 2020;45(2):98–106.

56. Huang P, Lin CT, Li Y, et al. Prediction of lung cancer risk at follow-up screening with low-dose CT: a training and validation study of a deep learning method. Lancet Digital Health. 2019;1(7):e353–62.

57. Wang D, Zhang T, Li M, et al. 3D deep learning based classification of pulmonary ground glass opacity nodules with automatic segmentation. Comput Med Imaging Graphics. 2020;101814.

58. Ciompi F, Chung K, van Riel SJ, et al. Towards automatic pulmonary nodule management in lung cancer screening with deep learning. Scientific Rep 2017;7(1):46479.

59. Raghu G. Epidemiology, survival, incidence and prevalence of idiopathic pulmonary fibrosis in the USA and Canada. Eur Respir J 2017;49(1): 1602384.

60. Watadani T, Sakai F, Johkoh T, et al. Interobserver variability in the CT assessment of honeycombing in the lungs. Radiology 2013;266(3):936–44.

61. Walsh SL, Calandriello L, Sverzellati N, et al. Interobserver agreement for the ATS/ERS/JRS/ALAT

criteria for a UIP pattern on CT. Thorax. 2016;71(1): 45–51.

62. Chen A, Karwoski RA, Gierada DS, et al. Quantitative CT analysis of diffuse lung disease. RadioGraphics. 2020;40(1):28–43.

63. Chassagnon G, Vakalopoulou M, Régent A, et al. Deep learning–based approach for automated assessment of interstitial lung disease in systemic sclerosis on CT images. Radiol Artif Intelligence. 2020;2(4):e190006.

64. Humphries SM, Notary AM, Centeno JP, et al. Deep learning enables automatic classification of emphysema pattern at CT. Radiology 2020; 294(2):434–44.

65. Sørensen L, Nielsen M, Petersen J, et al. Chronic obstructive pulmonary disease quantification using CT texture analysis and densitometry: results from the Danish Lung Cancer Screening Trial. AJR Am J Roentgenol 2020;214(6):1269–79.

66. Kim GB, Jung KH, Lee Y, et al. Comparison of shallow and deep learning methods on classifying the regional pattern of diffuse lung disease. J Digit Imaging 2018;31(4):415–24.

67. Walsh SLF, Calandriello L, Silva M, et al. Deep learning for classifying fibrotic lung disease on high-resolution computed tomography: a case-cohort study. Lancet Respir Med 2018;6(11): 837–45.

68. Gao M, Bagci U, Lu L, et al. Holistic classification of CT attenuation patterns for interstitial lung diseases via deep convolutional neural networks. Comput Methods Biomech Biomed Eng Imaging Vis 2018; 6(1):1–6.

69. Christe A, Peters AA, Drakopoulos D, et al. Computer-aided diagnosis of pulmonary fibrosis using deep learning and CT images. Invest Radiol 2019;54(10):627–32.

70. Lambin P, Leijenaar RTH, Deist TM, et al. Radiomics: the bridge between medical imaging and personalized medicine. Nat Rev Clin Oncol 2017; 14(12):749–62.

71. Lu MT, Ivanov A, Mayrhofer T, et al. Deep learning to assess long-term mortality from chest radiographs. JAMA Netw Open 2019;2(7):e197416.

72. González G, Ash SY, Vegas-Sánchez-Ferrero G, et al. Disease staging and prognosis in smokers using deep learning in chest computed tomography. Am J Respir Crit Care Med 2018;197(2): 193–203.

73. Vaidya P, Bera K, Gupta A, et al. CT derived radiomic score for predicting the added benefit of adjuvant chemotherapy following surgery in stage I, II resectable non-small cell lung cancer: a retrospective multicohort study for outcome prediction. Lancet Digit Health. 2020;2(3):e116–28.

74. Zhu X, Dong D, Chen Z, et al. Radiomic signature as a diagnostic factor for histologic subtype classification of non-small cell lung cancer. Eur Radiol 2018;28(7):2772–8.

75. Jia TY, Xiong JF, Li XY, et al. Identifying EGFR mutations in lung adenocarcinoma by noninvasive imaging using radiomics features and random forest modeling. Eur Radiol 2019;29(9):4742–50.

76. Khorrami M, Khunger M, Zagouras A, et al. Combination of peri- and intratumoral radiomic features on baseline CT scans predicts response to chemotherapy in lung adenocarcinoma. Radiol Artif Intell 2019;1(2):e180012.

77. Xu Y, Hosny A, Zeleznik R, et al. Deep learning predicts lung cancer treatment response from serial medical imaging. Clin Cancer Res 2019;25(11): 3266–75.

78. Summers RM. Artificial intelligence of COVID-19 imaging: a hammer in search of a nail. Radiology 2020;298(3):E162–4.

79. Zhang R, Tie X, Qi Z, et al. Diagnosis of COVID-19 pneumonia using chest radiography: value of artificial intelligence. Radiology 2020;202944.

80. Bai HX, Wang R, Xiong Z, et al. Artificial intelligence augmentation of radiologist performance in distinguishing COVID-19 from pneumonia of other origin at chest CT. Radiology 2020;296(3):E156–65.

81. Bernheim A, Mei X, Huang M, et al. Chest CT findings in Coronavirus Disease-19 (COVID-19): relationship to duration of infection. Radiology 2020; 295(3):200463.

82. Prokop M, Everdingen WV, Vellinga TVR, et al. CO-RADS: a categorical CT assessment scheme for patients suspected of having COVID-19—definition and evaluation. Radiology 2020;296(2):E97–104.

83. Lessmann N, Sánchez CI, Beenen L, et al. Automated assessment of COVID-19 reporting and data system and chest CT severity scores in patients suspected of having COVID-19 using artificial intelligence. Radiology 2021;298(1):E18–28.

84. Pu J, Leader JK, Bandos A, et al. Automated quantification of COVID-19 severity and progression using chest CT images. Eur Radiol 2021;31(1): 436–46.

85. Li Z, Zhong Z, Li Y, et al. From community-acquired pneumonia to COVID-19: a deep learning-based method for quantitative analysis of COVID-19 on thick-section CT scans. Eur Radiol 2020;30(12): 6828–37.

86. Wang Y, Chen Y, Wei Y, et al. Quantitative analysis of chest CT imaging findings with the risk of ARDS in COVID-19 patients: a preliminary study. Ann Transl Med 2020;8(9):594.

87. Lanza E, Muglia R, Bolengo I, et al. Quantitative chest CT analysis in COVID-19 to predict the need for oxygenation support and intubation. Eur Radiol 2020;30(12):6770–8.

88. Yue H, Yu Q, Liu C, et al. Machine learning-based CT radiomics method for predicting hospital stay in

patients with pneumonia associated with SARS-CoV-2 infection: a multicenter study. Ann translational Med 2020;8(14):859.

89. Mushtaq J, Pennella R, Lavalle S, et al. Initial chest radiographs and artificial intelligence (AI) predict clinical outcomes in COVID-19 patients: analysis of 697 Italian patients. Eur Radiol 2020;31(3):1770–9.

90. Li MD, Arun NT, Gidwani M, et al. Automated assessment and tracking of COVID-19 Pulmonary disease severity on chest radiographs using convolutional Siamese neural networks. Radiol Artif Intelligence. 2020;2(4):e200079.

91. Gupta A, Madhavan MV, Sehgal K, et al. Extrapulmonary manifestations of COVID-19. Nat Med 2020;26(7):1017–32.

92. Lenchik L, Heacock L, Weaver AA, et al. Automated segmentation of tissues using CT and MRI: a systematic review. Acad Radiol 2019;26(12):1695–706.

93. Humpire-Mamani GE, Bukala J, Scholten ET, et al. Fully automatic volume measurement of the spleen at CT using deep learning. Radiol Artif Intelligence. 2020;2(4):e190102.

94. Küstner T, Hepp T, Fischer M, et al. Fully automated and standardized segmentation of adipose tissue compartments via deep learning in 3D whole-body MRI of epidemiologic cohort studies. Radiol Artif Intelligence. 2020;2(6):e200010.

95. Burns JE, Yao J, Chalhoub D, et al. A machine learning algorithm to estimate sarcopenia on abdominal CT. Acad Radiol 2020;27(3):311–20.

96. Elton D, Sandfort V, Pickhardt P, et al. Accurately identifying vertebral levels in large datasets, 11314. Houston, TX, February 15-20, 2020.

97. Wang K, Mamidipalli A, Retson T, et al. Automated CT and MRI liver segmentation and biometry using a generalized convolutional neural network. Radiol Artif Intell 2019;1(2):180022.

98. Jackson P, Hardcastle N, Dawe N, et al. Deep learning renal segmentation for fully automated radiation dose estimation in unsealed source therapy. Front Oncol 2018;8:215.

99. Zhang Z, Zhao T, Gay H, et al. ARPM-net: A novel CNN-based adversarial method with Markov random field enhancement for prostate and organs at risk segmentation in pelvic CT images. Med Phys 2020;48(1):227–37.

100. Nemoto T, Futakami N, Yagi M, et al. Simple low-cost approaches to semantic segmentation in radiation therapy planning for prostate cancer using deep learning with non-contrast planning CT images. Phys Med 2020;78:93–100.

101. Diniz JOB, Ferreira JL, Diniz PHB, et al. Esophagus segmentation from planning CT images using an atlas-based deep learning approach. Comput Methods Programs Biomed 2020;197:105685.

102. Kumar H, DeSouza SV, Petrov MS. Automated pancreas segmentation from computed tomography and magnetic resonance images: a systematic review. Comput Methods Programs Biomed 2019;178:319–28.

103. Roth HR, Lu L, Lay N, et al. Spatial aggregation of holistically-nested convolutional neural networks for automated pancreas localization and segmentation. Med Image Anal 2018;45:94–107.

104. Kurata Y, Nishio M, Kido A, et al. Automatic segmentation of the uterus on MRI using a convolutional neural network. Comput Biol Med 2019;114:103438.

105. Cardenas CE, Yang J, Anderson BM, et al. Advances in auto-segmentation. Semin Radiat Oncol 2019;29(3):185–97.

106. Shin SY, Lee S, Elton D, Gulley JL, Summers RM. Deep small bowel segmentation with cylindrical topological constraints. Paper presented at: Medical Image Computing and Computer Assisted Intervention – MICCAI. Lima, Peru, October 4-8, 2020. p. 207-15.

107. Roth HR, Oda H, Zhou X, et al. An application of cascaded 3D fully convolutional networks for medical image segmentation. Comput Med Imaging Graphics. 2018;66:90–9.

108. Chen Y, Ruan D, Xiao J, et al. Fully automated multiorgan segmentation in abdominal magnetic resonance imaging with deep neural networks. Med Phys 2020;47(10):4971–82.

109. Kitrungrotsakul T, Han XH, Iwamoto Y, et al. VesselNet: A deep convolutional neural network with multi pathways for robust hepatic vessel segmentation. Comput Med Imaging Graph 2019;75:74–83.

110. Tian J, Liu L, Shi Z, Xu F. Automatic Couinaud Segmentation from CT Volumes on Liver Using GLC-UNet. Paper presented at: Machine Learning in Medical Imaging. Shenzhen, China, October 13, 2019. p. 274-82.

111. Ivashchenko OV, Rijkhorst EJ, Ter Beek LC, et al. A workflow for automated segmentation of the liver surface, hepatic vasculature and biliary tree anatomy from multiphase MR images. Magn Reson Imaging 2020;68:53–65.

112. Zabihollahy F, Schieda N, Krishna Jeyaraj S, et al. Automated segmentation of prostate zonal anatomy on T2-weighted (T2W) and apparent diffusion coefficient (ADC) map MR images using U-Nets. Med Phys 2019;46(7):3078–90.

113. Abdalla A, Ahmed N, Dakua S, Balakrishnan S, Abinahed J. A surgical-oriented liver segmentation approach using deep learning. Paper presented at: 2020 IEEE International Conference on Informatics, IoT, and Enabling Technologies (ICIoT). Doha, Qatar, February 2-5, 2020. p. 318-22.

114. Zhang C, Shu H, Yang G, et al. HIFUNet: multi-class segmentation of uterine regions from MR

images using global convolutional networks for HIFU surgery planning. IEEE Trans Med Imaging 2020;39(11):3309–20.

115. Liu Y, Lei Y, Wang T, et al. CBCT-based synthetic CT generation using deep-attention cycleGAN for pancreatic adaptive radiotherapy. Med Phys 2020;47(6):2472–83.

116. Ghavami N, Hu Y, Gibson E, et al. Automatic segmentation of prostate MRI using convolutional neural networks: Investigating the impact of network architecture on the accuracy of volume measurement and MRI-ultrasound registration. Med Image Anal 2019;58:101558.

117. Gotra A, Sivakumaran L, Chartrand G, et al. Liver segmentation: indications, techniques and future directions. Insights Imaging. 2017;8(4):377–92.

118. Pickhardt PJ, Blake GM, Graffy PM, et al. Liver steatosis categorization on contrast-enhanced CT using a fully-automated deep learning volumetric segmentation tool: evaluation in 1,204 heathy adults using unenhanced CT as reference standard. AJR Am J Roentgenol 2021;217(2):359–67.

119. Choi KJ, Jang JK, Lee SS, et al. Development and validation of a deep learning system for staging liver fibrosis by using contrast agent-enhanced CT images in the liver. Radiology 2018;289(3):688–97.

120. Pickhardt PJ, Graffy PM, Zea R, et al. Automated CT biomarkers for opportunistic prediction of future cardiovascular events and mortality in an asymptomatic screening population: a retrospective cohort study. Lancet Digital Health. 2020;2(4):e192–200.

121. Tang Y, Tang Y, Zhu Y, et al. E2Net: An edge enhanced network for accurate liver and tumor segmentation on CT scans. Paper presented Int Conf Med Image Comput Computer-Assisted Intervention2020.

122. Türk F, Lüy M, Kidney BN, et al. Segmentation using a hybrid V-Net-based model. Mathematics 2020;8(10):1772.

123. Zabihollahy F, Ukwatta E, Krishna S, et al. Fully automated localization of prostate peripheral zone tumors on apparent diffusion coefficient map MR images using an ensemble learning method. J Magn Reson Imaging 2020;51(4):1223–34.

124. Wang H, Wang H, Song L, Guo Q. Automatic diagnosis of rectal cancer based on CT images by deep learning method. Paper presented at: 2019 12th International Congress on Image and Signal Processing, BioMedical Engineering and Informatics (CISP-BMEI). Huaqiao, China, October 19-21, 2019. p. 1-5.

125. Chun-ming T, Dong L, Xiang Y. MRI image segmentation system of uterine fibroids based on AR-Unet network. Am Scientific Res J Eng Technol Sci (Asrjets) 2020;71(1):1–10.

126. Zhang L, Shi Y, Yao J, et al. Robust pancreatic ductal adenocarcinoma segmentation with multi-institutional multi-phase partially-annotated CT Scans. Paper presented at: Medical Image Computing and Computer Assisted Intervention – MICCAI. Lima, Peru, October 4-8, 2020. p. 491-500.

127. Lin YC, Lin CH, Lu HY, et al. Deep learning for fully automated tumor segmentation and extraction of magnetic resonance radiomics features in cervical cancer. Eur Radiol 2020;30(3):1297–305.

128. Vorontsov E, Cerny M, Régnier P, et al. Deep learning for automated segmentation of liver lesions at CT in patients with colorectal cancer liver metastases. Radiol Artif Intelligence. 2019;1(2):180014.

129. Ouhmich F, Agnus V, Noblet V, et al. Liver tissue segmentation in multiphase CT scans using cascaded convolutional neural networks. Int J Comput Assist Radiol Surg 2019;14(8):1275–84.

130. Zhang F, Yang J, Nezami N, et al. Liver tissue classification using an auto-context-based deep neural network with a multi-phase training framework. Patch Based Tech Med Imaging (. . 2018;2018(11075):59–66.

131. Näppi J, Uemura T, Kim SH, et al. Comparative performance of 3D machine-learning and deeplearning models in the detection of small polyps in dual-energy CT colonography, 11314. Houston, TX, February 15-20, 2020.

132. Graffy PM, Liu J, O'Connor S, et al. Automated segmentation and quantification of aortic calcification at abdominal CT: application of a deep learning-based algorithm to a longitudinal screening cohort. Abdom Radiol (Ny) 2019;44(8):2921–8.

133. Summers RM, Elton DC, Lee S, et al. Atherosclerotic plaque burden on abdominal CT: automated assessment with deep learning on noncontrast and contrast-enhanced scans. Acad Radiol 2020. https://doi.org/10.1016/j.acra.2020.08.022.

134. Dreizin D, Zhou Y, Fu S, et al. A multiscale deep learning method for quantitative visualization of traumatic hemoperitoneum at CT: assessment of feasibility and comparison with subjective categorical estimation. Radiol Artif Intelligence. 2020;2(6):e190220.

135. Taubmann O, Li J, Denzinger F, et al. Automatic detection of free intra-abdominal air in computed tomography. Paper presented at: Medical Image Computing and Computer Assisted Intervention – MICCAI. Lima, Peru, October 4-8, 2020. p. 232-41.

136. Parakh A, Lee H, Lee JH, et al. Urinary stone detection on CT images using deep convolutional neural networks: evaluation of model performance and generalization. Radiol Artif Intelligence. 2019;1(4):e180066.

137. Tang Y-B, Oh S, Tang Y-X, Xiao J, Summers RM. CT-realistic data augmentation using generative

adversarial network for robust lymph node segmentation. Paper presented at: Medical Imaging 2019: Computer-Aided Diagnosis. San Diego, CA, February 16-21, 2019. 109503V.

138. Tang Y-B, Yan K, Tang Y-X, Liu J, Xiao J, Summers RM. ULDor: A universal lesion detector for CT scans with pseudo masks and hard negative example mining. Paper presented at: 2019 IEEE 16th International Symposium on Biomedical Imaging. Venice, Italy, April 8-11, 2019. p. 833-6.

139. Yan K, Tang Y, Peng Y, et al. Mulan: Multitask universal lesion analysis network for joint lesion detection, tagging, and segmentation. Paper presented at: International Conference on Medical Image Computing and Computer-Assisted Intervention. Shenzhen, China, October 13-17, 2019. p. 194-202.

140. Byra M, Styczynski G, Szmigielski C, et al. Transfer learning with deep convolutional neural network for liver steatosis assessment in ultrasound images. Int J Comput Assist Radiol Surg 2018;13(12): 1895–903.

141. Wang J, Wu CJ, Bao ML, et al. Machine learning-based analysis of MR radiomics can help to improve the diagnostic performance of PI-RADS v2 in clinically relevant prostate cancer. Eur Radiol 2017;27(10):4082–90.

142. Schelb P, Kohl S, Radtke JP, et al. Classification of cancer at prostate MRI: deep learning versus clinical PI-RADS assessment. Radiology 2019;293(3): 607–17.

143. Homayounieh F, Singh R, Nitiwarangkul C, et al. Semiautomatic segmentation and radiomics for dual-energy CT: a pilot study to differentiate benign and malignant hepatic lesions. AJR Am J Roentgenol 2020;215(2):398–405.

144. Xi IL, Zhao Y, Wang R, et al. Deep learning to distinguish benign from malignant renal lesions based on routine MR imaging. Clin Cancer Res 2020; 26(8):1944–52.

145. Yao Z, Dong Y, Wu G, et al. Preoperative diagnosis and prediction of hepatocellular carcinoma: Radiomics analysis based on multi-modal ultrasound images. BMC Cancer. 2018;18(1):1089.

146. Liu KL, Wu T, Chen PT, et al. Deep learning to distinguish pancreatic cancer tissue from non-cancerous pancreatic tissue: a retrospective study with cross-racial external validation. Lancet Digit Health. 2020;2(6):e303–13.

147. Ho LM, Samei E, Mazurowski MA, et al. Can texture analysis be used to distinguish benign from malignant adrenal nodules on unenhanced CT, contrast-enhanced CT, or in-phase and opposed-phase MRI? AJR Am J Roentgenol 2019;212(3):554–61.

148. Zabihollahy F, Schieda N, Krishna S, et al. Automated classification of solid renal masses on

contrast-enhanced computed tomography images using convolutional neural network with decision fusion. Eur Radiol 2020;30(9):5183–90.

149. Jose M Castillo T, Arif M, Niessen WJ, Schoots IG, et al. Automated classification of significant prostate cancer on MRI: a systematic review on the performance of machine learning applications. Cancers. 2020;12(6):1606.

150. Song XL, Ren JL, Zhao D, et al. Radiomics derived from dynamic contrast-enhanced MRI pharmacokinetic protocol features: the value of precision diagnosis ovarian neoplasms. Eur Radiol 2021;31(1): 368–78.

151. Urushibara A, Saida T, Mori K, et al. Diagnosing uterine cervical cancer on a single T2-weighted image: comparison between deep learning versus radiologists. Eur J Radiol 2021;135:109471.

152. Wang CJ, Hamm CA, Savic LJ, et al. Deep learning for liver tumor diagnosis part II: convolutional neural network interpretation using radiologic imaging features. Eur Radiol 2019;29(7):3348–57.

153. Sanford T, Harmon SA, Turkbey EB, et al. Deep-learning-based artificial intelligence for PI-RADS classification to assist multiparametric prostate MRI interpretation: a development study. J Magn Reson Imaging 2020;52(5):1499–507.

154. Kocak B, Kaya OK, Erdim C, et al. Artificial intelligence in renal mass characterization: a systematic review of methodologic items related to modeling, performance evaluation, clinical utility, and transparency. AJR Am J Roentgenol 2020;215(5):1113–22.

155. Cui EM, Lin F, Li Q, et al. Differentiation of renal angiomyolipoma without visible fat from renal cell carcinoma by machine learning based on whole-tumor computed tomography texture features. Acta Radiol 2019;60(11):1543–52.

156. Midya A, Chakraborty J, Pak L, et al. Deep convolutional neural network for the classification of hepatocellular carcinoma and intrahepatic cholangiocarcinoma, 10575. Houston, TX, February 10-15, 2015.

157. Wu M, Krishna S, Thornhill RE, et al. Transition zone prostate cancer: logistic regression and machine-learning models of quantitative ADC, shape and texture features are highly accurate for diagnosis. J Magn Reson Imaging 2019;50(3):940–50.

158. Chen F, Zhou Y, Qi X, et al. Radiomics-assisted presurgical prediction for surgical portal vein-superior mesenteric vein invasion in pancreatic ductal adenocarcinoma. Front Oncol 2020;10:523543.

159. Jiang X, Li J, Kan Y, et al. MRI based radiomics approach with deep learning for prediction of vessel invasion in early-stage cervical cancer. IEEE/ACM Trans Comput Biol Bioinform 2020; 18(3):995–1002.

160. Stanzione A, Cuocolo R, Cocozza S, et al. Detection of extraprostatic extension of cancer on

biparametric MRI combining texture analysis and machine learning: preliminary results. Acad Radiol 2019;26(10):1338–44.

161. Chen F, Ma X, Li S, et al. MRI-based radiomics of rectal cancer: assessment of the local recurrence at the site of anastomosis. Acad Radiol 2020. https://doi.org/10.1016/j.acra.2020.09.024.

162. Mokrane FZ, Lu L, Vavasseur A, et al. Radiomics machine-learning signature for diagnosis of hepatocellular carcinoma in cirrhotic patients with indeterminate liver nodules. Eur Radiol 2020;30(1): 558–70.

163. Oyama A, Hiraoka Y, Obayashi I, et al. Hepatic tumor classification using texture and topology analysis of non-contrast-enhanced three-dimensional T1-weighted MR images with a radiomics approach. Sci Rep 2019;9(1):8764.

164. Khalili K, Lawlor RL, Pourafkari M, et al. Convolutional neural networks versus radiologists in characterization of small hypoattenuating hepatic nodules on CT: a critical diagnostic challenge in staging of colorectal carcinoma. Scientific Rep 2020;10(1):15248.

165. Park JJ, Kim KA, Nam Y, et al. Convolutional-neural-network-based diagnosis of appendicitis via CT scans in patients with acute abdominal pain presenting in the emergency department. Scientific Rep 2020;10(1):9556.

166. Xue LY, Jiang ZY, Fu TT, et al. Transfer learning radiomics based on multimodal ultrasound imaging for staging liver fibrosis. Eur Radiol 2020;30(5): 2973–83.

167. Kuo CC, Chang CM, Liu KT, et al. Automation of the kidney function prediction and classification through ultrasound-based kidney imaging using deep learning. NPJ Digit Med 2019;2:29.

168. Athavale AM, Hart PD, Itteera M, et al. Deep learning to predict degree of interstitial fibrosis and tubular atrophy from kidney ultrasound images - an artificial intelligence approach. medRxiv. 2020; 2020. 2008.2017.20176958.

169. Zheng Y, Liu X, Zhong Y, et al. A preliminary study for distinguish hormone-secreting functional adrenocortical adenoma subtypes using multiparametric CT radiomics-based machine learning model and nomogram. Front Oncol 2020;10:570502.

170. Corral JE, Hussein S, Kandel P, et al. Deep learning to classify intraductal papillary mucinous neoplasms using magnetic resonance imaging. Pancreas. 2019;48(6):805–10.

171. Lopes Vendrami C, McCarthy RJ, Villavicencio CP, et al. Predicting common solid renal tumors using machine learning models of classification of radiologist-assessed magnetic resonance characteristics. Abdom Radiol 2020;45(9):2797–809.

172. Luo Y, Chen X, Chen J, et al. Preoperative prediction of pancreatic neuroendocrine neoplasms grading based on enhanced computed tomography imaging: validation of deep learning with a convolutional neural network. Neuroendocrinology. 2020;110(5):338–50.

173. Lu H, Arshad M, Thornton A, et al. A mathematical-descriptor of tumor-mesoscopic-structure from computed-tomography images annotates prognostic- and molecular-phenotypes of epithelial ovarian cancer. Nat Commun 2019;10(1):764.

174. Lu CQ, Wang YC, Meng XP, et al. Diabetes risk assessment with imaging: a radiomics study of abdominal CT. Eur Radiol 2019;29(5):2233–42.

175. Ji GW, Zhu FP, Xu Q, et al. Machine-learning analysis of contrast-enhanced CT radiomics predicts recurrence of hepatocellular carcinoma after resection: a multi-institutional study. EBioMedicine. 2019;50:156–65.

176. Zhang Z, Jiang H, Chen J, et al. Hepatocellular carcinoma: radiomics nomogram on gadoxetic acid-enhanced MR imaging for early postoperative recurrence prediction. Cancer Imaging. 2019; 19(1):22.

177. Shayesteh SP, Alikhassi A, Farhan F, et al. Prediction of response to neoadjuvant chemoradiotherapy by MRI-based machine learning texture analysis in rectal cancer patients. J Gastrointest Cancer 2020;51(2):601–9.

178. Abdollahi H, Mofid B, Shiri I, et al. Machine learning-based radiomic models to predict intensity-modulated radiation therapy response, Gleason score and stage in prostate cancer. Radiol Med 2019;124(6):555–67.

179. Meier A, Veeraraghavan H, Nougaret S, et al. Association between CT-texture-derived tumor heterogeneity, outcomes, and BRCA mutation status in patients with high-grade serous ovarian cancer. Abdom Radiol (Ny) 2019;44(6):2040–7.

180. Liu W, Zargaria A, Thai T, et al. Utilizing deep learning technology to develop a novel CT image marker for categorizing cervical cancer patients at early stage, 10879. San Diego, CA, February 16-21, 2019.

181. Yang JQ, Zeng R, Cao JM, et al. Predicting gastro-oesophageal variceal bleeding in hepatitis B-related cirrhosis by CT radiomics signature. Clin Radiol 2019;74(12):976.e1-9.

182. Cao JM, Yang JQ, Ming ZQ, et al. A radiomics model of liver CT to predict risk of hepatic encephalopathy secondary to hepatitis B related cirrhosis. Eur J Radiol 2020;130:109201.

183. Liu J, Wu T, Peng Y, et al. Grade prediction of bleeding volume in cesarean section of patients with pernicious placenta previa based on deep learning. Front Bioeng Biotechnol 2020;8:343.

184. Park SH, Han K. Methodologic guide for evaluating clinical performance and effect of artificial intelligence technology for medical diagnosis and prediction. Radiology 2018;286(3):800–9.

185. Morris MA, Saboury B, Burkett B, et al. Reinventing radiology: big data and the future of medical imaging. J Thorac Imaging 2018;33(1).

186. Paul A, Tang YX, Shen TC, et al. Discriminative ensemble learning for few-shot chest x-ray diagnosis. Med Image Anal 2020;68:101911.

187. Colin Jacobs AAAS, Alberto Traverso, Bram van Ginneken. LUng Nodule Analysis. 2016. Available at: https://luna16.grand-challenge.org/. Accessed February 1, 2021.

188. Bilic P, Christ P, Vorontsov E, et al. The Liver Tumor Segmentation Benchmark (LiTS). arXiv: 1901.04056. 2019.

189. Meyer M, Ronald J, Vernuccio F, et al. Reproducibility of CT radiomic features within the same patient: influence of radiation dose and CT reconstruction settings. Radiology 2019;293(3):583–91.

190. Buch K, Kuno H, Qureshi MM, et al. Quantitative variations in texture analysis features dependent on MRI scanning parameters: a phantom model. J Appl Clin Med Phys 2018;19(6):253–64.

191. Greer MD, Lay N, Shih JH, et al. Computer-aided diagnosis prior to conventional interpretation of prostate mpMRI: an international multi-reader study. Eur Radiol 2018;28(10):4407–17.

192. Vivanti R, Joskowicz L, Lev-Cohain N, et al. Patient-specific and global convolutional neural networks for robust automatic liver tumor delineation in follow-up CT studies. Med Biol Eng Comput 2018; 56(9):1699–713.

Clinical Artificial Intelligence Applications in Radiology: Neuro

Felipe Campos Kitamura, MD, MSc, PhD[a,b,*], Ian Pan, MD[a,c,1], Suely Fazio Ferraciolli, MD[a,2], Kristen W. Yeom, MD[d,3], Nitamar Abdala, MD, PhD[b,4]

KEYWORDS

- Neuroradiology • Machine learning • Deep learning • Artificial intelligence • Clinical applications

KEY POINTS

- The most recent advances of AI in neuroradiology are presented.
- These include applications related to differential diagnosis, image acquisition, prediction of genetic mutations, lesion quantification, identification of critical findings, prognostication, and others.
- A brief review of machine learning competitions in neuroradiology is given.
- The first case of reimbursement for an AI algorithm is described.

INTRODUCTION

Radiologists have been at the forefront of the digitization process in medicine.[1] Artificial intelligence (AI) is a promising area of innovation, particularly in medical imaging.[1] Thus, it is no surprise that the number of publications on this topic has increased more than 6-fold from 2007 to 2017.[1] More than one-third of these articles relate to the central nervous system (CNS).[1] The number of applications of AI in neuroradiology has also grown.[2] This article illustrates some of these applications.

Machine learning (ML) competitions are a different approach to problem-solving in science. One of the advantages of ML challenges over classical hypothesis-driven research is that they encourage global collaboration. The result is often a set of out-of-the-box solutions that achieves state-of-the-art performance for the specified problem.[3] Many societies have launched ML challenges across almost all radiology subspecialties.[4–10] This article reviews those related to neuroradiology.[11–31]

The first approval of reimbursement for an AI algorithm by the Centers for Medicare and Medicaid Services (CMS) was announced at the end of 2020, covering a stroke software for early detection of large vessel occlusion (LVO), which is discussed at the end of this article.[32,33]

NEURORADIOLOGY EXAMPLES

The number of AI applications in neuroradiology is increasing every day, which include differential diagnosis of diseases, improvements in image acquisition (both quality and time), prediction of genetic mutations from MR imaging, segmentation of anatomy to guide interventional procedures, segmentation to quantify CNS lesions, identification of critical findings to shorten notification

[a] Dasalnova, Diagnósticos da América SA (Dasa), São Paulo, São Paulo, Brazil; [b] Universidade Federal de São Paulo, São Paulo, São Paulo, Brazil; [c] Brigham and Woman's Hospital, Boston, MA, USA; [d] Department of Radiology, Stanford University, CA, USA
[1] Present address: 75 Francis St, Mellins Library, Boston, MA 02115, USA
[2] Present address: Rua Rua Gilberto Sabino, 215, 3rd floor, Pinheiros, São Paulo, São Paulo CEP: 05425-020, Brazil
[3] Present address: 725 Welch Road G516, Palo Alto, CA 94304, USA
[4] Present address: Rua Napoleaão de Barros, 800, Vila Clementino, São Paulo, São Paulo CEP: 04024-002, Brazil
* Corresponding author. Rua Rua Gilberto Sabino, 215, 3rd floor, Pinheiros, São Paulo, São Paulo CEP: 05425-020, Brazil.
E-mail address: kitamura.felipe@gmail.com

Radiol Clin N Am 59 (2021) 1003–1012
https://doi.org/10.1016/j.rcl.2021.07.002

time, prognostication of diseases, quality assurance of patient position during image acquisition, and many others. This section presents notable examples of these applications.

Differential Diagnosis

Some papers focus on diagnosis of a single disease, including psychiatric and behavioral disorders, such as attention-deficit/hyperactivity disorder (ADHD). In "A Multichannel Deep Neural Network Model Analyzing Multiscale Functional Brain Connectome Data for Attention Deficit Hyperactivity Disorder Detection," the investigators use resting-state functional MR imaging to generate connectome maps in different scales, using these data to train a deep neural network to identify patients with ADHD, achieving an area under the curve (AUC) of 0.74 (95% confidence interval, 0.73, 0.76).[34] There are also many articles about cognitive diseases, with "A Deep Learning Model to Predict a Diagnosis of Alzheimer Disease by Using 18 F-FDG PET of the Brain" as an example for Alzheimer disease (AD), in which an Inception-V3 convolutional neural network (CNN) was trained on nuclear medicine images, achieving 100% sensitivity and 82% specificity in predicting the final diagnosis of AD, an average of 75.8 months before the diagnosis, outperforming reader performance.[35] Models like this may aid in the early diagnosis of these diseases, which may be difficult to pinpoint in the initial clinical stages, allowing patient selection for clinical trials looking for early treatment.

Algorithms used for differential diagnosis are also well known, including articles that compare their ability and performance to radiologists and neuroradiologists. In "Deep Learning for Pediatric Posterior Fossa Tumor Detection and Classification: A Multi-Institutional Study," the investigators trained a ResNeXt-50 CNN model to detect and classify pediatric posterior fossa tumors, achieving an area under the receiver operating characteristic curve of 0.99 for tumor detection and an accuracy of 92% (F1-score of .80) for classification, which was higher than two of four radiologists in the study.[36] A seminal paper "Neuroradiologist-level Differential Diagnosis Accuracy at Brain MRI" described an innovative way to use deep learning (DL) and Bayesian networks to diagnose 19 common and rare CNS diseases using only a few cases, comparing its performance to radiologists with different levels of training. The paper demonstrated a unique approach to creating models that make the differential diagnosis with just a few cases, breaking the established concept that AI requires large amounts of data.[37] The follow-up to this study is the article "Subspecialty-Level Deep Gray Matter Differential Diagnoses with Deep Learning and Bayesian Networks on Clinical Brain MRI: A Pilot Study" in which they used a similar approach to diagnose deep gray matter disease, with the same performance as neuroradiologists. The investigators demonstrated how integrating DL and Bayesian networks can be applied to other diseases.[38] These examples show us the capacity of a DL model to achieve a performance similar to neuroradiologists for some specific diseases, even complex and rare ones. The examples may aid the neuroradiologist in the differential diagnosis of some difficult cases and help radiology/neuroradiology fellows in their learning progress.

There are also some ML algorithms that may improve pathology detection, which may be used to increase radiologist's detection rate and also for automated peer review or peer learning. One example is "Deep Learning for MR Angiography: Automated Detection of Cerebral Aneurysms," where the investigators developed an aneurysm detection tool that improved the sensitivity in the external test set by 13% when compared with the initial reports, achieving 93% sensitivity at the cost of 6 false-positives per scan.[39] One company has also developed a product that uses AI to help create a structured radiology report. Their product characterizes tumors in terms of localization, size, signal intensity in each MR imaging sequence, and other features; automatically populates editable combo boxes; and generates a structured report with the most likely differential diagnoses. If the radiologist disagrees with any of the features, they can be adjusted, and a new report is automatically generated.[40] This approach could improve turnaround time and consistency of results for common diseases.

Image Acquisition

A separate article of this series was dedicated to improving image acquisition with AI. We briefly list some examples related to neuroimaging, such as techniques for imaging quality improvement. As shown in "Improving the Quality of Synthetic FLAIR Images with Deep Learning Using a Conditional Generative Adversarial Network for Pixel-by-Pixel Image Translation," a conditional generative adversarial network was used to improve the quality of synthetic fluid-attenuated inversion recovery (FLAIR) images (SyMRI version 8.0; SyntheticMR, Linköping, Sweden), with increment in image contrast and fewer granular/swelling artifacts, while preserving lesion contrast.[41] Another example is "Improving Arterial

Spin Labeling by Using Deep Learning," which leveraged a CNN to generate higher-quality perfusion images, with 40% lower mean squared error than the conventional method. The reconstructed images also had less noise and motion artifacts ($P<.001$).[42]

Gadolinium-based contrast media are part of the cost of some MR imaging examinations, and there is also an increasing concern regarding gadolinium deposition in the brain.[43] In "Deep Learning Enables Reduced Gadolinium Dose for Contrast-Enhanced Brain MRI," a DL model was trained to generate a full-dose T1-weighted sequence from the same sequence with only 10% of the conventional contrast dose. The results are promising, and the investigators continue to improve the model with more data.[44]

Many researchers have focused on generating one MR imaging sequence from another or generating computed tomography (CT) from MR imaging, and vice versa. Although the feasibility and reliability of some of these applications remain uncertain, generating a CT scan from MR imaging to plan radiotherapy seems to hold promise; this happens because there is no need to perfectly characterize the texture of bone lesions, but only to map the electron density of the head of the patients, which is highly dependent on the shape and thickness of the skull, as shown on "Generation of Synthetic CT Images from MRI for Treatment Planning and Patient Positioning Using a 3-Channel U-Net Trained on Sagittal Images."[45]

In "3D Deep Learning Angiography (3D-DLA) from C-Arm Conebeam CT," the model accurately generated the vasculature of 3D rotational angiography without a mask, reducing radiation exposure and misregistration artifacts.[46] Also, in "A Deep Learning-Based Approach to Reduce Rescan and Recall Rates in Clinical MRI Examinations," the DL model was able to identify MR imaging sequences with motion artifacts to avoid rescan and recall. The investigators estimate savings of $24,000 per scanner per year if the model is used in clinical practice.[47]

All these examples show how these algorithms may aid in reducing both the physical exposure of the patients and the financial costs in radiology departments, which may improve the quality of the medical care.

Prediction of Genetic Features from MR Imaging

Recent discoveries have shown MR imaging contains information predictive of genetic mutation in CNS tumors, such as high specificity of the T2-FLAIR mismatch sign for isocitrate dehydrogenase-mutant astrocytomas,[48] raising the possibility that DL could play a role in predicting tumor genomics. In "Predicting Deletion of Chromosomal Arms 1p/19q in Low-Grade Gliomas from MR Images Using Machine Intelligence," the investigators show that a multiscale CNN architecture was trained on T2 and postcontrast T1-weighted images, achieving 87.7% accuracy in predicting 1p/19q codeletion in low-grade gliomas.[49] In the paper "Residual Deep Convolutional Neural Network Predicts MGMT Methylation Status," a ResNet50 was trained to predict O6-methylguanine methyltransferase (MGMT) methylation status from routine T2-weighted images, with simpler preprocessing steps, achieving an accuracy of 94.9% $\pm$ 3.92%.[50] Chang and colleagues[51] used T2, FLAIR and T1-weighted precontrast and postcontrast images of both high- and low-grade gliomas to train a CNN to predict IDH1 status, MGMT promoter methylation, and 1p/19q codeletion, achieving 94%, 83%, and 92% accuracy, respectively. The important clinical implication of all these examples is that image-based predictors of tumor genomics might offer prognostic information or even identify tumor subgroups amenable to targeted therapies or eligible for new drug therapy clinical trials, which may improve the clinical outcome of these patients.

Applications of Segmentation

Segmentation is a pixelwise classification. It is useful to delineate lesions and measure their area and volume. In the past years, many applications have been designed for segmentation in neuroradiology, some of them already assimilated in everyday use, whereas others only in the research field.

Some articles emphasize the time reduction of such algorithms. One of them is "Deep Learning-Based Automatic Segmentation of Lumbosacral Nerves on CT for Spinal Intervention: A Translational Study," where the researchers developed and validated a segmentation model for the 3D reconstruction of the safe triangle and the Kambin triangle, which are targeted areas for transforaminal epidural steroid injection, primarily at the L5/S1 level. By automating this task, it could be feasibly applied in clinical practice because manual segmentation is time consuming.[52] Another example is "Deep Learning for Automated Delineation of Pediatric Cerebral Arteries on Pre-operative Brain Magnetic Resonance Imaging," in which a U-Net was modified to segment cerebral arteries in nonangiographic MR imaging sequences. Usually, manual delineation of critical structures is required by intraoperative navigation systems to avoid complications during surgery. This DL model achieved a Dice score of 0.75, and its inference time was around 8 seconds per patient, whereas manual segmentation took about 1 to 2 hours.[53]

Many articles showed ML algorithms that could be useful tools to aid neuroradiologists in their clinical practice, such as "Three-Plane–Assembled Deep Learning Segmentation of Gliomas," in which a U-Net was trained on the 2018 Multimodal Brain Tumor Segmentation Challenge (BraTS) Dataset using the axial, sagittal, and coronal planes to segment the enhancing tumor, tumor core, and whole tumor, achieving mean Dice scores of 0.80, 0.84, and 0.91, respectively. This model also could be implemented in clinical practice to assist radiologists or neuro-oncologists to better characterize the tumors.[54] In "Fully Automated Segmentation of Head CT Neuroanatomy Using Deep Learning," a U-Net was trained to segment 11 intracranial structures, achieving Dice scores comparable to neuroradiologists, even in external test sets with idiopathic normal pressure hydrocephalus.[55] Also, in "Artificial Intelligence for Automatic Cerebral Ventricle Segmentation and Volume Calculation: A Clinical Tool for the Evaluation of Pediatric Hydrocephalus," a U-Net was modified to segment the ventricles in T2-weighted images, achieving a Dice score of 0.901, and generalized to an external dataset. This model could be used to provide real-time clinical comparison and improve workflow, because the ventricular volume estimation can be used to objectively compare serial imaging in patients with hydrocephalus.[56]

The segmentation calculated by the AI model could also be used as a biomarker to estimate clinical symptoms, as shown in "Convolutional Neural Network-Based Automated Segmentation of the Spinal Cord and Contusion Injury: Deep Learning Biomarker Correlates of Motor Impairment in Acute Spinal Cord Injury." In this article, the segmentation models were trained on T2-weighted images of patients with spinal cord injuries and the automated volume estimate had a correlation with motor impairment in the acute phase.[57] Another well-known use of AI is to increase radiologist's performance with the use of ML algorithms. In "Deep Learning-Assisted Diagnosis of Cerebral Aneurysms Using the HeadXNet Model," a 3D CNN was trained to segment cerebral aneurysms and the performance of clinicians was compared with and without AI. There were statistically significant improvements in sensitivity, accuracy, and interrater agreement in the group augmented by AI.[58]

In "Improved Segmentation and Detection Sensitivity of Diffusion-weighted Stroke Lesions with Synthetically Enhanced Deep Learning," the investigators compared the performance of segmentation of stroke lesions on diffusion-weighted imaging when training with real and synthetic data. The best Dice was achieved with the training set comprising real and synthetic images. The idea of using synthetic data is not new, but this article proves it works for this use-case.[59] Use of synthetic data paves the way to the improvement of other segmentation models where annotated datasets are scarce.

Identification of Critical Findings

A well-established application of DL in medical imaging is the prioritization of studies with critical findings. In this section, we describe 2 seminal papers in this area. The first is "Automated Critical Test Findings Identification and Online Notification System Using Artificial Intelligence in Imaging," which may be the first use of DL to prioritize critical findings. Two CNNs were trained, one to identify suspected acute infarct (SAI) and the other to detect hemorrhage, mass effect, and hydrocephalus (HMH) at noncontrast head CT. The SAI model achieved 62% sensitivity and 96% specificity, whereas the HMH model reached 90% sensitivity and 85% specificity. The main conclusion of this article was that AI holds promise for detecting critical findings, supporting further investigation with a prospective trial.[60] The second paper is "Deep Learning Algorithms for Detection of Critical Findings in Head CT Scans: A Retrospective Study." The models created in this work are able to identify all types of intracranial hemorrhage, skull fractures, midline shift, and mass effect. The models used a large dataset from India comprising 313,318 CT scans, achieving AUCs greater than 0.90 in most of the test sets.[61]

Prognostication

Some studies have shown that DL can aid in determining the prognosis in a variety of diseases. Many articles were published trying to predict the prognosis of patients with brain tumor. One example is the "Multi-Channel 3D Deep Feature Learning for Survival Time Prediction of Brain Tumor Patients Using Multi-Modal Neuroimages," in which multiple MR imaging sequences and demographic data were used to train a DL model that achieved 90.66% accuracy in predicting survival time of patients with high-grade gliomas, which was better than the standard of care.[62]

Another hot topic is related to stroke characterization, patient treatment, and prognosis. In "Automated Calculation of the Alberta Stroke Program Early CT score: Feasibility and Reliability," the investigators compared an automated ASPECTS calculator to 2 neuroradiologists and found that the software showed a higher correlation with expert consensus than each neuroradiologists individually[63]; this could help the treatment decision based on a more accurate score. In "Prediction of Tissue Outcome and Assessment of Treatment Effect in Acute Ischemic Stroke Using Deep Learning," the DL model was better than other methods in predicting the final outcome (follow-up FLAIR image) based on the treatment and the MR imaging at admission, achieving an AUC of 0.88.[64]

Patients with multiple sclerosis (MS) were also the focus of some studies, because they are subjected to frequent administration of gadolinium-based contrasts during their life. In "Deep Learning for Predicting Enhancing Lesions in Multiple Sclerosis from Noncontrast MRI," the investigators aimed to identify active (enhancing) MS lesions from noncontrast MR imaging sequences, achieving a sensitivity of 72% and a specificity of 70%. Although this proof-of-concept study is insufficient to avoid contrast administration as of yet, it shows that noncontrast MR imaging contains information that can identify active MS lesions.[65]

MACHINE LEARNING COMPETITIONS

ML challenges are complementary to hypothesis-driven research. Various ML competitions in the health care domain have occurred on many platforms, with Kaggle.com and Grand-challenge.org being the most well-known platforms. The Medical Image Computing and Computer Assisted Intervention Society has organized most ML competitions in neuroimaging. The Radiological Society of North America has launched competitions with the largest, publicly available, expertly annotated datasets comprising images from international research centers. **Box 1** provides a list of the competitions related to neuroimaging.

The important contribution by many researchers who have collated the datasets and organized the competitions, as well as remarkable participation among radiologists, some of whom have won medals in these health care ML challenges, is noteworthy.

CENTERS FOR MEDICARE AND MEDICAID SERVICES APPROVAL

At the end of 2020, the CMS granted Viz.ai the first New Technology Add-on Payment (NTAP) for its LVO detection algorithm. Medicare will pay up to $1040 per use in patients with stroke. The decision was based on prospective evidence that the tool

---

> **Box 1**
> **List of the main machine learning competitions in neuroimaging, with references containing the hyperlinks to the respective Web sites**
>
> The RSNA Intracranial Hemorrhage Detection Challenge[6]
>
> QUBIQ: Quantification of Uncertainties in Biomedical Image Quantification Challenge[11]
>
> AutoImplant: Cranial Implant Design Challenge[12]
>
> Automatic Intervertebral Disc Localization and Segmentation from 3D Multi-modality MR (M3) Images[13]
>
> MR Brain Segmentation[14]
>
> ISLES: Ischemic Stroke Lesion Segmentation[15]
>
> VerSe'20: Large Scale Vertebrae Segmentation Challenge[16]
>
> WMH: White Matter Hyperintensity Segmentation Challenge[17]
>
> 6-month Infant Brain MRI Segmentation[18]
>
> MTOP: Mild Traumatic Brain Injury Outcome Prediction[19]
>
> MS: Multiple Sclerosis segmentation challenge[20]
>
> Computer-aided diagnosis of dementia based on structural MRI data[21]
>
> NEATBRAINS: Adult and neonatal brain differences[22]
>
> NeoBrainS12: Neonatal brain segmentation[24]
>
> CADA-RRE: Cerebral Aneurysm Rupture Risk Estimation[23]
>
> CADA: Cerebral Aneurysm Detection[25]
>
> CADA-AS: Cerebral Aneurysm Segmentation[26]
>
> Head and Neck Tumor segmentation challenge (HECKTOR)[27]
>
> AccelMR Prediction Challenge[28]
>
> MRI White Matter Reconstruction[29]
>
> ABCD Neurocognitive Prediction Challenge[30]
>
> Multi-shell Diffusion MRI Harmonisation Challenge 2018 (MUSHAC)[31]

---

improves clinical and financial outcomes, such as shortening the time to treatment and length of stay.[66] However, the modified Rankin Scale (mRS) at discharge had no statistically significant improvement in this study.[66] Another study (pre-print) showed that the LVO algorithm led to statistically significant improvement in the 5-day NIH Stroke Scale, the discharge mRS, and the median 90-day mRS.[67]

Although the approval was granted to a specific company, other similar technologies can also be categorized under the same NTAP status.[32] This first case of reimbursement for AI use in clinical practice paves the way for reimbursement of other AI software that has been proved to improve outcomes.

Fig. 1 shows the empirical perception of the distribution of evidence for AI software in neuroradiology, which can be extended to AI in medical imaging at large. Randomized clinical trials are the rarest studies with the strongest evidence, with approximately 200 ongoing/completed studies registered in ClinicalTrials.gov (DL in health care generally, not only in neuroimaging).

REVIEWS

Interested readers are invited to read other published reviews, which keep growing in number every month.[2,68–75] One of the first, "Machine Learning Studies on Major Brain Diseases: 5-Year Trends of 2014-2018," summarizes the evidence and current limitations of 209 articles published between 2014 and 2018 and emphasizes the limited sample size in most papers.[68] Another good review to start with is "Deep Learning in Neuroradiology," which outlines methods used to develop and test DL models. This review discusses many applications, such as imaging

logistics, image acquisition and improvement, image transformation, lesion detection and segmentation, DL for diagnosis, and the impact of DL on neuroradiology practice.[69] Also, in "Deep Learning in Neuroradiology: A Systematic Review of Current Algorithms and Approaches for the New Wave of Imaging Technology," the investigators studied 155 DL neuroradiology articles published through September 2019. The investigators concluded that, although the results are promising, there is a lack of external and clinical validation and inconsistency in implementation methods and metrics.[70] A more recent review is "Artificial Intelligence in Neuroradiology: Current Status and Future Directions." This white paper reviews AI applications in neuroradiology and provides many arguments (referenced in the literature) that fear of AI in radiology is overstated. On the other hand, our clinical practice may benefit from many improvements made possible by AI. Everyone, whether tech-savvy or tech-illiterate, will need to learn how to use AI.[71] There is also "Promises of Artificial Intelligence in Neuroradiology: A Systematic Technographic Review." This broad technographic review assesses the availability of neuroradiology AI products in the market between 2017 and 2019 and discusses their maturity level. The most important conclusions are that scientific validation is not as developed as regulatory approval and that most of the algorithms in the market have functionalities to "support" or "extend" the neuroradiologists' work, by aiding in particular tasks or providing quantitative information about pathologic findings.[2]

Many other review articles have been published so far. For neuro-oncology use-cases, we recommend the paper by Rudie and colleagues.[72] For management of intracranial aneurysms, Shi and colleagues[76] give a recent overview of the topic. For AI in acute stroke imaging, Soun and colleagues[74] is the most recent reference. Kaka and Zhang[73] review 7 AI applications, including spine imaging and multiple sclerosis. Zeng and colleagues[77] review approaches for segmentation of MS on brain MR imaging.

CLINICS CARE POINTS

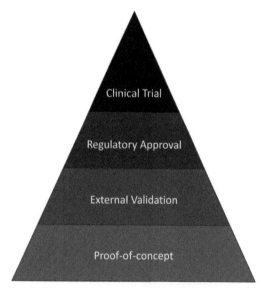

Fig. 1. The number of articles decreases as the strength of evidence increases. Most articles found in the literature show a proof of concept for an AI application in neuroradiology. Less research demonstrates external validation and regulatory approval. Even rarer are prospective trials with improved outcome.

- There are countless use-cases of AI in neuroradiology, most of which show no proper external validation.
- Both external validation and prospective clinical trials demonstrating improved outcomes are lacking for neuroradiology AI software.

- Some models have regulatory approval, but this is not a guarantee of model performance in real-world clinical settings or better health care outcomes.
- CMS approved the first case of reimbursement for AI software, an LVO identification software that was shown to reduce time to treatment and improve patients' outcomes, leading to clinical and financial gains.

SUMMARY

In this article, many promising use-cases of AI in neuroradiology are presented. However, there is a large gap between proof of concept and robust, prospectively validated algorithms. Most AI applications in neuroradiology fall in the former group. Although external validation is increasingly required for medical AI journal publication, this is just the first step toward safe and meaningful use of AI, which requires prospective trials. Regulatory approval does not guarantee model performance in real-world clinical settings or better health care outcomes. The recent CMS approval of an LVO detection software is an example that bridged the gap prospectively demonstrating better patient outcomes and a reduction in health care costs.

Despite current hurdles, there are important opportunities for AI clinical implementation including augmenting radiologists' performance by reducing reading time, improving consistency, bridging knowledge gaps, and reducing errors. Automation of quantitative analytics can foster precision medicine and enhance efficient workflows.

DISCLOSURE

F.C. Kitamura and I. Pan are consultants for MD.ai. F.C. Kitamura is a speaker for GE Healthcare. The other authors have nothing to disclose.

REFERENCES

1. Pesapane F, Codari M, Sardanelli F. Artificial intelligence in medical imaging: threat or opportunity? Radiologists again at the forefront of innovation in medicine. Eur Radiol Exp 2018;2(1). https://doi.org/10.1186/s41747-018-0061-6.
2. Olthof AW, van Ooijen PMA, Rezazade Mehrizi MH. Promises of artificial intelligence in neuroradiology: a systematic technographic review. Neuroradiology 2020. https://doi.org/10.1007/s00234-020-02424-w.
3. Prevedello LM, Halabi SS, Shih G, et al. Challenges Related to Artificial Intelligence Research in Medical Imaging and the Importance of Image Analysis Competitions. Radiol Artif Intell 2019;1(1): e180031.
4. Colak E, Kitamura FC, Hobbs SB, et al. The RSNA Pulmonary Embolism CT (RSPECT) Dataset. Radiol Artif Intell. 2021;0(ja):e200254. doi:10.1148/ryai.2021200254
5. Johnson AEW, Pollard TJ, Greenbaum NR, et al. MIMIC-CXR-JPG, a large publicly available database of labeled chest radiographs. arXiv 2019;14: 1–7.
6. Flanders AE, Prevedello LM, Shih G, et al. Construction of a Machine Learning Dataset through Collaboration: The RSNA 2019 Brain CT Hemorrhage Challenge. Radiol Artif Intell 2020;2(3):e190211.
7. Halabi SS, Prevedello LM, Kalpathy-Cramer J, et al. The RSNA Pediatric Bone Age Machine Learning Challenge 2018;290(2):498–503.
8. Shih G, Wu CC, Halabi SS, et al. Augmenting the National Institutes of Health Chest Radiograph Dataset with Expert Annotations of Possible Pneumonia. Radiol Artif Intell 2019;1(1):e180041.
9. Tsai EB, Simpson S, Lungren MP, et al. The RSNA International COVID-19 Open Radiology Database(R-ICORD). research-article. Radiology 2021;0(0): 203957. https://doi.org/10.1148/radiol.2021203957.
10. Challenge G. Grand Challenge. 2020. Available at: https://grand-challenge.org/challenges/. Accessed on July 29, 2021.
11. MICCAI. Quantification of Uncertainties in Biomedical Image Quantification Challenge - Grand Challenge. 2020. Available at: https://qubiq.grand-challenge.org/. Accessed on July 29, 2021.
12. MICCAI. AutoImplant - Grand Challenge. 2020. Available at: https://autoimplant.grand-challenge.org/. Accessed on July 29, 2021.
13. MICCAI. Automatic Intervertebral Disc Localization and Segmentation from 3D Multi-modality MR (M3). 2018. Available at: http://ivdm3seg.weebly.com/. Accessed on July 29, 2021.
14. MICCAI. Grand Challenge on MR Brain Segmentation at MICCAI 2018. 2018. Available at: https://mrbrains18.isi.uu.nl/. Accessed on July 29, 2021.
15. MICCAI. Isles Challenge - Ischemic Stroke Lesion Segmentation. Grand Challenge. 2018. Available at: http://www.isles-challenge.org. Accessed on July 29, 2021.
16. MICCAI. VerSe'20: Large Scale Vertebrae Segmentation Challenge. Grand Challenge. 2020. Available at: https://verse2020.grand-challenge.org/Home/. Accessed on July 29, 2021.
17. MICCAI. WMH Segmentation Challenge. Grand Challenge. 2020. Available at: https://wmh.isi.uu.nl/. Accessed on July 29, 2021.
18. MICCAI. Grand Challenge on 6-month Infant Brain MRI Segmentation from Multiple Sites. 2019. Available at: https://iseg2019.web.unc.edu/. Accessed on July 29, 2021.

19. MICCAI. MTOP - Mild Traumatic Brain Injury Outcome Prediction. Grand Challenge. 2016. Available at: https://tbichallenge.wordpress.com/. Accessed on July 29, 2021.

20. MICCAI. MS segmentation challenge. Grand Challenge. 2016. Available at: https://portal.fli-iam.irisa.fr/msseg-challenge/overview. Accessed on July 29, 2021.

21. MICCAI. Computer-Aided Diagnosis of Dementia based on structural MRI data. Grand Challenge. 2020. Available at: https://caddementia.grand-challenge.org/Home/. Accessed on July 29, 2021.

22. ISBI. NEATBRAINS. Grand Challenge. 2015. Available at: https://www.isi.uu.nl/research/challenges/neatbrains/. Accessed on July 29, 2021.

23. MICCAI. CADA - RRE - Cerebral Aneurysm Rupture Risk Estimation. Grand Challenge. 2020. Available at: https://cada-rre.grand-challenge.org/Overview/. Accessed on July 29, 2021.

24. MICCAI. NeoBrainS12 - Neonatal Brain Segmentation. Grand Challenge. 2012. Available at: https://neobrains12.isi.uu.nl/. Accessed on July 29, 2021.

25. MICCAI. Cerebral Aneurysm Detection. Grand Challenge. 2020. Available at: https://cada.grand-challenge.org/. Accessed on July 29, 2021.

26. MICCAI. Cerebral Aneurysm Segmentation. Grand Challenge. 2020. Available at: https://cada-as.grand-challenge.org/. Accessed on July 29, 2021.

27. MICCAI. HEad and neCK TumOR segmentation challenge (HECKTOR). Grand Challenge. 2020. Available at: https://www.aicrowd.com/challenges/hecktor. Accessed on July 29, 2021.

28. MICCAI. AccelMR Prediction Challenge. Grand Challenge. 2020. Available at: https://accelmrorg.wordpress.com/about/. Accessed on July 29, 2021.

29. MICCAI. MRI White Matter Reconstruction. Grand Challenge. 2020. Available at: https://my.vanderbilt.edu/memento/. Accessed on July 29, 2021.

30. MICCAI. ABCD Neurocognitive Prediction Challenge. 2020. Available at: https://sibis.sri.com/abcd-np-challenge/. Accessed on July 29, 2021.

31. MICCAI. Multi-shell Diffusion MRI Harmonisation Challenge 2018 (MUSHAC). Grand Challenge. 2018. Available at: https://projects.iq.harvard.edu/cdmri2018/challenge. Accessed on July 29, 2021.

32. Walach E. CMS Approves Reimbursement Opportunity for AI - Aidoc. 2020. 2020. Available at: https://www.aidoc.com/blog/cms-approves-reimbursement-ai/. Accessed on July 29, 2021.

33. Crotti N. Viz.ai stroke software lands Medicare 'new technology' coverage. Medical Design and Outsourcing. Available at: https://www.medicaldesignandoutsourcing.com/viz-ai-stroke-software-lands-medicare-new-technology-coverage/#:~:text=The%20Centers%20for%20Medicare%20and,software%2C%20the%20company%20announced%20today.

&text=Medicare%20will%20now%20pay%20up,in%20patients%20with%20suspected%20strokes. Accessed on July 29, 2021.

34. Chen M, Li H, Wang J, et al. A Multichannel Deep Neural Network Model Analyzing Multiscale Functional Brain Connectome Data for Attention Deficit Hyperactivity Disorder Detection. Radiol Artif Intell 2019;2(1):e190012.

35. Ding Y, Sohn JH, Kawczynski MG, et al. A Deep Learning Model to Predict a Diagnosis of Alzheimer Disease by Using 18 F-FDG PET of the Brain. Radiology 2019;290(2). https://doi.org/10.1148/radiol.2018180958.

36. Quon JL, Bala W, Chen LC, et al. Deep Learning for Pediatric Posterior Fossa Tumor Detection and Classification: A Multi-Institutional Study. AJNR Am J Neuroradiol 2020. https://doi.org/10.3174/ajnr.A6704.

37. Rauschecker AM, Rudie JD, Xie L, et al. Artificial Intelligence System Approaching Neuroradiologist-level Differential Diagnosis Accuracy at Brain MRI. Radiology 2020;295(3). https://doi.org/10.1148/radiol.2020190283.

38. Rudie JD, Rauschecker AM, Xie L, et al. Subspecialty-level deep gray matter differential diagnoses with deep learning and Bayesian networks on clinical brain MRI: a Pilot study. Radiology 2020. https://doi.org/10.1148/ryai.2020190146.

39. Ueda D, Yamamoto A, Nishimori M, et al. Deep learning for MR angiography: Automated detection of cerebral aneurysms. Radiology 2019;290(1):187–94.

40. Biomind. BioMind Website. Available at: https://www.biomind.ai/. Accessed on July 29, 2021.

41. Hagiwara XA, Otsuka XY, Hori XM, et al. Improving the Quality of Synthetic FLAIR Images with Deep Learning Using a Conditional Generative Adversarial Network for Pixel-by-Pixel Image Translation. AJNR Am J Neuroradiol 2019;40(2). https://doi.org/10.3174/ajnr.A5927.

42. Kim KH, Choi SH, Park SH. Improving Arterial Spin Labeling by Using Deep Learning. Radiology 2018;287(2). https://doi.org/10.1148/radiol.2017171154.

43. Ramalho J, Ramalho M, AlObaidy M, et al. T1 Signal-Intensity Increase in the Dentate Nucleus after Multiple Exposures to Gadodiamide: Intraindividual Comparison between 2 Commonly Used Sequences. AJNR Am J Neuroradiol 2016;37(8). https://doi.org/10.3174/ajnr.A4757.

44. Gong E, Pauly JM, Wintermark M, et al. Deep learning enables reduced gadolinium dose for contrast-enhanced brain MRI. J Magn Reson Imaging 2018;48(2). https://doi.org/10.1002/jmri.25970.

45. Gupta D, Kim M, Vineberg KA, et al. Generation of Synthetic CT Images From MRI for Treatment

Planning and Patient Positioning Using a 3-Channel U-Net Trained on Sagittal Images. Front Oncol 2019; 9. https://doi.org/10.3389/fonc.2019.00964.

46. Montoya JC, Li Y, Strother C, et al. 3D Deep Learning Angiography (3D-DLA) from C-arm Cone-beam CT. AJNR Am J Neuroradiol 2018;39(5). https://doi.org/10.3174/ajnr.A5597.

47. Sreekumari A, Shanbhag D, Yeo D, et al. A Deep Learning-Based Approach to Reduce Rescan and Recall Rates in Clinical MRI Examinations. AJNR Am J Neuroradiol 2019;40(2). https://doi.org/10.3174/ajnr.A5926.

48. Deguchi S, Oishi T, Mitsuya K, et al. Clinicopathological analysis of T2-FLAIR mismatch sign in lower-grade gliomas. Scientific Rep 2020;10(1). https://doi.org/10.1038/s41598-020-67244-7.

49. Akkus Z, Ali I, Sedlář J, et al. Predicting Deletion of Chromosomal Arms 1p/19q in Low-Grade Gliomas from MR Images Using Machine Intelligence. J Digit Imaging 2017;30(4). https://doi.org/10.1007/s10278-017-9984-3.

50. Korfiatis P, Kline TL, Lachance DH, et al. Residual Deep Convolutional Neural Network Predicts MGMT Methylation Status. J Digit Imaging 2017; 30(5). https://doi.org/10.1007/s10278-017-0009-z.

51. Chang XP, Grinband J, Weinberg XBD, et al. Deep-learning convolutional neural networks accurately classify genetic mutations in gliomas. AJNR Am J Neuroradiol 2018;39(7):1201–7.

52. Fan XG, Liu XH, Wu XZ, et al. Deep Learning-Based Automatic Segmentation of Lumbosacral Nerves on CT for Spinal Intervention: A Translational Study. AJNR Am J Neuroradiol 2019;40(6). https://doi.org/10.3174/ajnr.A6070.

53. Quon JL, Chen LC, Kim L, et al. Deep Learning for Automated Delineation of Pediatric Cerebral Arteries on Pre-operative Brain Magnetic Resonance Imaging. Front Surg 2020;7. https://doi.org/10.3389/fsurg.2020.517375.

54. Wu S, Li H, Quang D, et al. Three-Plane–assembled Deep Learning Segmentation of Gliomas. Radiol Artif Intell 2020;2(2):10.

55. Cai JC, Akkus Z, Philbrick KA, et al. Fully Automated Segmentation of Head CT Neuroanatomy Using Deep Learning. Radiol Artif Intell 2020;2(5):12.

56. Quon JL, Han M, Kim LH, et al. Artificial intelligence for automatic cerebral ventricle segmentation and volume calculation: a clinical tool for the evaluation of pediatric hydrocephalus. J Neurosurg Pediatr 2020;c:1–8.

57. Mccoy XDB, Dupont XSM, Gros XC, et al. Convolutional Neural Network-Based Automated Segmentation of the Spinal Cord and Contusion Injury: Deep Learning Biomarker Correlates of Motor Impairment in Acute Spinal Cord Injury. AJNR Am J Neuroradiol 2019;40(4). https://doi.org/10.3174/ajnr.A6020.

58. Park A, Chute C, Rajpurkar P, et al. Deep Learning-Assisted Diagnosis of Cerebral Aneurysms Using the HeadXNet Model. JAMA Netw open 2019;2(6). https://doi.org/10.1001/jamanetworkopen.2019.5600.

59. Federau C, Christensen S, Scherrer N, et al. Improved Segmentation and Detection Sensitivity of Diffusion-weighted Stroke Lesions with Synthetically Enhanced Deep Learning. Radiol Artif Intell 2020;2(5):8.

60. Prevedello LM, Erdal BS, Ryu JL, et al. Automated Critical Test Findings Identification and Online Notification System Using Artificial Intelligence in Imaging. Radiology 2017;285(3). https://doi.org/10.1148/radiol.2017162664.

61. Chilamkurthy S, Ghosh R, Tanamala S, et al. Deep learning algorithms for detection of critical findings in head CT scans: a retrospective study. Lancet 2018;392(10162). https://doi.org/10.1016/S0140-6736(18)31645-3.

62. Nie D, Lu J, Zhang H, et al. Multi-Channel 3D Deep Feature Learning for Survival Time Prediction of Brain Tumor Patients Using Multi-Modal Neuroimages. Scientific Rep 2019;9(1):1–14.

63. Maegerlein C, Fischer J, Mönch S, et al. Automated Calculation of the Alberta Stroke Program Early CT Score: Feasibility and Reliability. Radiology 2019;291(1). https://doi.org/10.1148/radiol.2019181228.

64. Nielsen A, Hansen MB, Tietze A, et al. Prediction of Tissue Outcome and Assessment of Treatment Effect in Acute Ischemic Stroke Using Deep Learning. Stroke 2018;49(6). https://doi.org/10.1161/STROKEAHA.117.019740.

65. Narayana PA, Coronado I, Sujit SJ, et al. Deep Learning for Predicting Enhancing Lesions in Multiple Sclerosis from Noncontrast MRI. Radiology 2020;294(2). https://doi.org/10.1148/radiol.2019191061.

66. Hassan AE, Ringheanu VM, Rabah RR, et al. Early experience utilizing artificial intelligence shows significant reduction in transfer times and length of stay in a hub and spoke model. Interv Neuroradiol 2020;8. https://doi.org/10.1177/1591019920953055.

67. Morey JR, Fiano E, Yaeger KA, et al. Impact of Viz LVO on Time-to-Treatment and Clinical Outcomes in Large Vessel Occlusion Stroke Patients Presenting to Primary Stroke Centers. medRxiv 2020;2–7. https://doi.org/10.1101/2020.07.02.20143834.

68. Sakai K, Yamada K. Machine learning studies on major brain diseases: 5-year trends of 2014-2018. Jpn J Radiol 2019;37(1). https://doi.org/10.1007/s11604-018-0794-4.

69. Zaharchuk G, Gong E, Wintermark M, et al. Deep Learning in Neuroradiology. AJNR Am J Neuroradiol 2018;39(10). https://doi.org/10.3174/ajnr.A5543.

70. Yao AD, Cheng DL, Pan I, et al. Deep Learning in Neuroradiology: A Systematic Review of Current Algorithms and Approaches for the New Wave of Imaging Technology. Radiol Artif Intell 2020;2(2): e190026.

71. Lui YW, Chang PD, Zaharchuk G, et al. Artificial Intelligence in Neuroradiology: Current Status and Future Directions. AJNR Am J Neuroradiol 2020; 41(8). https://doi.org/10.3174/ajnr.A6681.

72. Rudie JD, Rauschecker AM, Bryan RN. Emerging Applications of Artificial Intelligence in Neuro-Oncology. Radiology 2019;290(3). https://doi.org/10.1148/radiol.2018181928.

73. Kaka H, Zhang E. Artificial Intelligence and Deep Learning in Neuroradiology: Exploring the New Frontier. Can Assoc Radiol J 2021;72(1). https://doi.org/10.1177/0846537120954293.

74. Soun JE, Chow DS, Nagamine M, et al. Artificial Intelligence and Acute Stroke Imaging. AJNR Am J Neuroradiol 2021;42(1). https://doi.org/10.3174/ajnr.A6883.

75. Attyé A, Ognard J, Rousseau F, et al. Artificial neuroradiology: Between human and artificial networks of neurons? J Neuroradiol 2019;46(5). https://doi.org/10.1016/j.neurad.2019.07.001.

76. Shi Z, Hu B, Schoepf UJ, et al. Artificial Intelligence in the Management of Intracranial Aneurysms: Current Status and Future Perspectives. AJNR Am J Neuroradiol 2020;41(3). https://doi.org/10.3174/ajnr.A6468.

77. Zeng C, Gu L, Liu Z, et al. Review of Deep Learning Approaches for the Segmentation of Multiple Sclerosis Lesions on Brain MRI. Front neuroinformatics 2020;14. https://doi.org/10.3389/fninf.2020.610967.

Clinical Artificial Intelligence Applications
Musculoskeletal

Simukayi Mutasa, MD[a],*, Paul H. Yi, MD[b]

KEYWORDS

- Musculoskeletal ● Bone ● Joint ● Sports imaging ● Deep learning ● Machine learning
- Artificial intelligence ● Clinical applications

KEY POINTS

- Deep learning for MSK imaging can be difficult because of the subtlety of pathology, the intricate biomechanical interplay of structures in diseases requiring clinical intuition to fully diagnose, and the overall breadth of the specialty.
- There are several built-in advantages to deep learning for MSK imaging. These include ease of co-registration and localization due to the inherent rigidity of osseous structures and the ease of obtaining high-quality images owing to the widespread use of surface coils and overall patient comfort when scanning extremities.
- Most deep learning models for musculoskeletal radiology tackle diagnosing and classifying injuries of the osseous structures.
- Many time-consuming tasks in MSK imaging, such as measuring limb length, bone age assessment, and quantifying muscle volumes, are accelerated by deep learning.
- As in other subspecialties, deep learning can aid in nonimaging interpretation aspects of MSK imaging including accelerating study acquisition, allowing for modality-to-modality conversion, and improving the quality of images with regard to signal-to-noise ratio.

INTRODUCTION

Unique Challenges of Musculoskeletal Radiology Artificial Intelligence

Musculoskeletal (MSK) radiology is a subspecialty of radiology that involves the interpretation of advanced medical images for the diagnosis of disorders of the osseous structures, joints, and their associated soft tissues along with the performance of minimally invasive imaging-guided procedures targeted to treat the disorders thereof. While we have seen many applications of artificial intelligence (AI) targeting disorders of other organ systems, MSK disorders present several unique challenges that have limited the rapid development of AI solutions. These difficulties involved not only the broad range of subtle diseases inherent to bone radiology but also the complex interplay of biomechanics that requires learned intuition.

The first obstacle relates to one of the largest current limitations of AI as it pertains to replacing human radiologists; each trained algorithm can only consider one or a very limited number of diagnoses at any one time. Unfortunately, the subject of MSK radiology involves a large number of differential diagnoses, spanning a large proportion of the total known diagnoses in the entire specialty. One popular online radiology encyclopedia (Radiopaedia) boasts over 55,000 radiology

a Department of Diagnostic Radiology, Division of Musculoskeletal Imaging, Thomas Jefferson University Medical Center, 111 South 11th Street, Third Floor, Philadelphia, PA 19107, USA; b Department of Diagnostic Radiology and Nuclear Medicine, University of Maryland Intelligent Imaging Center, University of Maryland School of Medicine, 22 South Greene Street, First Floor, Baltimore, MD 21201, USA
* Corresponding author.
E-mail address: stmutasa@gmail.com

Radiol Clin N Am 59 (2021) 1013–1026
https://doi.org/10.1016/j.rcl.2021.07.011
0033-8389/21/© 2021 Elsevier Inc. All rights reserved.

articles and cases, of which over 15,000 (28%) are categorized under MSK imaging. It is apparent the act of entirely replacing the duties of an MSK radiologist with the current technology would involve employing a prohibitive number of different algorithms.

Another obstacle involves the often subtle abnormalities in several significant MSK diseases or injuries, a problem that is compounded by the relatively large number of other structures that are unrelated to these subtle abnormalities. For example, when considering an elbow MR imaging in a professional pitcher, a partial tear of their single most important ligament, the ulnar collateral ligament, could lead to debilitating elbow instability and downstream degenerative changes that could prematurely end their career if not addressed. Detection of this partial tear may be limited to detecting less than a handful of abnormal voxels adjacent to the sublime tubercle of the ulnar bone on one view out of the tens of millions of voxels that compromise the entire study (**Fig. 1**). This is a problem because contemporary deep learning techniques are based on statistical modeling. One intuitive way is to think of subtle abnormalities having exceedingly small signal-to-noise ratio (SNR), where the "signal" is the abnormality of interest and the "noise" is any other pixel or voxel. Additionally, this is a problem because most pipelines involve downsampling of original resolution volumes and images, thereby further reducing the amount of "signal" present in these subtle abnormalities.

A final challenge for the development of AI for MSK imaging tasks is that rendering diagnoses in MSK imaging often requires an understanding and integration of the underlying biomechanics of an injury with the imaging findings. The bones, joints, ligaments, muscles, and tendons of the skeletal system are a complex interdependent collective of levers, hinges, and wedges whose function depends on the normal function of proximal and adjacent parts of the system. As such, when one part of the system is damaged, there is often a cascade of interrelated injuries resulting from the subsequent malfunctioning of that specific link in the chain. Human radiologists learn the intuition necessary to use these principles when searching out injuries of the MSK system, which often significantly augments their ability to find corresponding diagnoses. The current state of deep learning technology possesses no ability to form an intuition and cannot extrapolate findings based on prior domain knowledge. One example

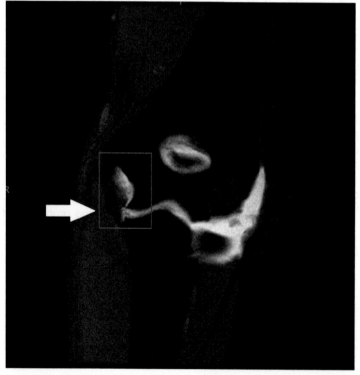

Fig. 1. Coronal MR imaging of the elbow showing tear of the ulnar collateral ligament (UCL) and the relatively small area of the image that the tear comprises.

sometimes encountered is that of a tertius (posterior malleolus) fracture. When an expert radiologist identifies an isolated finding of a posterior malleolus of the ankle fracture, they understand that the biomechanics of such an injury almost invariably preclude the absence of another fracture elsewhere in the lower extremity due to the biomechanical stresses that result in such a fracture, namely supination-external rotation forces. This triggers an automatic search for other, more subtle fractures, such as a distal fibular fracture or medial malleolus fracture, and a request for further imaging, such as a stress view of the mortise to evaluate for potentially associated deltoid ligament injury. A computer cannot be easily taught such intuition, and accordingly, AI's ability to function in the same capacity as a radiologist is limited.

Benefits of Working with Musculosketal Radiology Artificial Intelligence

Although we have outlined several hurdles that impede the rapid development of AI toward fully replacing or automating the tasks of an MSK radiologist, there are several uniquely beneficial features of bone and joint disease that present tremendous opportunities toward automating his or her workflow and tasks that take advantage of some of the unique features of the MSK system. These involve the general rigidity of bone and joint structures, the ease of obtaining MSK studies for the patient and radiologist, and the ability to use surface coils focused on the structures of interest.

Many deep learning problems require the coregistration of different imaging acquisitions. Often when radiologists desire to consolidate the information inside multiple sequences of the same or different patients, such as an MR imaging obtained with T2 and T1 weighted sequences or a computed tomography (CT) scan containing a separate PET acquisition, they run into issues when the images contain separate coordinate systems or spatial resolutions. This issue can be addressed using image coregistration. Image coregistration is a broad subfield of study in computer vision that involves spatially aligning the features that are common in multiple acquisitions so that this and other common features overlap their footprints on any other images in all the sequences. Coregistration is typically one of the initial preprocessing steps in computer vision with medical imaging, as this obviates the requirement of keeping track of each voxels' differing spatial coordinates when we aspire to use the information from multiple acquisitions simultaneously. Broadly speaking, coregistration of rigid structures such as the cranial vault is far easier from a compute and technical know-how

requirement point of view than coregistration of elastic structures that deform and move during acquisitions such as the heart or any structure subject to respiratory motion artifact in the abdomen or chest. With few exceptions, MSK imaging involves body parts that suffer minimal to no respiratory motion, and when they do, they undergo motion in rigid, locally congruent ways. In reality, numerous MSK acquisitions suffer such little motion or movement between sequences that coregistration is not always needed. The patella, for example, remains at the same spatial coordinate in the MR imaging scanner during the entire patient's scan, regardless of whether we are acquiring the T1, T2, or proton density sequence, with the rare exception of dynamic or kinematic CT or MR imaging.

Imaging of the extremities typically involves placing patients in relatively comfortable positions when compared to those required for imaging of internal organs or neurologic structures. A large percentage of extremity imaging is performed in extremely comfortable, extremity scanners that eliminate the issue of claustrophobia (Fig. 2). This significantly reduces the potential artifacts one may face when performing imaging that is related to patient comfort, particularly motion artifacts. This not only assists with image preprocessing as discussed but is also beneficial for regularization during AI model training, as the reduction in artifacts present in MSK studies may

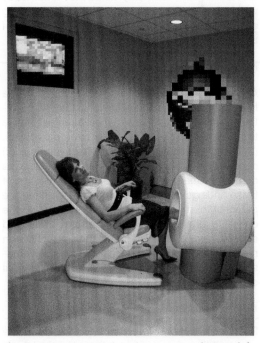

Fig. 2. Extremity MR imaging scanner designed for patient comfort.

reduce potential confounding factors in the imaging that can reduce a given algorithm's ability to generalize to new data.

Increasingly, MR imaging is obtained using arrays of small surface coils placed at or near the body part of interest to be imaged. These have the advantage of dramatically increasing the SNR of the regions of interest while dramatically decreasing the signal contribution from a structure outside the region of interest in a type of "vignette" effect. When training classical imaging recognition neural networks on input images with a relatively small area of important signal, it often takes several steps of training for the neural network to "learn" to ignore structures outside the critical region of interest. For example, suppose we would like to train a neural network to segment the pancreas on a typical imaging slice through the upper abdomen. This slice will contain only a relatively small number of pixels that correspond to the pancreas and a large number of pixels that correspond to unimportant "noise" such as the liver, spleen, kidney, or vertebral body. It may take several hundred-thousand training "steps" comprised of forward propagation and backpropagation before the neural network learns to ignore the spurious background pixels corresponding to other abdominal organs. Furthermore, this learned irrelevance may be defective. Performing imaging with surface coils in MSK MR imaging allows us to narrow in on a much smaller and focused region of anatomy inside the human body while decreasing the signal from surrounding areas without heavy reliance on prelocalization of data.

GENERAL TASKS

AI models can help perform basic tasks that a MSK radiologist is responsible for in the interpretation of imaging studies. At their simplest, these tasks can be broken down into three categories: (1) detection of a disease or image finding, (2) quantification of the severity or degree of a disease or relevant image, and finally (3) characterization of these findings or diseases. These tasks have the potential to augment radiologists by reducing the cognitive efforts required to perform them and allowing radiologists to focus their attention on more sophisticated mental tasks, such as synthesis of image findings to generate a differential diagnosis.

Detection of Disease or Condition

Perhaps the most fundamental of tasks in the interpretation of an imaging study is simply detecting the presence of disease or injury, which AI and

deep learning are well primed to perform. Toward this task, there are two main approaches. The first is to train an image classifier that analyzes an entire image and outputs a single diagnosis based on what the classifier was trained to identify. For example, a binary classifier for the detection of a hip dislocation would analyze a single hip radiograph and predict whether or not a dislocation is or is not present (**Fig. 3**, top row). An important limitation of this approach is the lack of a localizer to help guide human interpretation or verification of the findings. Computational techniques, such as class activation mapping, have been developed toward this goal to create "heatmaps" showing the areas of the image most emphasized by the classifier in making its decision, although such methods have shown variable utility for the localization of diseases in medical imaging.[1] The second main approach is to train an object-detection model that analyzes an entire image and outputs bounding boxes around parts of the image that the model thinks has the disease or condition of interest. For example, an object-detection model for hip dislocation would output bounding boxes around a dislocated hip with the label "dislocation" (**Fig. 3**, bottom row). Such models have the benefit of localization of the disease of interest to aid a radiologist, as well as inherent explainability in its decision to predict whether or not the disease or condition of interest is present. The primary limitation of such a model involves the need for images with annotation at the structure level, requiring manual placement of bounding boxes on the disease or condition of interest, a time-consuming task.

Regardless of the approach taken, deep learning models have tremendous potential to automate the detection of diseases and conditions across all age groups and settings. In the pediatric population, deep learning classifiers have been developed to identify elbow effusions, supracondylar humerus fractures, and other acute elbow fractures on radiographs with areas under the receiver operating characteristic curve (AUC) greater than 0.97.[2–4] In the adult population, deep learning models have similarly been developed to identify fractures of both the upper and lower extremities on radiographs using both classifiers[5–8] and object detectors[9] on radiographs, with some studies showing performance of AI models exceeding that of human experts.[10] Beyond trauma, deep learning models have been used extensively for the detection of degenerative joint diseases, including osteoarthritis in both the hip[11–13] and knee[14–17] on radiographs, and internal derangement of the knee, including meniscus tears and anterior cruciate ligament tears[18–21] on knee MR imaging and rotator

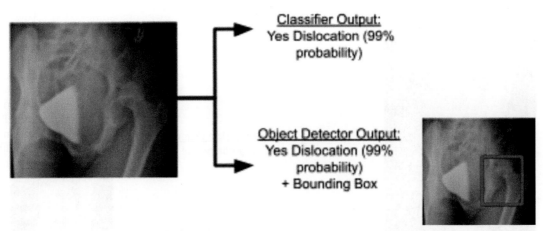

Fig. 3. Schematic of left hip dislocation classifier model (*top row*) versus object detector (*bottom row*) output. Note that the classifier outputs only a prediction with probability of that prediction, while an object detector outputs both the prediction, as well as a bounding box around the object of interest (in this case, a hip dislocation).

cuff tears on shoulder MR imaging.[22] Although the initial use cases for deep learning in MSK disease or condition identification have largely focused on trauma, degenerative joint disease, and internal derangement, any relevant finding that a radiologist is tasked with identifying could potentially be automated using AI and deep learning.

Quantification

Once a disease or condition is identified, one of the next steps for the MSK radiologist is to quantify the severity or degree of disease burden. As for disease or condition identification, a few approaches exist. First, a classifier can be trained to categorize an image into one of two or more severity categories. The benefit of this approach is that labels are only necessary on an image-level basis. Second, a deep learning regression model (**Fig. 4**, top row) can be trained to directly output a quantitative score or measurement of disease burden or severity of a disease. This approach can be difficult to perform because it requires quantitative measurements of a disease or condition, such as angulation of a specific osseous deformity. Third, a segmentation model can be trained to directly outline a disease or condition of interest, which can then, in turn, be used to calculate various quantities, including the area or volume of a lesion and the angle of a particular anatomic relationship, such as fracture angulation (**Fig. 4**, bottom row).

Deep learning classifiers have been trained to quantify severity or subtype of disease, ranging from the grading of rotator cuff tears on shoulder MR imaging[22] and ACL tears on knee MR imaging[23] to specific subtype of calcaneal fractures

on CT.[24] Deep learning regression models have been used in MSK imaging toward quantification tasks such as bone mineral density prediction[25] from CT and measurement of alpha angle on hip radiographs. Perhaps the most widely known type of deep learning regression models used for quantification of the MSK "condition" is for bone age prediction, which was the topic of the first Radiological Society of North America AI Challenge in 2017, in which the top-performing model achieved accurate bone age predictions with a mean absolute difference of 4.2 months compared to radiologist ground-truth,[26] which have been improved even further using ensembles of the top submissions to that competition.[27] Deep learning segmentation models have been used extensively to directly quantify the degree or severity of cartilage disease or defects[28,29] on MR imaging of the knee, the volume of the anterior cruciate ligament in both native and surgically reconstructed ligaments,[30,31] and body composition (eg, cross-sectional areas of fat vs muscle on CT).[32] Segmentation models have also been used to identify anatomic landmarks, from which certain measurements of skeletal anatomy have been performed, such as spinal deformity on radiographs.[33,34]

Characterization

An additional basic task the MSK radiologist is tasked with once they have identified a relevant disease or condition of interest is to further characterize that disease. The specific characteristics of that disease or condition will depend on the specific treatment paradigms. For example, characterization of degenerative joint disease will

Lateral wrist radiograph
shows dorsally tilted distal
radius fracture.

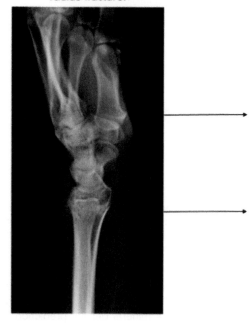

Regression Output:
5 degrees dorsal tilt

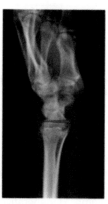

Segmentation Output:
Deformity calculation
based on segmentation =
5 degrees dorsal tilt

Fig. 4. Schematic of distal radius fracture deformity regression model (*top row*) versus segmentation model followed by direct calculation of deformity based on segmentation of anatomic landmarks (*bottom row*). Note that the regression model directly outputs a number without any segmentation of anatomic landmarks, while the segmentation model outputs segmentation of landmarks, allowing for human verification of appropriate localization of the measurement of interest.

require description and breakdown of what features of disease are present (Are there osteophytes, joint space narrowing, or subchondral cysts?),[12] while characterization of a bone lesion or tumor will require description of whether or not the lesion is aggressive or malignant versus not aggressive or benign, both of which are characterization tasks that have been performed using deep learning.[35] The approaches toward characterization of disease are similar to those used for identification of disease and quantification and can theoretically be used to characterize disease to any level of granularity provided that there are enough labeled data with high-quality annotations.

CHANGE DETECTION AND PREDICTION

Beyond the basic tasks described in the preceding sections, the MSK radiologist is responsible for comparing the current image to prior images to evaluate for change in disease or condition. Such a task is more complex than simply detecting, quantifying, or characterizing disease because it requires processing of two pieces of data from two separate time points. Nevertheless, comparing images for change is crucial when evaluating treatment responses. Advanced deep learning techniques have been developed that expand on the approaches described in the preceding section to be able to not only quantify or grade the severity of disease but also to evaluate for change. A recent study by Li and colleagues used a special type of convolutional neural network called a "Siamese" neural network that can compare two knee radiographs to each other and output a continuous measure of change in osteoarthritis severity scoring (**Fig. 5**), thereby allowing for detection of change of disease over time. Although this is a proof of concept that has been applied to this single use case in MSK imaging, this approach could be applied to other clinical scenarios the MSK radiologist may face, such as evaluating change in fracture alignment or healing over time. An alternative approach also evaluated by Li and colleagues is outputting quantitative severity scores for osteoarthritis and directly comparing those scores.

A related but slightly different task that a MSK radiologist may be tasked with is predicting if a patient is at risk for a complication or worsening of disease in the future (prognostication). For example, when evaluating skeletal tumors for risk

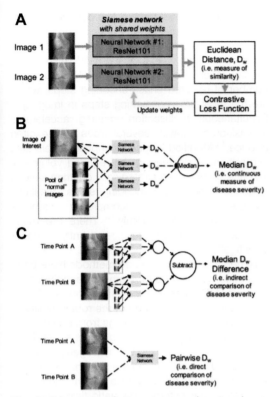

Fig. 5. Schematic of Siamese neural network approaches for evaluating disease severity and change on a continuous spectrum. (*A*) Schematic of the Siamese neural network architecture, which takes two images as inputs and outputs the Euclidean distance between the two images (ie, a measure of similarity). (*B*) Schematic of evaluating a single image for disease severity on a continuous spectrum. (*C*) Schematic of two approaches for evaluating longitudinal images for disease severity on a continuous spectrum. Dw refers to the Euclidean distance. (Reprinted under a Creative Commons Attribution 4.0 International License (https://creativecommons.org/licenses/by/4.0/) from Li, M.D., Chang, K., Bearce, B. et al. Siamese neural networks for continuous disease severity evaluation and change detection in medical imaging. npj Digit. Med. 3, 48 (2020). No changes were made to this figure.)

of pathologic fracture, radiologists will use features such as the severity of endosteal scalloping or cortical thinning to communicate to patients and providers whether or not a patient is at risk of developing a pathologic fracture. Theoretically, one could train deep learning classifiers or object detectors to identify such endosteal scalloping or cortical thinning and thereby help predict if a patient is at risk of developing pathologic fracture. Although this example is theoretic, other similar use cases have been described using deep learning, including prediction of the need for total knee arthroplasty on MR imaging of the knee in

patients without osteoarthritis on radiographs.[36] Such prediction of progression of disease is still new but is promising for the hope of identifying patients at risk for disease and intervening to prevent the onset of these conditions.

TASK ASSISTANCE

AI and deep learning have the potential to assist with tasks certainly for radiologists but also for clinicians who are the ordering providers of MSK imaging. By automating these tasks, many of which can be tedious, workflows can become more efficient and free up time and mental energy of these parties toward tasks of higher value.

For Radiologists

As discussed previously, AI and deep learning can assist with automating many parts of the radiology image interpretation workflow, including identification, quantification or severity grading, and characterization of diseases or conditions, which are tasks that can be mentally taxing but do not necessarily provide as much value as synthesizing these imaging features into a differential diagnosis. Accordingly, the assistance of a radiologist in these tasks could be tremendously helpful in aiding other radiologists to deliver expert-level care at faster rates. Particularly boring and time-consuming tasks that are intellectually unsatisfying and can be automated include leg length measurements and bone age prediction.[26,27,37]

For Clinicians

For clinicians who are the ordering providers and "customers" of the MSK radiology workflow, AI and deep learning models can aid in several tasks. First, for providers who regularly review their own images, such as orthopedic surgeons, deep learning models can provide aid for tasks that they are often tasked with that are not necessarily within the radiologist's set of responsibilities. For example, orthopedic surgeons often are tasked with not only simply identifying the presence of a hip or knee arthroplasty but also to identify the specific implant model to plan for revision surgery, as patients will not infrequently be referred to a surgical center without prior operative notes with an estimated 10% of implants not identified before surgery. Accordingly, deep learning models have been developed to identify specific implant models and manufacturers for the knee, hip, and shoulder.[38–45] Second, for providers who may or may not regularly review their own images, deep learning models can provide "preliminary" results for imaging before radiologist review, which could be particularly helpful in time-sensitive settings, such as the emergency department, or in the outpatient setting where on-site radiologists may not be available regularly. In this regard, one prior study showed that a deep learning model for wrist fracture detection improved emergency physicians' ability to identify wrist fractures.[7] Third, for communication with patients, AI and deep learning models could potentially translate radiology reports into layman's terms or "plain language," which could aid clinicians in explaining radiology results. Although such a natural language processing approach has not yet been applied to MSK radiology, prior models have been developed for general medical notes.[46]

TECHNICAL ASSISTANCE

The practice of obtaining patient imaging for the bones and joints involves many technically demanding aspects for the human specialist, be it a radiologist, technologist, or department physicist, that happen long before a doctor begins to interpret the images themselves. These include difficulties in physically obtaining the study for the technologists such as inability to recognize important or small structures in ultrasound, slow acquisition times leading to greater potential for mistakes in MR imaging, overcoming challenges in patients who are unable to obtain the standard-of-care imaging modalities over another such as the patient unable to get an MR imaging because of a pacemaker, and overcoming artifacts in any modality. Overcoming these challenges not only promises to improve the overall quality and consistency of imaging but may also allow us to obtain more information. These challenges differ based on the acquisition modality of choice for the given study; however, many of them are common to all modalities.

Accelerated Acquisitions

Introduced in the 1970s, MR imaging rapidly became the established standard for diagnosing and treating disorders of almost every joint in the MSK system. This owes to superior contrast when assessing a wide range of soft-tissue and osseous pathologies including disorders of the articular cartilage, bone marrow, muscles, ligaments, and tendons. It is an invaluable tool for noninvasive imaging of bone and joint disorders.

An important limitation in MR imaging involves the relatively long acquisition time, often requiring patients to maintain painful positioning for prolonged periods.[47] While CT imaging of bones and joints typically takes seconds, MR imaging can take several minutes. To overcome this, many techniques have been developed over the last few decades to optimize acquisition speed and are now commercially available. Parallel imaging takes advantage of the knowledge of the spatial location and sensitivity of several receiver coils to dramatically reduce the number of required phase-encoding steps, which are the most time-consuming steps in imaging.[48] Simultaneous multisection imaging accelerates acquisition by allowing several slices to be excited at once.[49] Modified k-space sampling accelerates acquisition by decreasing the required volume of k-space obtained via strategically omitting several frequency and phase-encoding steps. Similarly, compressed sensing incompletely samples k-space, but semi-randomly.[50] There are many experimental techniques currently under investigation.

Recently, various research methods have been proposed to use deep learning techniques to improve MR imaging acquisition times. These techniques take advantage of the robust ability of deep learning to learn mappings from one domain to another. Briefly, MR imaging works by applying a strong magnetic field to the hydrogen protons in the imaged volume forcing the protons to precess about the external field with a net magnetization oriented to the external magnetic field. The precessing protons exist in a slightly imbalanced state whereby a portion of them are in a higher energy state and another proportion of them in the lower energy state. A separate magnetic field is subsequently applied that minimizes this imbalance and turns it into a phase coherence whereby the hydrogen protons are rotating together with a net magnetization that is oriented perpendicular to the external magnetic field. It is this rotating charge that produces a signal whose amplitude is spatially mapped to a Fourier region referred to as "k-space" whereby the x and y coordinates represent different phases and frequencies, and the pixel intensity represents the amplitude of each wave. To convert this into an image, classically a reverse Fourier transform is applied to the raw k-space data. The basis for deep learning–based MR imaging reconstruction involves plugging in a deep neural network into this reverse transformation step to either replace the reverse Fourier transform or augment it in some manner. When combined with incomplete K-space sampling techniques such as radial acquisition or compressed sensing, this has the promise of achieving significant speed increases. The idea being that a neural network trained in a data-driven manner to perform K-space reconstruction would be robust to the missing K-space data, as it has some latent knowledge of the typical Fourier space amplitudes in the given context.

Various methods have been proposed for this task in the literature which typically involves performing this task as either a supervised learning task or a semi-supervised task. Many examples of the former method exist in the literature, typically using a baseline fully connected neural network architecture. One such example is described by Zhu and colleagues[51] where they reimagined the task of converting raw k-space data to diagnostic images as a data-driven supervised learning task using a deep neural network they coined "AUTOMAP". The methods usually involve using a U-Net architecture to directly perform the k-space to image reconstruction. A second paradigm for deep learning–based MR imaging image reconstruction revolves around the concept of using semi-supervised conditional generative adversarial networks (GANs) to perform the mapping whereby the k-space data are used as the conditional input. One such technique was described by Yang and colleagues[52] where they combined compressed sensing MR imaging acquisition with a GAN. Their GAN used a typical U-Net architecture as the generator and a novel loss function for the discriminator.

As it is rare for institutions to store their k-space data for long periods, research into deep learning-based MR imaging reconstruction is significantly aided by institutions who chose to release large data sets containing medical images and their corresponding k-space data. The largest such data set specifically targeting MSK imaging was released publicly by New York University[53] and is comprised of 1594 fully sampled knee examinations with k-space data and over 10,000 clinical knee examinations without coil data.

Noise Reduction

Medical imaging has often been plagued with various artifacts that compromise the diagnostic information available in the acquisitions. Every imaging modality uses various techniques for improving image quality that centers on increasing the SNR. Prior research has focused on improving SNR, while more recent research has begun to explore methods that maintain the current SNR standards while seeking to improve on other imaging parameters. These include reducing radiation dose to the patient in the case of CT and acquisition which uses techniques that invariably decrease SNR and decreasing acquisition time in the case of magnetic resonance imaging which uses techniques discussed previously that decrease SNR. In addition to methods that decrease SNR, various modalities suffer from artifacts that are hardware-related, such as magnetic

field inhomogeneity and aliasing; patient-induced, such as motion degradation or signal degradation from the presence of foreign bodies; or environment-related such as external interference from radiofrequency spikes. Because of its dependence on statistical modeling, deep learning has a robust ability to marginalize the noise of various sources. To put it simply, neural networks are trained to predict the most likely output for a given input using knowledge obtained on numerous training examples. This gives them an ability to recognize when certain inputs such as noise are abnormal for a given domain and subsequently ignore their contributions to the final output.

Image denoising involves removing the noise component of images while maintaining the signal component. Several authors have explored image denoising using deep learning, commonly using a modified fully connected U-Net as the architecture of choice.[54] The typical problem setup involves feeding a noise-filled image into the U-Net and having it output the same image but without noise. The idea is that the network learns to predict which pixels can be classified as noise and replaces them with what it thinks the proper noise-free pixel value is. In MR imaging acquisition, time can be reduced, and in CT scanning, radiation exposure is mitigated. Authors differ in minor details such as how they generate their noisy and noise-free images, and what loss functions are used. Chen and colleagues[55] trained their U-Net by using real images added to a random Poisson noise matrix as their "noisy" image inputs and the original real image as the desired output, a common technique. Hong and colleagues[56] reimagined this paradigm, however, and defined the problem differently. They instead had their U-Net try to generate an image of the noise present in the image itself, as opposed to trying to predict the denoised image. For training, the input was a noisy image, and the output was a picture of the noise in the input image. This picture of the noise was subtracted from the original input image to generate a picture with less noise. Zhang and colleagues[57] tackled the task of metal reduction in CT imaging by creating images with synthetically implanted metals as the input and the original image as the output. Wolterink and colleagues[58] used a completely different technique. They added the generator in a GAN to their pipeline trained to transform low-dose CT images into routine-dose CT images and trained the discriminator to distinguish the output of the generator from routine-dose CT images.

The most concerning drawback of deep learning–based noise reduction is an issue intrinsic to their function. Fundamentally, the algorithms are looking at low-quality images and "guessing" what the high-quality image looks like by filling in the missing portions. This guess is based on statistically evaluating the most likely output for each given input based on what was available in the training data. As such, outputs tend to represent the most statistically likely high-quality image, as opposed to the actual underlying information. This is particularly noticeable when the algorithm encounters anatomy, noise, or artifact it has not encountered before. Currently, the only way to mitigate this is by increasing training data size and diversity.

Modality Conversion

When seeking to maximize the sensitivity and specificity of a study for obtaining an appropriate diagnosis for each patient, radiologists generally refer to the American College of Radiology appropriateness criteria. These contain a listing of the ideal study to obtain for the most common presentations based on factors such as general availability, cost, and minimizing the harm done to the patient. In general, when compared to MR imaging, CT scans are faster to obtain, more widespread, and more comfortable for the patient. In contrast, MR imaging scans provide more soft-tissue contrast and do not impart ionizing radiation into the patient. There are many patient-dependent or reader-dependent situations where one modality is preferred over another, for example, patients with non–MR imaging-compatible implants such as pacemakers or patients who decline to receive ionizing radiation for one reason or another. Often in MSK imaging, it may be beneficial or necessary to obtain both CT and magnetic resonance imaging of the same anatomy for a patient. One example of this is the infamous "six-pack" preoperative spine MR imaging in patients with scoliosis. The study, a favorite of junior MSK radiology faculty everywhere, involves obtaining both CT and MR images of the cervical, thoracic, and lumbar spine simultaneously for preoperative planning. Another example is cross-sectional studies obtained for quantifying femoroacetabular impingement, where some institutions use MR imaging and others use CT. In these situations, the ability to convert MR imaging to CT would be helpful because the simultaneously obtained CT sequences are only useful for gross osseous structural information and surgical measurements as opposed to fine detail. Also, radiologists are often more comfortable performing some measurements such as alpha angle, glenoid version, or lateral center edge on CT images as opposed to MR images given the superior osseous contrast resolution. This makes

the ability to generate a CT series automatically during an MR imaging acquisition valuable.

Converting MR imaging to CT using deep learning has been accomplished with high fidelity, both by using fully supervised techniques and by using domain-to-domain semi-supervised learning. Xiang and colleagues[59] investigated a method to convert T1-weighted MR imaging scans into CT scans by using coregistered MR imaging and CT scans as training data for a fully supervised CNN architecture. Alternatively, Yucheng and colleagues used a semi-supervised method based on a 2.5-dimensional context-aware conditional GAN to generate synthetic shoulder CT images from T1 MR images of the same shoulders. Each desired output slice used the image from the slice above and below each input slice as a separate channel, hence the 2.5 dimensions.

Modality conversion deep learning techniques suffer from several drawbacks. As of this writing, it has not been shown possible to a high level of accuracy to generate MR images from input CT images. This is perhaps intuitively understood as CT scans contain far less inherent signal than MR imaging. Additionally, modality converted images universally suffer from signal infidelity in the converted images. Neural networks are not perfect at recreating the exact CT scan that would be generated normally, as the two technologies fundamentally operate on different physics principles, forcing the algorithms to "guess" the desired output based on prior training statistics as described in the noise-reduction segment. This significantly limits their diagnostic use, as the signal intensities generated cannot be fully relied upon to represent true pathology. They remain useful for the gross evaluation of structure and for the aforementioned task of making measurements.

OUTCOME PREDICTION AND RISK STRATIFICATION

Perhaps unsurprisingly, one of the most difficult tasks to train a neural network to perform is predicting the future. This has not stopped researchers from exploring methods to leverage this technology for this task. Researchers have investigated topics ranging from predicting the prognosis of patients diagnosed with sarcomas to forecasting clinical outcomes in patients with rheumatoid arthritis, to stratifying the fracture risk of patients based on baseline imaging. The desire to predict outcomes and stratify risks is not new. Researchers, societies, and commercial entities have been doing this for decades to help personalize medical treatment. Current tools are imperfect, and many commercially available options are only marginally better than guesses. Deep learning, however, offers the ability to combine currently available tools with a powerful new technology that promises to help us take the next step forward in personalized medicine.

Outcome Prediction

When patients are newly diagnosed with a disease, one of the most immediate goals of the treatment team involves attempting to get a handle on the most likely potential outcome of the patient's condition. This allows the physicians to titrate how aggressive the monitoring and treatment plan for the patient should be. For many diseases, monitoring and treatment are based on decades of empirical data. Recently for cancer treatment, statistical models for survival analysis and treatment outcome based on clinical data and related outcomes are increasingly being used. One of the most widely used survival models is the Cox proportional hazard regression model (CoxPHR).[60,61] While statistical models such as CoxPHR have achieved good accuracy on the prediction of patient survival for many types of cancer, relatively rare cancers such as those encountered in MSK radiology are difficult for such models secondary to the difficulty of identifying time-dependent variables that influence overall survival. Statistical models also suffer when forecasting outcomes based on electronic health record (EHR) data owing to the large amounts of missing data and the inconsistent number of data points among patients.

For predicting survival in patients with synovial sarcomas, Han and colleagues[62] used a hybrid approach wherein they manually selected important variables using Kaplan-Meier survival analysis and the log-rank test as the majority of the input into a feed-forward neural network along with a yearly updating risk score. Their investigative cross-validation scores were able to show an improved AUC for predicting survival of 0.814 (95% confidence interval [CI]: 0.813–0.823) when compared to a Cox prediction model with an AUC of 0.629 (95% CI: 0.471–0.77).

For predicting outcomes in patients with rheumatoid arthritis, Norgeot and colleagues[63] obtained structured clinical data from the electronic medical records of 820 patients at two institutions to predict the disease activity at the next clinical appointment to a high level of accuracy. They extracted over 20 variables with time-dependent interactions that were known to be clinically important for disease activity prediction and settled on a gated recurrent neural network for analysis.

Because of its end-to-end nature, deep learning has a robust ability to make connections between inputs and outputs that are otherwise imperceptible to human beings. The three studies mentioned previously have the drawback of resorting to hand-selected features that fail to appropriately leverage this ability of neural networks.

Risk Stratification

In contrast to outcome prediction, risk stratification involves attempting to predict future disease in patients who are currently healthy. Knowledge of a patient's risk of disease compared to their peers allows primary care physicians to intervene early to alter the course of a patient's life or to personalize their follow-up. Currently, risk stratification is based on knowledge of clinically important variables about the patient and how they contribute to long-term outcomes. Besides, for many disease states in MSK radiology, risk stratification is not currently available. Several tools have been proposed in this field, the most common type being the prediction of the development of fractures in the future. The tools available today such as the FRAX assessment tool[64] use various manually selected clinical risk factors to predict long-term risk. The main drawback to risk-stratification models is a generally low level of accuracy. This leads to misclassifying patients into the incorrect grouping, leading to improper treatment and follow-up. Subsequently, risk stratification models are best evaluated with large longitudinal analyses.

Almog and colleagues[65] proposed a risk fracture algorithm based on deep learning to identify the risk of osteoporotic fractures within the next 2 years. Dubbed "Crystal Bone," their system analyzed vectorized ICD-10 codes in the EHRs of over 1 million patients with a recurrent neural network to predict whether a patient's future trajectory may contain a fracture event. Their model achieved a high AUC of 0.81.

SUMMARY

AI promises to augment every aspect of the imaging chain, from easing the acquisition of high-quality imaging, classifying disease severity, to stratifying patients at risk for fracture. Although much of the initial working on developing AI and deep learning in MSK radiology has focused on the diagnosis of orthopedic trauma, internal joint derangement, and degenerative joint disease on radiographs and MR imaging, the concepts that have been used for these use cases can be applied toward any other disease process and imaging modality.

DISCLOSURE

The authors have nothing to disclose.

REFERENCES

1. Zhou B, Khosla A, Lapedriza A, et al. Learning deep features for discriminative localization. arXiv [csCV]; 2015. Available at: http://arxiv.org/abs/1512.04150.
2. England JR, Gross JS, White EA, et al. Detection of traumatic pediatric elbow joint effusion using a deep convolutional neural network. AJR Am J Roentgenol 2018;211(6):1361–8.
3. Rayan JC, Reddy N, Kan JH, et al. Binomial classification of pediatric elbow fractures using a deep learning multiview approach emulating radiologist decision making. Radiol Artif Intelligence 2019; 1(1):e180015.
4. Choi JW, Cho YJ, Lee S, et al. Using a dual-input convolutional neural network for automated detection of pediatric supracondylar fracture on conventional radiography. Invest Radiol 2020;55(2):101–10.
5. Jones RM, Sharma A, Hotchkiss R, et al. Assessment of a deep-learning system for fracture detection in musculoskeletal radiographs. NPJ Digit Med 2020;3(1):144.
6. Chen H-Y, Hsu BW-Y, Yin Y-K, et al. Application of deep learning algorithm to detect and visualize vertebral fractures on plain frontal radiographs. PLoS One 2021;16(1):e0245992.
7. Lindsey R, Daluiski A, Chopra S, et al. Deep neural network improves fracture detection by clinicians. Proc Natl Acad Sci U S A 2018;115(45):11591–6.
8. Krogue JD, Cheng KV, Hwang KM, et al. Automatic hip fracture identification and functional subclassification with deep learning. Radiol Artif Intelligence 2020;2(2):e190023.
9. Thian YL, Li Y, Jagmohan P, et al. Convolutional neural networks for automated fracture detection and localization on wrist radiographs. Radiol Artif Intelligence 2019;1(1):e180001.
10. Langerhuizen DWG, Janssen SJ, Mallee WH, et al. What are the applications and limitations of artificial intelligence for fracture detection and classification in orthopaedic trauma imaging? a systematic review. Clin Orthop Relat Res 2019;477(11):2482–91.
11. Üreten K, Arslan T, Gültekin KE, et al. Detection of hip osteoarthritis by using plain pelvic radiographs with deep learning methods. Skeletal Radiol 2020; 49(9):1369–74.
12. von Schacky CE, Sohn JH, Liu F, et al. Development and validation of a multitask deep learning model for severity grading of hip osteoarthritis features on radiographs. Radiology 2020;295(1):136–45.
13. Xue Y, Zhang R, Deng Y, et al. A preliminary examination of the diagnostic value of deep learning in hip osteoarthritis. PLoS One 2017;12(6):e0178992.
14. Thomas KA, Kidziński Ł, Halilaj E, et al. Automated classification of radiographic knee osteoarthritis severity using deep neural networks. Radiol Artif Intell 2020;2(2):e190065.
15. Schwartz AJ, Clarke HD, Spangehl MJ, et al. Can a convolutional neural network classify knee osteoarthritis on plain radiographs as accurately as fellowship-trained knee arthroplasty surgeons? J Arthroplasty 2020;35(9):2423–8.
16. Leung K, Zhang B, Tan J, et al. Prediction of total knee replacement and diagnosis of osteoarthritis by using deep learning on knee radiographs: data from the osteoarthritis initiative. Radiology 2020; 296(3):584–93.
17. Tiulpin A, Thevenot J, Rahtu E, et al. Automatic knee osteoarthritis diagnosis from plain radiographs: a deep learning-based approach. Sci Rep 2018;8(1): 1727.
18. Bien N, Rajpurkar P, Ball RL, et al. Deep-learning-assisted diagnosis for knee magnetic resonance imaging: development and retrospective validation of MRNet. PLoS Med 2018;15(11):e1002699.
19. Liu F, Guan B, Zhou Z, et al. Fully automated diagnosis of anterior cruciate ligament tears on knee MR images by using deep learning. Radiol Artif Intell 2019;1(3):180091.
20. Zhang L, Li M, Zhou Y, et al. Deep learning approach for anterior cruciate ligament lesion detection: evaluation of diagnostic performance using arthroscopy as the reference standard. J Magn Reson Imaging 2020;52(6):1745–52.
21. Chang PD, Wong TT, Rasiej MJ. Deep learning for detection of complete anterior cruciate ligament tear. J Digit Imaging 2019;32(6):980–6.
22. Shim E, Kim JY, Yoon JP, et al. Automated rotator cuff tear classification using 3D convolutional neural network. Sci Rep 2020;10(1):15632.
23. Namiri NK, Flament I, Astuto B, et al. Deep learning for hierarchical severity staging of anterior cruciate ligament injuries from MRI. Radiol Artif Intell 2020; 2(4):e190207.
24. Aghnia Farda N, Lai J-Y, Wang J-C, et al. Sanders classification of calcaneal fractures in CT images with deep learning and differential data augmentation techniques. Injury 2020. https://doi.org/10.1016/j.injury.2020.09.010.
25. Fang Y, Li W, Chen X, et al. Opportunistic osteoporosis screening in multi-detector CT images using deep convolutional neural networks. Eur Radiol 2020. https://doi.org/10.1007/s00330-020-07312-8.
26. Halabi SS, Prevedello LM, Kalpathy-Cramer J, et al. The RSNA pediatric bone age machine learning challenge. Radiology 2019;290(2):498–503.

27. Pan I, Thodberg HH, Halabi SS, et al. Improving automated pediatric bone age estimation using ensembles of models from the 2017 RSNA machine learning challenge. Radiol Artif Intell 2019;1(6):e190053.

28. Lange T, Taghizadeh E, Knowles BR, et al. Quantification of patellofemoral cartilage deformation and contact area changes in response to static loading via high-resolution MRI with prospective motion correction. J Magn Reson Imaging 2019;50(5):1561–70.

29. Eckstein F, Chaudhari AS, Fuerst D, et al. A deep learning automated segmentation algorithm accurately detects differences in longitudinal cartilage thickness loss - data from the FNIH biomarkers study of the osteoarthritis initiative. Arthritis Care Res 2020. https://doi.org/10.1002/acr.24539.

30. Flannery SW, Kiapour AM, Edgar DJ, et al. Automated magnetic resonance image segmentation of the anterior cruciate ligament. J Orthop Res 2020. https://doi.org/10.1002/jor.24926.

31. Flannery SW, Kiapour AM, Edgar DJ, et al. A transfer learning approach for automatic segmentation of the surgically treated anterior cruciate ligament. J Orthop Res 2021. https://doi.org/10.1002/jor.24984.

32. Magudia K, Bridge CP, Bay CP, et al. Population-Scale CT-based body composition analysis of a large outpatient population using deep learning to derive age-, sex-, and race-specific reference curves. Radiology 2021;298(2):319–29.

33. Galbusera F, Niemeyer F, Wilke H-J, et al. Fully automated radiological analysis of spinal disorders and deformities: a deep learning approach. Eur Spine J 2019;28(5):951–60.

34. Schwartz JT, Cho BH, Tang P, et al. Deep learning automates measurement of spinopelvic parameters on lateral lumbar radiographs. Spine 2020. https://doi.org/10.1097/BRS.0000000000003830.

35. He Y, Pan I, Bao B, et al. Deep learning-based classification of primary bone tumors on radiographs: a preliminary study. EBioMedicine 2020;62:103121.

36. Tolpadi AA, Lee JJ, Pedoia V, et al. Deep learning predicts total knee replacement from magnetic resonance images. Sci Rep 2020;10(1):6371.

37. Zheng Q, Shellikeri S, Huang H, et al. Deep learning measurement of leg length discrepancy in children based on radiographs. Radiology 2020;296(1):152–8.

38. Wilson NA, Jehn M, York S, et al. Revision total hip and knee arthroplasty implant identification: implications for use of Unique Device Identification 2012 AAHKS member survey results. J Arthroplasty 2014;29(2):251–5.

39. Yi PH, Wei J, Kim TK, et al. Automated detection & classification of knee arthroplasty using deep learning. Knee 2020;27(2):535–42.

40. Karnuta JM, Luu BC, Roth AL, et al. Artificial intelligence to identify arthroplasty implants from radiographs of the knee. J Arthroplasty 2020. https://doi.org/10.1016/j.arth.2020.10.021.

41. Murphy M, Killen C, Burnham R, et al. Artificial intelligence accurately identifies total hip arthroplasty implants: a tool for revision surgery. Hip Int 2021. 1120700020987526.

42. Borjali A, Chen AF, Bedair HS, et al. Comparing the performance of a deep convolutional neural network with orthopaedic surgeons on the identification of total hip prosthesis design from plain radiographs. Med Phys 2021. https://doi.org/10.1002/mp.14705.

43. Karnuta JM, Haeberle HS, Luu BC, et al. Artificial intelligence to identify arthroplasty implants from radiographs of the hip. J Arthroplasty 2020. https://doi.org/10.1016/j.arth.2020.11.015.

44. Kang Y-J, Yoo J-I, Cha Y-H, et al. Machine learning-based identification of hip arthroplasty designs. J Orthop Translat 2020;21:13–7.

45. Urban G, Porhemmat S, Stark M, et al. Classifying shoulder implants in X-ray images using deep learning. Comput Struct Biotechnol J 2020;18:967–72.

46. Bala S, Keniston A, Burden M. Patient perception of plain-language medical notes generated using artificial intelligence software: pilot mixed-methods study. JMIR Form Res 2020;4(6):e16670.

47. Kozak BM, Jaimes C, Kirsch J, et al. MRI techniques to decrease imaging times in children. Radiographics 2020;40(2):485–502.

48. Hamilton J, Franson D, Seiberlich N. Recent advances in parallel imaging for MRI. Prog Nucl Magn Reson Spectrosc 2017;101:71–95.

49. Li X, Peng Z, Sun Y, et al. Is simultaneous multisection turbo spin echo ready for clinical MRI? A feasibility study on fast imaging of knee lesions. Clin Radiol 2020;75(3):238.e21–30.

50. Jaspan ON, Fleysher R, Lipton ML. Compressed sensing MRI: a review of the clinical literature. Br J Radiol 2015;88(1056):20150487.

51. Zhu B, Liu JZ, Cauley SF, et al. Image reconstruction by domain-transform manifold learning. Nature 2018;555(7697):487–92.

52. Yang G, Yu S, Dong H, et al. DAGAN: deep de-aliasing generative adversarial networks for fast compressed sensing MRI reconstruction. IEEE Trans Med Imaging 2018;37(6):1310–21.

53. Zbontar J, Knoll F, Sriram A, et al. fastMRI: an open dataset and benchmarks for accelerated MRI. arXiv [csCV]; 2018. Available at: http://arxiv.org/abs/1811.08839.

54. Ronneberger O, Fischer P, Brox T. U-Net: convolutional networks for biomedical image segmentation. In: Medical image computing and computer-assisted intervention – MICCAI 2015. Springer International Publishing; 2015. p. 234–41.

55. Chen H, Zhang Y, Zhang W, et al. Low-dose CT via convolutional neural network. Biomed Opt Express 2017;8(2):679–94.

56. Hong JH, Park EA, Lee W, et al. Incremental image noise reduction in coronary CT angiography using a deep learning-based technique with iterative reconstruction. Korean J Radiol 2020;21(10): 1165–77.

57. Zhang K, Zuo W, Chen Y, et al. Beyond a gaussian denoiser: residual learning of deep CNN for image denoising. IEEE Trans Image Process 2017;26(7): 3142–55.

58. Wolterink JM, Leiner T, Viergever MA, et al. Generative adversarial networks for noise reduction in low-dose CT. IEEE Trans Med Imaging 2017;36(12): 2536–45.

59. Xiang L, Wang Q, Nie D, et al. Deep embedding convolutional neural network for synthesizing CT image from T1-weighted MR image. Med Image Anal 2018;47:31–44.

60. Lee JG, Moon S, Salamatian K. Modeling and predicting the popularity of online contents with Cox proportional hazard regression model. Neurocomputing 2012;76(1):134–45.

61. Peng Y, Bi L, Guo Y, et al. Deep multi-modality collaborative learning for distant metastases predication in PET-CT soft-tissue sarcoma studies. Conf Proc IEEE Eng Med Biol Soc 2019;2019:3658–88.

62. Han I, Kim JH, Park H, et al. Deep learning approach for survival prediction for patients with synovial sarcoma. Tumour Biol 2018;40(9). 1010428318799264.

63. Norgeot B, Glicksberg BS, Trupin L, et al. Assessment of a deep learning model based on electronic health record data to forecast clinical outcomes in patients with rheumatoid arthritis. JAMA Netw Open 2019;2(3):e190606.

64. Kanis JA, Oden A, Johansson H, et al. FRAX® and its applications to clinical practice. Bone 2009; 44(5):734–43.

65. Almog YA, Rai A, Zhang P, et al. Deep learning with electronic health records for short-term fracture risk identification: crystal bone algorithm development and validation. J Med Internet Res 2020;22(10): e22550.

Clinical Artificial Intelligence Applications
Breast Imaging

Qiyuan Hu, BA, Maryellen L. Giger, PhD*

KEYWORDS

- Breast cancer • Medical imaging • Computer-aided diagnosis • Deep learning • Screening
- Diagnosis • Machine learning • Treatment response

KEY POINTS

- AI in breast imaging is expected to impact both interpretation efficacy and workflow efficiency in radiology as it is applied to imaging examinations being routinely obtained in clinical practice.
- AI algorithms, including human-engineered radiomics algorithms and deep learning methods, have been under development for multiple decades.
- AI can have a role in improving breast cancer risk assessment, detection, diagnosis, prognosis, assessing response to treatment, and predicting recurrence.
- Currently the main use of AI algorithms is in decision support, where computers augment human decision-making as opposed to replacing radiologists.

INTRODUCTION

Breast cancer is the most commonly diagnosed cancer and the second leading cause of cancer death among women in the United States, with over 281,000 estimated new cases and 43,000 estimated deaths in 2021.[1] Owing to its high prevalence, the advancement of clinical practice and basic research to predict the risk, detect and diagnose the disease, and predict response to therapy has a high potential impact. Over the course of many decades, medical imaging modalities have been developed and used in routine clinical practice for these purposes in several capacities, including detection through screening programs, staging when a cancer is found, and planning and monitoring treatment. Screening with mammography is associated with a 20% – 40% reduction in breast cancer deaths.[2] However, screening with mammography alone may be insufficient for women at high risk of breast cancer.[3] For example, cancers can be missed at mammography in women with dense breasts because of the camouflaging effect.[4] The need for more effective assessment strategies has led to the emergence of newer imaging techniques for supplemental screening and diagnostic, prognostic, and treatment purposes, including full-field digital mammography (FFDM), multiparametric magnetic resonance imaging (MRI), digital breast tomosynthesis (DBT), and automated breast ultrasound (ABUS).[2,5]

While imaging technologies have expanding roles in breast cancer and have provided radiologists with multimodality diagnostic tools applied to various clinical scenarios, they have also led to an increased need for interpretation expertise and reading time. The desire to improve the efficacy and efficiency of clinical care continues to drive innovations, including artificial intelligence (AI). AI offers the opportunity to optimize and streamline the clinical workflow as well as aid in many of the clinical decision-making tasks in image interpretations. AI's capacity to recognize

Funded by: NIHHYB. Grant number(s): U01CA195564.
Committee on Medical Physics, Department of Radiology, The University of Chicago, 5841 S Maryland Avenue, MC2026, Chicago, IL 60637, USA
* Corresponding author.
E-mail address: qhu@uchicago.edu

Radiol Clin N Am 59 (2021) 1027–1043
https://doi.org/10.1016/j.rcl.2021.07.010

radiologic.theclinics.com

complex patterns in images, even those that are not noticeable or detectable by human experts, transforms image interpretation into a more quantitative and objective process. AI also excels at processing the sheer amount of information in multimodal data, giving it the potential to integrate not only multiple radiographic imaging modalities but also genomics, pathology, and electronic health records to perform comprehensive analyses and predictions.

AI-assisted systems, such as computer-aided detection (CADe), diagnosis (CADx), and triaging (CADt), have been under development and deployment for clinical use for decades and have accelerated in recent years with the advancement in computing power and modern algorithms.[6-10] These AI methods extract and analyze large volumes of quantitative information from image data, assisting radiologists in image interpretation as a concurrent, secondary, or autonomous reader at various steps of the clinical workflow. It is worth noting that while AI systems hold promising prospects in breast cancer image analysis, they also bring along challenges and should be developed and used with abundant caution.

It is important to note that in AI development, two major aspects need to be considered: (1) development of the AI algorithm and (2) evaluation of how it will be eventually used in practice. Currently, most AI systems are being developed and cleared by US Food and Drug Administration (FDA) to augment the interpretation of the medical image, as opposed to autonomous use. These computer-aided methods of implementation include a second reader, a concurrent reader, means to triage cases for reading prioritization, and methods to rule out cases that might not require a human read (a partial autonomous use). In the evaluation of such methods, the human needs to be involved as in dedicated reader studies to demonstrate effectiveness and safety. **Table 1** provides a list of AI algorithms cleared by the FDA for various use cases in breast imaging.[11]

Table 1
FDA-cleared AI algorithm for breast imaging

Product	Company	Modality	Use Case	Date Cleared
ClearView cCAD	ClearView Diagnostics Inc	US	Diagnosis	12/28/16
QuantX	Quantitative Insights, Inc	MRI	Diagnosis	7/19/17
Insight BD	Siemens Healthineers	FFDM, DBT	Breast density	2/6/18
DM-Density	Densitas, Inc	FFDM	Breast density	2/23/18
PowerLook Density Assessment Software	ICAD Inc	DBT	Breast density	4/5/18
DenSeeMammo	Statlife	FFDM	Breast density	6/26/18
Volpara Imaging Software	Volpara Health Technologies Limited	FFDM, DBT	Breast density	9/21/18
cmTriage	CureMetrix, Inc	FFDM	Triage	3/8/19
Koios DS	Koios Medical, Inc	US	Diagnosis	7/3/19
ProFound AI Software V2.1	ICAD Inc	DBT	Detection, Diagnosis	10/4/19
densitas densityai	Densitas, Inc	FFDM, DBT	Breast density	2/19/20
Transpara	ScreenPoint Medical B.V.	FFDM, DBT	Detection	3/5/20
MammoScreen	Therapixel	FFDM	Detection	3/25/20
HealthMammo	Zebra Medical Vision Ltd	FFDM	Triage	7/16/20
WRDensity	Whiterabbit.ai Inc	FFDM, DBT	Breast density	10/30/20
Genius AI Detection	Hologic, Inc	DBT	Detection, Diagnosis	11/18/20
Visage Breast Density	Visage Imaging GmbH	FFDM, DBT	Breast density	1/29/21

Abbreviations: US, ultrasound.
Data from FDA Cleared AI Algorithm. https://models.acrdsi.org.

This article focuses on the research and development of AI systems for clinical breast cancer image analysis, covering the role of AI in the clinical tasks of risk assessment, detection, diagnosis, prognosis, as well as treatment response monitoring and risk of recurrence. In addition to presenting applications by task, the article will start with an introduction to human-engineered radiomics and deep learning techniques and conclude with a discussion on current challenges in the field and future directions.

HUMAN-ENGINEERED ANALYTICS AND DEEP LEARNING TECHNIQUES

AI algorithms often use either human-engineered, analytical, or deep learning methods in the development of machine intelligence tasks. Human-engineered features are mathematical descriptors/model-driven analytics developed to characterize lesions or tissue in medical images.

These features quantify visually discernible characteristics, such as size, shape, texture, and morphology, collectively describing the phenotypes of the anatomy imaged. They can be automatically extracted from images of lesions using computer algorithms with analytical expressions encoded, and machine learning models, such as linear discriminant analysis and support vector machines, can be trained on the extracted features to produce predictions for clinical questions. The extraction of human-engineered features often requires a prior segmentation of the lesion from the parenchyma background. Such extraction of features has been conducted on mammography, tomosynthesis, ultrasound, and MRI.[8,12] For example, **Fig. 1** presents a CADx pipeline that automatically segments breast lesions and extracts six categories of human-engineered radiomic features from dynamic contrast-enhanced (DCE) MRI on a workstation.[13–18] Note that the extraction and interpretation of features

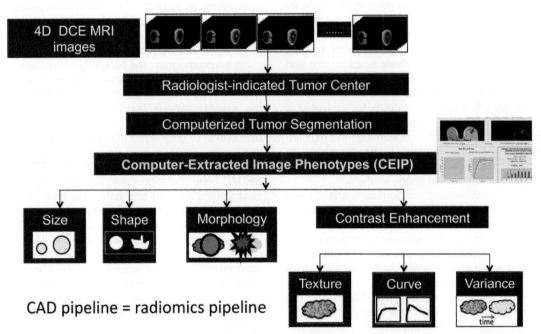

University of Chicago High-Throughput MRI Phenotyping System

Fig. 1. Schematic flowchart of a computerized tumor phenotyping system for breast cancers on DCE-MRI. The CAD radiomics pipeline includes computer segmentation of the tumor from the local parenchyma and computer-extraction of human-engineered radiomic features covering six phenotypic categories: (1) size (measuring tumor dimensions), (2) shape (quantifying the 3D geometry), (3) morphology (characterizing tumor margin), (4) enhancement texture (describing the heterogeneity within the texture of the contrast uptake in the tumor on the first postcontrast MRIs), (5) kinetic curve assessment (describing the shape of the kinetic curve and assessing the physiologic process of the uptake and washout of the contrast agent in the tumor during the dynamic imaging series, and (6) enhancement-variance kinetics (characterizing the time course of the spatial variance of the enhancement within the tumor). CAD, computer-aided diagnosis; DCE-MRI, dynamic contrast-enhanced MRI. (*From* Giger ML. Machine learning in medical imaging. J Am Coll Radiol. 2018;15(3):512-520; with permission.)

depend on the imaging modality and the clinical task required.

In addition, AI systems that use deep learning algorithms have been increasingly developed for health care applications in recent years.[19] Deep learning is a subfield of machine learning and has seen a dramatic resurgence recently, largely driven by increases in computational power and the availability of large data sets. Some of the greatest successes of deep learning have been in computer vision, which considerably accelerated AI applications of medical imaging. Numerous types of models, including convolutional neural networks (CNNs), recurrent neural networks (RNNs), autoencoders, generative adversarial networks, and reinforcement learning, have been developed for medical imaging applications, where they automatically learn features that optimally represent the data for a given task during the training process.[20,21] Medical images, nevertheless, pose a set of unique challenges to deep-learning-based computer vision methods, and breast imaging is no exception. For one, the high-dimensionality and large size of medical images allow them to contain a wealth of clinically useful information but make them not suitable for naive applications of standard CNNs developed for image recognition and object detection tasks in natural images. Furthermore, medical imaging data sets are usually relatively small in size and can have incomplete or noisy labels. The lack of interpretability is another hurdle in adopting deep-learning-based AI systems for clinical use. Transfer learning, fusion and aggregation methods, multiple-instance learning, and explainable AI methods continue to be developed to address these challenges in using deep learning algorithms for medical image analysis.[22–25]

Human-engineered radiomics and deep learning methods for breast imaging analysis both have advantages and disadvantages regarding computation efficiency, amount of data required, preprocessing, interpretability, and prediction accuracy. They should be chosen based on the specific tasks and can be potentially integrated to maximize the benefits of each.[26,27] The following sections will cover both of them for each clinical task when applicable.

ARTIFICIAL INTELLIGENCE IN BREAST CANCER RISK ASSESSMENT AND PREVENTION

Computer vision techniques have been developed to extract quantitative biomarkers from normal tissue that are related to cancer risk factors in the task of breast cancer risk assessment in AI-assisted breast image analysis. To improve upon the current one-size-fits-all screening programs, computerized risk assessment can potentially help estimate a woman's lifetime risk of breast cancer and, thus, recommend risk-stratified screening protocols and/or preventative therapies to reduce the overall risk. Risk models consider risk factors, including demographics, personal history, family history, hormonal status, and hormonal therapy, as well as image-based characteristics such as breast density and parenchymal pattern.

Breast density and parenchymal patterns have been shown to be strong indicators in breast cancer risk estimation.[28] Breast density refers to the amount of fibroglandular tissue relative to the amount of fatty tissue. These tissue types are distinguishable on FFDM because fibroglandular tissue attenuates x-ray beams much more than fatty tissue. Breast density has been assessed by radiologists using the four-category Breast Imaging Reporting and Data System (BI-RADS) density ratings, proposed by the American College of Radiology.[29] Computerized methods for assessing breast density include calculating the skewness of the gray-level histograms of FFDMs, as well as estimating volumetric density from the 2D projections on FFDMs.[8,30,31] Automated assessment of breast density on mammograms is now routinely performed using FDA-cleared clinical systems in breast cancer screening.

On a mammogram, the parenchymal pattern indicates the spatial distribution of dense tissue. To quantitatively evaluate the parenchymal pattern of the breast, various texture-based approaches have been investigated to characterize the spatial distribution of gray levels in FFDMs.[8] Such radiomic texture analyses have been conducted using data sets from high-risk groups (eg, BRCA1/BRCA2 gene mutation carriers and women with contralateral cancer) and data sets from low or average risk groups (eg, routine screening populations). Results have shown that women at high risk of breast cancer tend to have dense breasts with parenchymal patterns that are coarse and low in contrast.[32–34] Texture analysis on DBT images have also been conducted for risk assessment, with early results showing that texture features correlated with breast density better on DBT than on FFDM.[35]

Beyond FFDM and DBT, investigators have also assessed the background parenchymal enhancement (BPE) on DCE-MRI. It has been shown that quantitative measures of BPE are associated with the presence of breast cancer, and relative changes in BPE percentages are predictive of breast cancer development after risk-reducing salpingo-oophorectomy.[36] A more recent study shows that BPE is associated with an increased risk of breast cancer, and the risk is independent of breast density.[37]

Various deep learning methods for breast cancer risk assessment have been reported.[38,39] One of these methods has shown strong agreement with BI-RADS density assessments by radiologists.[40] Another deep learning approach has demonstrated superior performance to methods based on human-engineered features in assessing breast density on FFDMs, as deep learning algorithms can potentially extract additional information contained in FFDMs beyond features defined by human-engineered analytical expressions.[41] Moreover, studies have also compared and merged radiomic texture analysis and deep learning approaches in characterizing parenchymal patterns on FFDMs, showing that the combination yield improved results in predicting risk of breast cancer (**Fig. 2**).[39] Besides analyses of FFDM, a deep learning method based on U-Net has been developed to segment fibroglandular tissue on MRI to calculate breast density.[42]

ARTIFICIAL INTELLIGENCE IN BREAST CANCER SCREENING AND DETECTION

Detection of abnormalities in breast imaging is a common task for radiologists when reading screening images. Detection task refers to the localization of a lesion, including mass lesion, clustered microcalcifications, and architectural distortion, within the breast. One challenge when detecting abnormalities is that dense tissue can mask the presence of an underlying lesion at mammogram, resulting in missed cancers during breast cancer screening. In addition, radiologists' ability to detect lesions is also limited by inaccurate assessment of subtle or complex patterns, suboptimal image quality, and fatigue. Therefore, although screening programs have contributed to a reduction in breast cancer–related mortality,[43] this process tends to be costly, time-consuming, and error-prone. As a result, CADe methods have been in development for decades to serve a reader besides the radiologists in the task of finding suspicious lesions within images.

In the 1980s, CADe for clustered microcalcifications in digitized mammography was developed using a difference-image technique in which a signal-suppressed image was subtracted from a signal-enhanced image to remove the structured background.[44] Human-engineered features were extracted based on the understanding of the signal presentation on mammograms. With the introduction of FFDM, various radiomics methods have evolved and progressed over the years.[6–9,12] In 1994, a shift-invariant artificial neural network

was used for computerized detection of clustered microcalcifications in breast cancer screening, which was the first journal publication on the use of CNN in medical image analysis (**Fig. 3**).[45]

The ImageChecker M1000 system (version 1.2; R2 Technology, Los Altos, CA) was approved by the FDA in 1998, which marked the first clinical translation of mammographic CADe. The system was approved for use as a second reader, where the radiologist would first perform their own interpretation of the mammogram and would only view the CADe system output afterward. A potential lesion indicated by the radiologist but not by the computer output would not be eliminated, ensuring that the sensitivity would not be reduced with the use of CADe. Clinical adoption increased as CADe systems continued to improve. By 2008, CADe systems were used in 70% of screening mammography studies in hospital-based facilities and 81% of private offices[46] and stabilized at over 90% of digital mammography screening facilities in the US from 2008 to 2016.[47]

With the adoption of DBT in screening programs, the development of CADe methods for DBT images accelerated, first as a second reader and more recently as a concurrent reader.[48] A multireader, multi-case reader study evaluated a deep learning system developed to detect suspicious

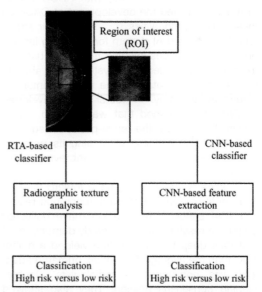

Fig. 2. Schematic of methods for the classification of ROIs using human-engineered texture feature analysis and deep convolutional neural network methods. ROI, region of interest. (*From* Li H. et al. Deep learning in breast cancer risk assessment: evaluation of convolutional neural networks on a clinical dataset of full-field digital mammograms. J Med Imaging 2017;**4**; with permission.)

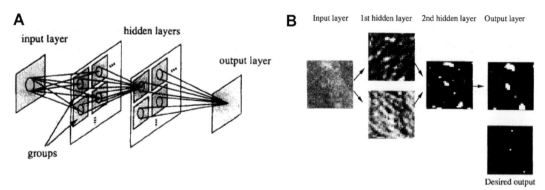

Fig. 3. Illustration of the first journal publication on the use of a convolutional neural network (CNN), that is, a shift-invariant neural network, in medical image analysis. The CNN was used in a computer-aided detection system to detect microcalcification on digitized mammograms and later on full-field digital mammograms. (A) A 2D shift-invariant neural network. (B) Illustration of input testing image, output image, desired output image, and responses in hidden layers. (*From* Zhang W. et al. Computerized detection of clustered microcalcifications in digital mammograms using a shift-invariant artificial neural network. Med Phys. 1994;21(4):517-524; with permission.)

soft-tissue and calcified lesions in DBT images and found that the concurrent use of AI improved cancer detection accuracy and efficiency as shown by the increased area under the receiver operating characteristic curve (AUC), sensitivity, and specificity, as well as the reduced recall rate and reading time.[49]

The recommendation for high-risk patients to receive additional screening with ABUS and/or MRI has motivated the development of CADe on these imaging modalities.[50–54] In a reader study, an FDA-approved AI system for detecting lesions on 3D ABUS images showed that when used as a concurrent reader, the system was able to reduce the interpretation time while maintaining diagnostic accuracy.[55] Another study developed a CNN-based method that was able to detect breast lesions on the early-phase images in DCE-MRI examinations, suggesting its potential use in screening programs with abbreviated MRI protocols.

Investigators continue working toward the ultimate goal of using AI as an autonomous reader in breast cancer screening and have delivered promising results.[56] A recent study demonstrated that their deep learning system yielded a higher AUC than the average AUC of six human readers and was noninferior to radiologists' double-reading consensus opinion. They also showed through simulation that the system could obviate double reading in 88% of UK screening cases while maintaining a similar level of accuracy to the standard protocol.[57] Another recent study proposed a deep learning model whose AUC was greater than the average AUC of 14 human readers, reducing the error approximately by half,

and combining radiologists' assessment and model prediction improved the average specificity by 6.3% compared to human readers alone (Fig. 4).[58] It is worth noting that similar to their predecessors, the new CADe systems require additional studies, especially prospective ones, to gauge their real-world performance, robustness, and generalizability before being introduced into the clinical workflow.

Furthermore, researchers are also investigating the use of AI for triaging and rule out in CADt systems. In a screening program with a CADt system implemented, a certain percentage of FFDMs would be deemed negative by the algorithm without having a radiologist read their mammograms, and those patients would be asked to return for their next screening after the regular screening interval (Fig. 5). In a simulation study, a deep learning approach was used to triage 20% of screening mammograms, and the results showed improvement in radiologist efficiency and specificity without sacrificing sensitivity.[59]

ARTIFICIAL INTELLIGENCE IN BREAST CANCER DIAGNOSIS AND PROGNOSIS

During the workup of a breast lesion, diagnosis and prognosis occur after the lesion has been detected by either screening mammography or other examinations. Lesion characterization occurs at this step, and thus, it is a classification task, leaving the radiologist to further assess the likelihood that the lesion is cancerous and determine if the patient should proceed to biopsy for pathologic confirmation. Oftentimes, multiple imaging modalities, including additional

A

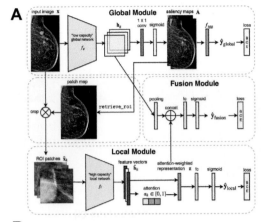

B

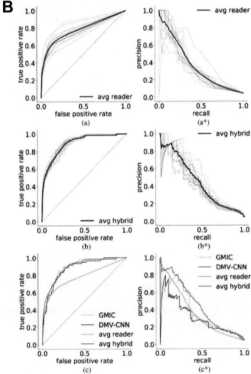

mammography, ultrasound, or MRI, are involved in this diagnostic step to better characterize the suspect lesion. When a cancerous tumor is diagnosed, additional imaging is usually conducted to assess the extent of the disease and determine patient management. Given its ability to quantitatively analyze complex patterns in images and process large amounts of information, AI is well suited for the tasks of breast cancer diagnosis and prognosis using image data.

Since the 1980s, investigators have been developing machine learning techniques for CADx in the task of distinguishing between malignant and benign breast lesions.[8] From the input image of a lesion, the AI algorithm either extracts human-engineered radiomic features or automatically learns predictive features in the case of deep learning and then outputs a probability of malignancy of the lesion. Algorithms should be trained using pathologically confirmed ground truth to ensure the quality of the data and, in turn, the predictions.

Over the decades, investigators have developed CADx methods that merge features into a tumor signature.[9,12,18] Although some radiomic features, such as size, shape, and morphology, can be extracted across various imaging modalities, others are dependent on the modality. For example, spiculation may be extracted from mammographic images of lesions with high spatial resolution, while kinetics-based features are special for DCE-MRI, which contains a temporal sequence of images that visualize the uptake and washout of the contrast agent in the breast.[13–17]

Fig. 4. (*A*) Overall architecture of the globally aware multiple instance classifier (GMIC), in which the patch map indicates positions of the region of interest patches (blue squares) on the input. (*B*) The receiver operating characteristic curves and precision-recall curves computed on the reader study set. (a, a*): Curves for all 14 readers. (b, b*): Curves for hybrid models with each single reader. The curve highlighted in blue indicates the average performance of all hybrids. (c, c*): Comparison among the GMIC, deep multiview convolutional neural network (DMV-CNN), the average reader, and average hybrid. (*From* Shen Y. et al. An interpretable classifier for high-resolution breast cancer screening images utilizing weakly supervised localization. Med Image Anal. 2021;**68**:101908; with permission. (For interpretation of the references to color in this figure legend, the reader is referred to the web version of this article.))

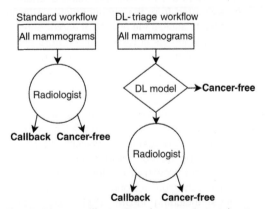

Fig. 5. Diagram illustrating the experimental setup for triage analysis (CADt). In the standard scenario, radiologists read all mammograms. In CADt (or rule-out), radiologists only read mammograms above the model's cancer-free threshold. (*From* Yala A. et al. A deep learning model to triage screening mammograms: a simulation study. Radiology 2019;**293**:38-46; with permission.)

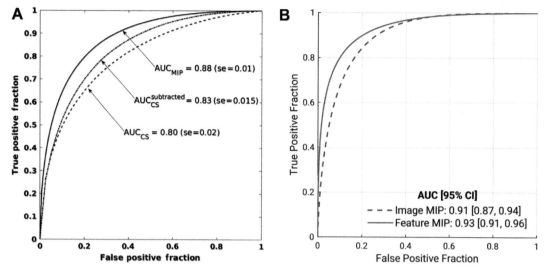

Fig. 6. Comparisons of classifier performance in distinguishing between benign and malignant breast lesions when different methods are used to incorporate volumetric information of breast lesions on DCE-MRI. (A) Using the maximum intensity projection (MIP) of the second postcontrast subtraction image outperformed using the central slice of both the second postcontrast subtraction images and the second-post contrast images. CS, central slice. (B) Feature MIP, that is, max pooling the feature space of all slices along the axial dimension, outperformed using image MIP at the input. (From [A] Antropova N, Abe H, Giger ML. Use of clinical MRI maximum intensity projections for improved breast lesion classification with deep convolutional neural networks. J Med Imaging 2018;5(1):14503; with permission. [B] Hu Q, et al. Improved Classification of Benign and Malignant Breast Lesions using Deep Feature Maximum Intensity Projection MRI in Breast Cancer Diagnosis using Dynamic Contrast-Enhanced MRI. Radiol Artif Intell. 2021:e200159; with permission.)

Moreover, when a feature defined by the same analytical expression is extracted from different imaging modalities, the phenotypes being quantified can be different. For example, texture features can be extracted from the enhancement patterns in DCE-MRI to assess the effects of angiogenesis, but these mathematical texture descriptors characterize different properties of the lesion when extracted from T2-weighted MRI or diffusion-weighted MRI because of the underlying differences between these MRI sequences.[60–62] There is also evidence that radiomic analysis on contralateral parenchyma, in addition to the lesion itself, may add value to breast lesion classification.[63]

Deep learning–based methods have also been developed and proven promising to differentiate benign and cancerous lesions on multiple imaging modalities, including FFDM, DBT, ABUS, and MRI.[64–67] Owing to the limited size of data sets in the medical imaging domain, transfer learning is often used where the deep network is initialized with weights pretrained on millions of natural images. As natural images are 2D color images, various approaches have been proposed to maximally use the information in high-dimensional (3D or 4D), gray-level medical images with the pretrained model architectures. For example, the maximum intensity projection of image slices or feature space as well as 3D CNNs has been used to incorporate volumetric information (Fig. 6), and subtraction images, RGB channels in pretrained CNNs, and RNNs have been used to incorporate temporal information (Fig. 7).[68–73]

-With the advancements in breast imaging technology, CADx methods continue to evolve to use the increasingly rich phenotypical information provided in the images and improve the diagnostic performance. For example, multiparametric MRI has been adopted for routine clinical use and has proven to improve clinical diagnostic performance for breast cancer because the different sequences in a multiparametric MRI examination provide complementary information.[5,74] AI methods that incorporate the multiple MRI sequences in an examination have been developed in recent years and have demonstrated improved diagnostic performance compared with using DCE-MRI alone (Fig. 8).[60,61,67,71] One of these studies investigated fusion strategies at various levels of the classification pipeline and found that latent feature fusion

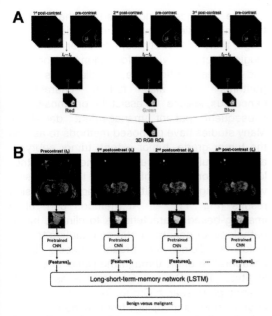

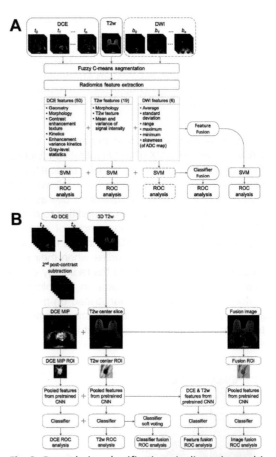

Fig. 7. Illustrations of image two approaches of using the temporal sequence of images in DCE-MRI in deep learning–based computer-aided diagnosis methods in distinguishing between benign and malignant breast lesions. (*A*) The same region of interest (ROI) is cropped from the first, second, and third postcontrast subtraction images and combined in the red, green, and blue (RGB) channels to form an RGB ROI. (*B*) Features extracted using a pretrained convolutional neural network (CNN) from all time points in DCE-MRI sequences are analyzed by a long short-term memory (LSTM) network to predict the probability of malignancy. (*From* [A] Hu Q. et al. Improved Classification of Benign and Malignant Breast Lesions using Deep Feature Maximum Intensity Projection MRI in Breast Cancer Diagnosis using Dynamic Contrast-Enhanced MRI. Radiol Artif Intell. 2021:e200159; with permission. [B] Antropova N, et al. Breast lesion classification based on dynamic contrast-enhanced magnetic resonance images sequences with long short-term memory networks. J Med Imaging 2018;6(1):1-7; with permission.)

was superior to image fusion and classifier output fusion.[67] Notable disagreement was observed between the predictions from classifiers based on different MRI sequences, suggesting that incorporating multiple sequences would be valuable in predicting the probability of malignancy of a lesion (Fig. 9).[61,67]

CADx systems based on human-engineered radiomics and deep learning models have been compared and combined. It is worth noting that these two types of machine intelligence have achieved comparable performances and have shown synergistic improvements when combined across multiple modalities (Fig. 10).[26,65,75]

Fig. 8. Breast lesion classification pipeline using multiparametric MRI exams using (*A*) human-engineered radiomics and (*B*) deep learning. (*A*) Radiomic features are extracted from dynamic contrast-enhanced (DCE), T2-weighted (T2w), and diffusion-weighted (DWI) MRI sequences. Information from the three sequences is integrated using two fusion strategies: feature fusion, that is, concatenating features extracted from all sequences to train a classifier, and classifier fusion, that is, aggregating the probability of malignancy output from all single-parametric classifiers via soft voting. Parentheses contain the numbers of features extracted from each sequence. The dashed lines for DWI indicate that the DWI sequence is not available in all cases and is included in the classification process when it is available. (*B*) Information DCE and T2w MRI sequences are integrated using three fusion strategies: image fusion, that is, fusing DCE and T2w images to create RGB composite image, feature fusion as defined in (*A*), and classifier fusion as defined in (*A*). ADC, apparent diffusion coefficient; CNN, convolutional neural network; MIP, maximum intensity projection; ROI, region of interest; ROC, receiver operating characteristic; SVM, support vector machine. ([A] *From* Hu Q, Whitney HM, Giger ML. Radiomics methodology for breast cancer diagnosis using multiparametric magnetic resonance imaging. J Med Imaging. 2020;**7**(4):44502; with permission. [B] Adapted from Hu Q, Whitney HM,

The FDA cleared the first commercial breast CADx system (QuantX from Quantitative Insights, Chicago, IL; now Qlarity Imaging) for clinical translation in 2017,[76,77] and others have followed for various breast imaging modalities for use as secondary or concurrent readers. In addition to evaluating the diagnostic performance of the AI algorithms themselves, CADx systems have also been evaluated in reader studies when their predictions are incorporated into the radiology workflow as an aid. Improvement in radiologists' performance has been demonstrated on multiple imaging modalities in the task of distinguishing between benign and malignant breast lesions.[77–80]

Once a cancer is identified, further workup through biopsies provides information on the stage, molecular subtypes, and other histopathological factors to yield information on prognosis and treatment options. Beyond diagnosis, AI algorithms can also further characterize cancerous lesions to assist in prognosis and subsequent patient management decisions. Many studies have proposed methods to assess the tumor grade, tumor extent, tumor subtype, and molecular subtypes and other histopathological information of breast lesions using various imaging modalities and shown promising results (**Fig. 11**).[81–93] AI methods can relate imaging-based characteristics to clinical, histopathology, or genomic data, contributing to precision medicine for breast cancer. In a collaborative effort through the National Cancer Institute The Cancer Genome Atlas Breast Phenotype Research Group, for example, investigators studied mappings from image-based information of breast tumors extracted to clinical,

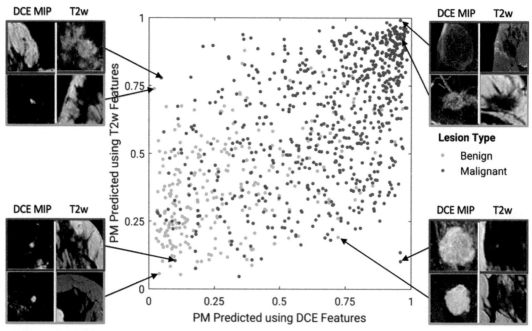

Fig. 9. A diagonal classifier agreement plot between the T2-weighted (T2w) and dynamic contrast-enhanced (DCE)-MRI single-sequence deep learning–based classifiers. The x-axis and y-axis denote the probability of malignancy (PM) scores predicted by the DCE classifier and the T2w classifier, respectively. Each point represents a lesion for which predictions were made. Points along or near the diagonal from bottom left to top right indicate high classifier agreement; points far from the diagonal indicate low agreement. A notable disagreement between the two classifiers is observed, suggesting that features extracted from the two MRI sequences provide complementary information, and it is likely valuable to incorporate multiple sequences in multiparametric MRI when making a computer-aided diagnosis prediction. Examples of lesions on which the two classifiers are in extreme agreement/disagreement are also included. (*From* Hu Q, Whitney HM, Giger ML. A deep learning methodology for improved breast cancer diagnosis using multiparametric MRI. Sci Rep. 2020;**10**(1):1-11; with permission. This article is licensed under a Creative Commons Attribution 4.0 International License: http://creativecommons.org/licenses/by/4.0/.)

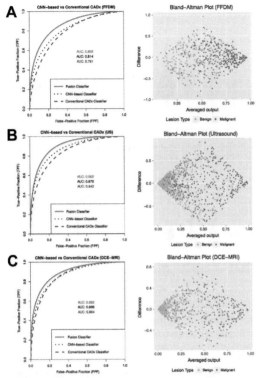

Fig. 10. *Left column*: Fitted binormal ROC curves comparing the performances of classifiers based on human-engineered radiomics, convolutional neural network (CNN), and fusion of the two on three imaging modalities. *Right column*: Associated Bland-Altman plots illustrating agreement between the classifiers based on human-engineered radiomics and CNN. Since the averaged output is used in the fusion classifier, these plots also help visualize potential decision boundaries for the fusion classifier. (*From* Antropova N, Huynh BQ, Giger ML. A deep feature fusion methodology for breast cancer diagnosis demonstrated on three imaging modality datasets. Med Phys 2017;**44**(10):5162-71; with permission.)

important role that tumor heterogeneity plays in the prognosis of cancerous lesions, AI-assisted analysis of images presents a strong potential impact on breast cancer prognosis.

ARTIFICIAL INTELLIGENCE IN BREAST CANCER TREATMENT RESPONSE AND RISK OF RECURRENCE

AI algorithms can also be used to assess tumor response to therapy and the risk of recurrence during the treatment of breast cancer. In one example, the size of the most enhancing voxels within the tumor, which was initially extracted from DCE-MRI using a fuzzy c-means method for CADx, has been found useful in assessing recurrence-free survival before or early on during neoadjuvant chemotherapy (NAC) and yielded a comparable performance as another semi-manual method on cases in the I-SPY1 trial.[95–97] Another recent study found that while pre-NAC tumor features generally appear uninformative in predicting response to therapy, some pre-NAC lymph node features are predictive.[98] Others have used CNNs to predict pathologic complete response (pCR) using the I-SPY1 database and yielded probability heatmaps that indicate regions within the tumors most strongly associated with pCR.[99] In another study, a long short-term memory network was able to predict recurrence-free survival in patients with breast cancer only using MRIs acquired early on during the NAC treatment.[99] Furthermore, in a study by the TCGA Breast Phenotype Research Group, breast MRIs were quantitatively mapped to research versions of gene assays and showed a significant association between the radiomics signatures and the multigene assay recurrence scores, demonstrating the potential of MRI-based biomarkers for predicting the risk of recurrence.[100]

Using AI to predict treatment response effectively serves as a "virtual biopsy" that can be conducted during multiple rounds of therapy to track the tumor over time when an actual biopsy is not practical. Such image-based signatures have the potential for increasing the precision in individualized patient management. Moreover, currently unknown correlations between observed phenotypes and genotypes may be discovered through the mappings between imaging data and genomic data, and the unveiled image-based biomarkers can be used in routine screening, prognosis, and monitoring in the future, providing possibilities to improve early detection and better management of the disease.

molecular, and genomic markers. Statistically significant associations were observed between enhancement texture features on DCE-MRI and molecular subtypes.[84] Associations between MRI and genomic data were also reported, shedding light on the genetic mechanisms that govern the development of tumor phenotypes, which formed a basis for the future development of noninvasive imaging-based techniques for accurate cancer diagnosis and prognosis (Fig. 12).[94]

Besides its noninvasiveness, such an imaging-based "virtual biopsy" can also provide the advantage of examining a tumor in its entirety, rather than only evaluating the biopsy samples that constitute small parts of a tumor. Given the

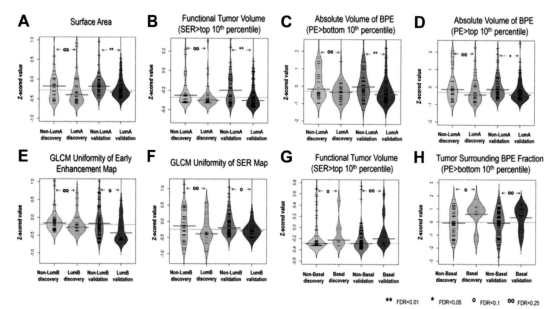

Fig. 11. Imaging features significantly associated with molecular subtypes (after correction for multiple testing) in both discovery and validation cohorts, (*A–D*) four features for distinguishing luminal A versus nonluminal A; (*E, F*) two features for distinguishing luminal B versus nonluminal B; and (*G, H*) two features for distinguishing basal-like versus nonbasal-like. Wilcoxon rank-sum test was implemented to investigate pairwise differences. Also, the FDR adjusted for multiple testing is reported. (*From* Wu J, Sun X, Wang J, et al. Identifying relations between imaging phenotypes and molecular subtypes of breast cancer: Model discovery and external validation. J Magn Reson Imaging. 2017;**46**(4):1017-1027; with permission.)

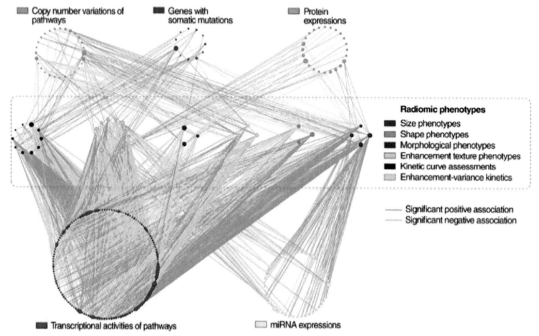

Fig. 12. Statistically significant associations between genomic features and radiomic features on MRI in breast carcinoma. Genomic features are organized into circles by data platform and indicated by different node colors. Genomic features without statistically significant associations are not shown. Radiomic phenotypes in six categories are also indicated by different node colors. The node size is proportional to its connectivity relative to other nodes in the category. (*From* Zhu Y. et al. Deciphering genomic underpinnings of quantitative MRI-based radiomic phenotypes of invasive breast carcinoma. Sci Rep 2015;**42**(6):3603; with permission.)

CHALLENGES IN THE FIELD AND FUTURE DIRECTIONS

Although many breast imaging AI publications are published each year, there are still only a few algorithms that are being translated to clinical care, hindered often by lack of large data sets, which are diverse and well-curated, for training and independent testing. Creating such large data sets will require a change in data-sharing culture allowing for medical institutions to contribute their medical images and data to common image repositories for the public good.

Furthermore, for AI methods to be translated ultimately to clinical care, the algorithms need to demonstrate high performance over a large range of radiological presentations of various breast cancer states on user-friendly interfaces.

In addition, AI methods can be perceived as a "black box" for medical tasks. More research is needed on the *explainability* of AI methods to help the developer and on the *interpretability* of AI methods to aid the user. It is interesting to contemplate when might AI be acceptable without giving reasons for its output. To reach such a stage will require high performance in the given clinical task along with high reproducibility and repeatability.

AI in breast imaging is expected to impact both interpretation efficacy and workflow efficiency in radiology as it is applied to imaging examinations being routinely obtained in clinical practice. Although there are more and more novel machine intelligence methods being developed, currently the main use will be in decision support, that is, computers will augment human decision-making as opposed to replacing radiologist decision-making.

CLINICS CARE POINTS

> - Radiologists need to understand the performance level and correct use of AI applications in medical imaging.

FUNDING INFORMATION

The authors are partially supported by NIH QIN Grant U01CA195564, NIH S10 OD025081 Shared Instrument Grant, the University of Chicago Comprehensive Cancer Center, and an RSNA/AAPM Graduate Fellowship.

DISCLOSURE

Q.Hu declares no competing interests. M.L. Giger is a stockholder in R2 technology/Hologic and QView; receives royalties from Hologic, GE Medical Systems, MEDIAN Technologies, Riverain Medical, Mitsubishi, and Toshiba; and is a cofounder of Quantitative Insights (now Qlarity Imaging). Following the University of Chicago Conflict of Interest Policy, the investigators disclose publicly actual or potential significant financial interest that would reasonably appear to be directly and significantly affected by the research activities.

REFERENCE

1. Siegel RL, Miller KD, Fuchs HE, et al. Cancer statistics, 2021. CA Cancer J Clin 2021;71(1):7–33.
2. Niell BL, Freer PE, Weinfurtner RJ, et al. Screening for breast cancer. Radiol Clin North Am 2017;55(6):1145–62.
3. ACR appropriateness criteria: breast cancer screening. American College of Radiology; 2017. Available at: https://acsearch.acr.org/docs/70910/Narrative. Accessed January 17, 2021.
4. Nelson HD, O'Meara ES, Kerlikowske K, et al. Factors associated with rates of false-positive and false-negative results from digital mammography screening: an analysis of registry data. Ann Intern Med 2016;164(4):226–35.
5. Mann RM, Cho N, Moy L. Breast MRI: state of the art. Radiology 2019;292(3):520–36.
6. Vyborny CJ, Giger ML. Computer vision and artificial intelligence in mammography. Am J Roentgenol 1994;162(3):699–708.
7. Vyborny CJ, Giger ML, Nishikawa RM. Computer-aided detection and diagnosis of breast cancer. Radiol Clin North Am 2000;38(4):725–40.
8. Giger ML, Karssemeijer N, Schnabel JA. Breast image analysis for risk assessment, detection, diagnosis, and treatment of cancer. Annu Rev Biomed Eng 2013;15:327–57.
9. El Naqa I, Haider MA, Giger ML, et al. Artificial Intelligence: reshaping the practice of radiological sciences in the 21st century. Br J Radiol 2020;93(1106):20190855.
10. Li H, Giger ML. Chapter 15 - Artificial intelligence and interpretations in breast cancer imaging. In: Xing L, Giger ML, Min JK, editors. Artificial intelligence in medicine. Cambridge (MA): Academic Press; 2021. p. 291–308.
11. FDA cleared AI algorithm. Available at: https://models.acrdsi.org. Accessed March 7, 2021.
12. Giger ML, Chan H-P, Boone J. Anniversary paper: history and status of CAD and quantitative image analysis: the role of medical physics and AAPM. Med Phys 2008;35(12):5799–820.
13. Gilhuijs KGA, Giger ML, Bick U. Computerized analysis of breast lesions in three dimensions using

dynamic magnetic-resonance imaging. Med Phys 1998;25(9):1647–54.

14. Chen W, Giger ML, Lan L, et al. Computerized interpretation of breast MRI: investigation of enhancement-variance dynamics. Med Phys 2004;31:1076–82.

15. Chen W, Giger ML, Bick U, et al. Automatic identification and classification of characteristic kinetic curves of breast lesions on DCE-MRI. Med Phys 2006;33(8):2878–87.

16. Chen W, Giger ML, Li H, et al. Volumetric texture analysis of breast lesions on contrast-enhanced magnetic resonance images. Magn Reson Med 2007;58(3):562–71.

17. Chen W, Giger ML, Newstead GM, et al. Computerized assessment of breast lesion malignancy using DCE-MRI: robustness study on two independent clinical datasets from two manufacturers. Acad Radiol 2010;17(7):822–9.

18. Giger ML. Machine learning in medical imaging. J Am Coll Radiol 2018;15(3):512–20.

19. Esteva A, Robicquet A, Ramsundar B, et al. A guide to deep learning in healthcare. Nat Med 2019;25(1):24–9.

20. Litjens G, Kooi T, Bejnordi BE, et al. A survey on deep learning in medical image analysis. Med Image Anal 2017;42:60–88.

21. Sahiner B, Pezeshk A, Hadjiiski LM, et al. Deep learning in medical imaging and radiation therapy. Med Phys 2019;46(1):e1–36.

22. Maron O, Lozano-Pérez T. A framework for multiple-instance learning. In: Kearns MJ, Solla SA, Cohn DA, editors. Advances in neural information processing systems. Cambridge (MA): The MIT Press; 1998. p. 570–6.

23. Tajbakhsh N, Shin JY, Gurudu SR, et al. Convolutional neural networks for medical image analysis: Full training or fine tuning? IEEE Trans Med Imaging 2016;35(5):1299–312.

24. Shin H-C, Roth HR, Gao M, et al. Deep convolutional neural networks for computer-aided detection: CNN architectures, dataset characteristics and transfer learning. IEEE Trans Med Imaging 2016;35(5):1285–98.

25. Zhang Q, Zhu S-C. Visual interpretability for deep learning: a survey. Front Inf Technol Electron Eng 2018;19(1):27–39.

26. Whitney HM, Li H, Ji Y, et al. Comparison of breast MRI tumor classification using human-engineered radiomics, transfer learning from deep convolutional neural networks, and fusion method. Proc IEEE 2019;108(1):163–77.

27. Truhn D, Schrading S, Haarburger C, et al. Radiomic versus convolutional neural networks analysis for classification of contrast-enhancing lesions at multiparametric breast MRI. Radiology 2019; 290(2):290–7.

28. Freer PE. Mammographic breast density: impact on breast cancer risk and implications for screening. RadioGraphics 2015;35(2):302–15.

29. D'Orsi C, Sickles E, Mendelson E, et al. ACR BI-RADS® atlas, breast imaging reporting and data system. Reston, VA, American College of Radiology; 2013.

30. Byng JW, Yaffe MJ, Lockwood GA, et al. Automated analysis of mammographic densities and breast carcinoma risk. Cancer 1997;80(1):66–74.

31. van Engeland S, Snoeren PR, Huisman H, et al. Volumetric breast density estimation from full-field digital mammograms. IEEE Trans Med Imaging 2006;25(3):273–82.

32. Li H, Giger ML, Olopade OI, et al. Power spectral analysis of mammographic parenchymal patterns for breast cancer risk assessment. J Digit Imaging 2008;21(2):145–52.

33. Li H, Giger ML, Olopade OI, et al. Fractal analysis of mammographic parenchymal patterns in breast cancer risk assessment. Acad Radiol 2007;14(5):513–21.

34. Huo Z, Giger ML, Olopade OI, et al. Computerized analysis of digitized mammograms of BRCA1 and BRCA2 gene mutation carriers. Radiology 2002;225(2):519–26.

35. Kontos D, Bakic PR, Carton A-K, et al. Parenchymal texture analysis in digital breast tomosynthesis for breast cancer risk estimation: a preliminary study. Acad Radiol 2009;16(3):283–98.

36. Wu S, Weinstein SP, DeLeo MJ, et al. Quantitative assessment of background parenchymal enhancement in breast MRI predicts response to risk-reducing salpingo-oophorectomy: preliminary evaluation in a cohort of BRCA1/2 mutation carriers. Breast Cancer Res 2015;17(1):67.

37. Arasu VA, Miglioretti DL, Sprague BL, et al. Population-based assessment of the association between magnetic resonance imaging background parenchymal enhancement and future primary breast cancer risk. J Clin Oncol 2019;37(12):954–63.

38. Gastounioti A, Oustimov A, Hsieh M-K, et al. Using convolutional neural networks for enhanced capture of breast parenchymal complexity patterns associated with breast cancer risk. Acad Radiol 2018;25(8):977–84.

39. Li H, Giger ML, Huynh BQ, et al. Deep learning in breast cancer risk assessment: evaluation of convolutional neural networks on a clinical dataset of full-field digital mammograms. J Med Imaging 2017;4(4):41304.

40. Lee J, Nishikawa RM. Automated mammographic breast density estimation using a fully convolutional network. Med Phys 2018;45(3):1178–90.

41. Li S, Wei J, Chan H-P, et al. Computer-aided assessment of breast density: comparison of

supervised deep learning and feature-based statistical learning. Phys Med Biol 2018;63(2):25005.

42. Dalmış MU, Litjens G, Holland K, et al. Using deep learning to segment breast and fibroglandular tissue in MRI volumes. Med Phys 2017;44(2):533–46.

43. Lauby-Secretan B, Scoccianti C, Loomis D, et al. Breast-cancer screening — viewpoint of the IARC Working Group. N Engl J Med 2015;372(24):2353–8.

44. Chan H-P, Doi K, Galhotra S, et al. Image feature analysis and computer-aided diagnosis in digital radiography. I. Automated detection of microcalcifications in mammography. Med Phys 1987;14(4):538–48.

45. Zhang W, Doi K, Giger ML, et al. Computerized detection of clustered microcalcifications in digital mammograms using a shift-invariant artificial neural network. Med Phys 1994;21(4):517–24.

46. Rao VM, Levin DC, Parker L, et al. How widely is computer-aided detection used in screening and diagnostic mammography? J Am Coll Radiol 2010;7(10):802–5.

47. Keen JD, Keen JM, Keen JE. Utilization of computer-aided detection for digital screening mammography in the United States, 2008 to 2016. J Am Coll Radiol 2018;15(1, Part A):44–8.

48. Geras KJ, Mann RM, Moy L. Artificial intelligence for mammography and digital breast tomosynthesis: current concepts and future perspectives. Radiology 2019;293(2):246–59.

49. Conant EF, Toledano AY, Periaswamy S, et al. Improving accuracy and efficiency with concurrent use of artificial intelligence for digital breast tomosynthesis. Radiol Artif Intell 2019;1(4):e180096.

50. Kuhl CK. Abbreviated breast MRI for screening women with dense breast: the EA1141 trial. Br J Radiol 2018;91(1090):20170441.

51. Supplemental screening for breast cancer in women with dense breasts: a systematic review for the U.S. preventive services task force. Ann Intern Med 2016;164(4):268–78.

52. Giger ML, Inciardi MF, Edwards A, et al. Automated breast ultrasound in breast cancer screening of women with dense breasts: reader study of mammography-negative and mammography-positive cancers. Am J Roentgenol 2016;206(6):1341–50.

53. Comstock CE, Gatsonis C, Newstead GM, et al. Comparison of abbreviated breast MRI vs digital breast tomosynthesis for breast cancer detection among women with dense breasts undergoing screening. JAMA 2020;323(8):746–56.

54. van Zelst JCM, Tan T, Clauser P, et al. Dedicated computer-aided detection software for automated 3D breast ultrasound; an efficient tool for the radiologist in supplemental screening of

women with dense breasts. Eur Radiol 2018;28(7):2996–3006.

55. Jiang Y, Inciardi MF, Edwards AV, et al. Interpretation time using a concurrent-read computer-aided detection system for automated breast ultrasound in breast cancer screening of women with dense breast tissue. Am J Roentgenol 2018;211(2):452–61.

56. Sechopoulos I, Mann RM. Stand-alone artificial intelligence - The future of breast cancer screening? Breast 2020;49:254–60.

57. McKinney SM, Sieniek M, Godbole V, et al. International evaluation of an AI system for breast cancer screening. Nature 2020;577(7788):89–94.

58. Shen Y, Wu N, Phang J, et al. An interpretable classifier for high-resolution breast cancer screening images utilizing weakly supervised localization. Med Image Anal 2021;68:101908.

59. Yala A, Schuster T, Miles R, et al. A deep learning model to triage screening mammograms: a simulation study. Radiology 2019;293(1):38–46.

60. Bhooshan N, Giger M, Lan L, et al. Combined use of T2-weighted MRI and T1-weighted dynamic contrast-enhanced MRI in the automated analysis of breast lesions. Magn Reson Med 2011;66(2):555–64.

61. Hu Q, Whitney HM, Giger ML. Radiomics methodology for breast cancer diagnosis using multiparametric magnetic resonance imaging. J Med Imaging 2020;7(4):44502.

62. Parekh VS, Jacobs MA. Integrated radiomic framework for breast cancer and tumor biology using advanced machine learning and multiparametric MRI. NPJ Breast Cancer 2017;3(1):43.

63. Li H, Mendel KR, Lan L, et al. Digital mammography in breast cancer: additive value of radiomics of breast parenchyma. Radiology 2019;291(1):15–20.

64. Huynh BQ, Li H, Giger ML. Digital mammographic tumor classification using transfer learning from deep convolutional neural networks. J Med Imaging 2016;3(3):34501.

65. Antropova N, Huynh BQ, Giger ML. A deep feature fusion methodology for breast cancer diagnosis demonstrated on three imaging modality datasets. Med Phys 2017;44(10):5162–71.

66. Samala RK, Chan H-P, Hadjiiski LM, et al. Evolutionary pruning of transfer learned deep convolutional neural network for breast cancer diagnosis in digital breast tomosynthesis. Phys Med Biol 2018;63(9):95005.

67. Hu Q, Whitney HM, Giger ML. A deep learning methodology for improved breast cancer diagnosis using multiparametric MRI. Sci Rep 2020;10(1):1–11.

68. Antropova N, Abe H, Giger ML. Use of clinical MRI maximum intensity projections for improved breast

lesion classification with deep convolutional neural networks. J Med Imaging 2018;5(1):14503.

69. Hu Q, Whitney HM, Giger ML. Transfer learning in 4D for breast cancer diagnosis using dynamic contrast-enhanced magnetic resonance imaging. arXiv Prepr arXiv191103022. 2019.

70. Hu Q, Whitney HM, Li H, et al. Improved classification of benign and malignant breast lesions using deep feature maximum intensity projection MRI in breast cancer diagnosis using dynamic contrast-enhanced MRI. Radiol Artif Intell 2021;3(3):e200159.

71. Dalmis MU, Gubern-Mérida A, Vreemann S, et al. Artificial intelligence–based classification of breast lesions imaged with a multiparametric breast MRI protocol with ultrafast DCE-MRI, T2, and DWI. Invest Radiol 2019;54(6):325–32.

72. Li J, Fan M, Zhang J, et al. Discriminating between benign and malignant breast tumors using 3D convolutional neural network in dynamic contrast enhanced-MR images. In: Cook TS, Zhang J, editors. medical imaging 2017: imaging Informatics for healthcare, research, and applications. vol. 10138. Bellingham (WA): SPIE Press; 2017: 1013808.

73. Antropova N, Huynh B, Li H, et al. Breast lesion classification based on dynamic contrast-enhanced magnetic resonance images sequences with long short-term memory networks. J Med Imaging 2018;6(1):1–7.

74. Leithner D, Wengert GJ, Helbich TH, et al. Clinical role of breast MRI now and going forward. Clin Radiol 2018;73(8):700–14.

75. Hu Q, Whitney HM, Edwards A, et al. Radiomics and deep learning of diffusion-weighted MRI in the diagnosis of breast cancer. In: Mori K, Hahn HK, editors. Medical imaging 2019: computer-aided diagnosis. vol. 10950. Bellingham (WA): SPIE Press; 2019:109504A.

76. Evaluation of Automatic Class III Designation (De Novo) Summaries. The Food and Drug Administration.

77. Jiang Y, Edwards AV, Newstead GM. Artificial intelligence applied to breast MRI for improved diagnosis. Radiology 2021;298(1):38–46.

78. Huo Z, Giger ML, Vyborny CJ, et al. Breast cancer: effectiveness of computer-aided diagnosis—observer study with independent database of mammograms. Radiology 2002;224(2):560–8.

79. Horsch K, Giger ML, Vyborny CJ, et al. Performance of computer-aided diagnosis in the interpretation of lesions on breast sonography. Acad Radiol 2004;11(3):272–80.

80. Shimauchi A, Giger ML, Bhooshan N, et al. Evaluation of clinical breast MR imaging performed with prototype computer-aided diagnosis breast MR imaging workstation: reader study. Radiology 2011; 258(3):696–704.

81. Loiselle C, Eby PR, Kim JN, et al. Preoperative MRI improves prediction of extensive occult axillary lymph node metastases in breast cancer patients with a positive sentinel lymph node biopsy. Acad Radiol 2014;21(1):92–8.

82. Schacht DV, Drukker K, Pak I, et al. Using quantitative image analysis to classify axillary lymph nodes on breast MRI: a new application for the Z 0011 Era. Eur J Radiol 2015;84(3):392–7.

83. Guo W, Li H, Zhu Y, et al. Prediction of clinical phenotypes in invasive breast carcinomas from the integration of radiomics and genomics data. J Med Imaging 2015;2(4):1–12.

84. Li H, Zhu Y, Burnside ES, et al. Quantitative MRI radiomics in the prediction of molecular classifications of breast cancer subtypes in the TCGA/TCIA data set. npj Breast Cancer 2016;2(1):16012.

85. Bhooshan N, Giger ML, Jansen SA, et al. Cancerous breast lesions on dynamic contrast-enhanced MR images. Breast Imaging 2010; 254(3):680–90.

86. Liu W, Cheng Y, Liu Z, et al. Preoperative prediction of Ki-67 status in breast cancer with multiparametric MRI using transfer learning. Acad Radiol 2021; 28(2):e44–53.

87. Liang C, Cheng Z, Huang Y, et al. An MRI-based radiomics classifier for preoperative prediction of Ki-67 status in breast cancer. Acad Radiol 2018; 25(9):1111–7.

88. Ma W, Zhao Y, Ji Y, et al. Breast cancer molecular subtype prediction by mammographic radiomic features. Acad Radiol 2019;26(2):196–201.

89. Leithner D, Mayerhoefer ME, Martinez DF, et al. Non-invasive assessment of breast cancer molecular subtypes with multiparametric magnetic resonance imaging radiomics. J Clin Med 2020;9(6): 1853.

90. Son J, Lee SE, Kim E-K, et al. Prediction of breast cancer molecular subtypes using radiomics signatures of synthetic mammography from digital breast tomosynthesis. Sci Rep 2020;10(1):21566.

91. Grimm LJ, Zhang J, Baker JA, et al. Relationships between MRI Breast Imaging-Reporting and Data System (BI-RADS) lexicon descriptors and breast cancer molecular subtypes: internal enhancement is associated with luminal B subtype. Breast J 2017;23(5):579–82.

92. Wu J, Sun X, Wang J, et al. Identifying relations between imaging phenotypes and molecular subtypes of breast cancer: model discovery and external validation. J Magn Reson Imaging 2017; 46(4):1017–27.

93. Burnside ES, Drukker K, Li H, et al. Using computer-extracted image phenotypes from tumors on breast magnetic resonance imaging to predict breast cancer pathologic stage. Cancer 2016;122(5):748–57.

94. Zhu Y, Li H, Guo W, et al. TU-CD-BRB-06: deciphering genomic underpinnings of quantitative MRI-based radiomic phenotypes of invasive breast carcinoma. Med Phys 2015;42(6Part32):3603.

95. Chen W, Giger ML, Bick U. A fuzzy c-means (FCM)-based approach for computerized segmentation of breast lesions in dynamic contrast-enhanced MR images. Acad Radiol 2006;13(1): 63–72.

96. Hylton NM, Gatsonis CA, Rosen MA, et al. Neoadjuvant chemotherapy for breast cancer: functional tumor volume by MR imaging predicts recurrence-free survival—results from the ACRIN 6657/CALGB 150007 I-SPY 1 TRIAL. Radiology 2016;279(1):44–55.

97. Drukker K, Li H, Antropova N, et al. Most-enhancing tumor volume by MRI radiomics predicts recurrence-free survival "early on" in neoadjuvant treatment of breast cancer. Cancer Imaging 2018;18(1):12.

98. Drukker K, Edwards AV, Doyle C, et al. Breast MRI radiomics for the pretreatment prediction of response to neoadjuvant chemotherapy in node-positive breast cancer patients. J Med Imaging 2019;6(3):34502.

99. Ravichandran K, Braman N, Janowczyk A, et al. A deep learning classifier for prediction of pathological complete response to neoadjuvant chemotherapy from baseline breast DCE-MRI. In: Petrick N, Mori K, editors. Medical imaging 2018: computer-aided diagnosis, vol. 10575. Bellingham (WA): SPIE; 2018. p. 79–88.

100. Li H, Zhu Y, Burnside ES, et al. Mr imaging radiomics signatures for predicting the risk of breast cancer recurrence as given by research versions of mammaprint, oncotype DX, and PAM50 gene assays. Radiology 2016;281(2):382–91.

Artificial Intelligence Enabling Radiology Reporting

Bernardo C. Bizzo, MD, PhD[a], Renata R. Almeida, MD, PhD[b],
Tarik K. Alkasab, MD, PhD[a],*

KEYWORDS

- Artificial intelligence • Machine learning • Deep learning • Radiology • Report • Structured
- Integration

KEY POINTS

- The radiology reporting process is beginning to incorporate structured data, including common data element identifiers for bringing a universal ontology to radiology reports.
- Artificial intelligence tools can assist with internal consistency, determine whether additional information is required, provide suggestions to make expert-like reports, and help with longitudinal tracking.
- A dynamic to-do list could be assembled by artificial intelligence tools to ensure that they are addressed by the current report.
- Radiologists will review and determine if artificial intelligence-generated data should be transmitted to the electronic health record, and generate feedback for monitoring and continuous tool improvement.
- Artificial intelligence has the potential to move the radiologists emphasis onto more advanced cognitive tasks while increasing the clinical relevance of reports for driving decision support and care pathways.

INTRODUCTION

The work product of radiology is the radiology report, which is still most typically a plain text, natural language description of the radiologists' observations, synthesized impressions of the clinical situation, and possibly recommendations for further management of the patient. As artificial intelligence (AI) plays an increasing role throughout medicine, the data-oriented nature of imaging has made it an early target for application. Because the radiology report is the end-product of the interpretation process, the reporting process is a natural place for the application of AI technologies. This situation creates certain challenges to overcome, but also presents important opportunities for improving the reporting process. The challenges primarily center around the process of incorporating data into the reporting process, whereas the opportunities can relate to long-standing obstacles in creating high-quality radiology reports.

The radiology report has traditionally been natural language text generated by a radiologist via voice dictation. In recent years, the standard practice has moved toward structured reporting,[1] but this practice has typically remained within the framework of plain text reports without associated structured data. This process presents a challenge to integrate results generated by AI tools into radiology results. Progress has been made in incorporating structured numeric and categorical data into

[a] Department of Radiology, Massachusetts General Hospital, Harvard Medical School, 55 Fruit Street, Founders 210, Boston, MA 02114, USA; [b] Department of Radiology, Brigham and Women's Hospital, Harvard Medical School, 75 Francis St, Boston, MA 02115, USA
* Corresponding author.
E-mail address: TALKASAB@mgh.harvard.edu

Radiol Clin N Am 59 (2021) 1045–1052
https://doi.org/10.1016/j.rcl.2021.07.004

the radiology reporting process and product. This process can manifest as a bilayered radiology report with a text layer resembling the current plain text radiology report along with a data layer, consisting of appropriately tagged structured data. The American College of Radiology (ACR) and the Radiological Society of North America have collaborated to create a registry of common data element identifiers for the purpose of bringing a universal ontology to this data layer.[2,3] Although these efforts are in an early stage, they will clearly form an important part of the foundation for incorporating AI tools into radiology reporting, and much of the further discussion will presuppose this kind of data structure underlying the radiology report.

Most of the progress toward implementing AI into radiology reporting in the recent past has been focused on leveraging simple sentences generated by AI imaging analysis tools and using natural language processing (NLP) tools for the annotation, summarization, or extraction of findings from reports.[4–7] The creation of radiology reporting tools integrating convolutional neural networks for image analysis alongside recurrent neural networks for NLP to integrate structured data as part of the radiology result is an area of growing research interest.[8] The new generation of AI-enabled NLP has made possible the extraction of structured data from the dictated text that radiologists are currently creating (or have previously created).[9] This development could lead to a more sophisticated reporting system in which as a radiologist describes a finding using voice dictation, an NLP-based system automatically recognizes what has been described (eg, a hepatic lesion) and encodes the relevant attributes of that entity (eg, size, location, enhancement characteristics) with semantic labels. This process could help radiologists to evolve their practice of reporting to one underpinned by structured data.

This process leads to an opportunity for AI to be applied to several important problems in radiology reporting, such as that of internal report consistency. For example, a radiologist may describe a tumor in the left kidney in the body of their report, but then in their impression, misplace the lesion in the right kidney.[10] Another common issue is the description of wrong-sex structures, such as the uterus in a man or a prostate in a woman. Once descriptions are captured as structured data, these descriptions can be analyzed for internal consistency and potential errors flagged for the radiologist to review before final signing. An even more common and dangerous scenario is radiologists describing the absence of a finding in the body of their report (or not describing a finding at all in the body of their

report) and then, through a dictation error, seeming to indicate that such a finding is present in the impression. For example, a radiologist might say that the pleural spaces are clear in the body of the report, intend to say, "No evidence of pneumothorax" in the impression of their report, but owing to a voice recognition error, have the impression read "Evidence of pneumothorax." With findings in both the body and the impression encoded by AI-enabled NLP using common data element-labeled data structures, separate AI-based tools could then assess for consistency and alert the radiologist to potential disagreements.

Specific report content may be expected in certain clinical scenarios. This content might include relevant characterizations or categorizations and possibly guideline-oriented recommendations for further work-up and management. AI tools can assess data-based descriptions of lesions and determine whether the descriptions would be considered complete or additional characterization or assessment is required. In addition, by encoding published guidelines for further management, these tools could lead to more guideline-compliant radiology reports. The open computer-assisted reporting/decision support (CAR/DS)[11] framework promulgated by the ACR provides a foundation for early assistance with such suggestions, but must be encoded manually. AI tools could take this even further by helping to "discover" new guidelines to assist radiologists to improve their reporting. For example, AI tools may examine what the reporting patterns are for specific clinical entities used by experts (ie, how experts characterize and assess the lesion, and what recommendations they make for further characterization). These tools could be deployed for less expert radiologists; when the AI tool recognizes the relevant clinical scenario from the underlying data structures, it can provide suggestions to readers as to how to make their report more like reports generated by experts.

An additional challenge AI tools could help address is the longitudinal reporting of lesions, which is especially important in oncologic imaging. Specifically, many radiology examinations are ordered to reassess findings seen on prior imaging examinations. An important issue then is how to compare the findings being described in the current examination with the findings from prior examinations. Currently, radiologists have been responsible for examining the prior report text, determine which lesions require follow-up, correlating the current findings with previous ones, and describing their evolution (in many cases by redictating measurements from prior reports). For complex cases with many lesions, this process can be quite tedious and time consuming. An AI tool could examine a data structural description of a lesion and compare it with lesions described in multiple previous reports and try to construct the sequence of measurements and assessments of a lesion on serial studies over time. This information could then be presented to the radiologist in a format such that the appropriateness of the associations created by the AI algorithm can be established, each lesion's current properties confirmed, and any time-based trend assessed. Such tables, automatically generated from the data associated with prior reports without the need for data reentry, could even then be included in the report and made available to ordering providers and other registries for automatic import into care management or research systems.

A recent challenge in radiology reporting has been to make radiology results more accessible to patients. Both recent trends and federal law changes have increased the availability of radiology reports to patients. Radiology reports have not traditionally been intended for patient consumption and tend to include language that is opaque to nonmedical professionals. Having radiologists manually create an additional work product exclusively intended for patient review is impractical. Thus, automated methods for making reports more comprehensible to laypeople would markedly improve the patient experience. AI tools could attack this problem in at least 2 ways. One would be direct natural language analysis of the report generated by the radiologist, providing links and definitions to annotate the original report that has been developed.[12] As more sophisticated NLP becomes available, the sophistication of this annotation could improve. Such annotation could also be markedly improved by leveraging associated structured data to create specific patient-oriented descriptions of the radiologist's findings.

CHALLENGES AND OPPORTUNITIES IN ARTIFICIAL INTELLIGENCE FOR REPORT PREPARATION, ASSEMBLY, AND CLINICAL INTEGRATION

Although radiology examinations are typically ordered to address a specific clinical question, every patient has numerous open questions at any given time. Each radiology examination presents an opportunity to address many of these questions. A tool integrated with the reporting system that can make the radiologist aware of the patient's open questions at the time of reporting and suggest how the current examination might help to provide relevant information for those questions could allow radiologists to markedly increase the clinical value of radiology reports. Such a tool would cross-reference the patient's given problem list against a knowledgebase of possible findings that might be seen on the given examination. That is, for each problem on the problem list, the tool would consult a list of potential imaging findings filtered by the type of examination being interpreted. Some of these findings might be flagged as potentially pertinent negative findings in a patient with a particular condition. The reporting system could then examination the data structures of the current report and prompt radiologists to note the specific absence of relevant findings that might be of concern. For example, when reporting on patients with genetic syndromes predisposing them to specific lesions, an AI-based system could recognize that the report did not mention those lesions in the current report and prompt the radiologist to consider describing their presence or absence. As another example, patients on immunotherapy-based oncology treatments are prone to agent-specific complications that might be seen on chest or abdominal computed tomography (CT) scans.[13] When a radiologist reports an abdomen CT scan in such a patient, an AI system could recognize that the radiologist has not described the presence or absence of those complications and bring that to the radiologist's attention (possibly including reference material on typical CT appearance of these complications). This means that, even though an examination was ordered for the specific condition, the resulting report can answer not only the main clinical question, but many more of the relevant clinical questions for the patient. A related phenomenon would be to help the radiologist by identifying findings and recommendations from prior radiology reports that are likely to be detected on the current examination. These could then be cross-referenced against the findings described in the current report to determine whether those issues had been addressed, and possibly point out to the radiologist the opportunity to describe them (or even insert an "unchanged" statement automatically). For example, if a patient with a history of an incidental pulmonary nodule has a chest CT scan to assess for pulmonary embolus in the emergency department, the radiologist might concentrate on the pulmonary vasculature and other acute findings and not comment on the previously seen pulmonary nodule. Such a tool could identify this opportunity for the radiologist, which might help to prevent future, unnecessary imaging. Extending this further, because NLP tools are applied to prior radiology reports, patterns can be identified that in aggregate provide insights that could be missed when seen in isolation. For example, intimate partner violence could be predicted with high specificity around 3 years before violence prevention program entry using such techniques on the basis of the distribution and imaging appearance of the patient's current and past injuries.[14,15]

Note that this interaction between the patient's broad clinical history and the imaging findings could also be bidirectional. As a radiologist (or an image-analyzing AI tool) identifies a specific finding, this information may suggest additional diagnoses that are not currently attached to the patient. These new diagnoses could possibly be corroborated by other results (prior imaging results, previous laboratory results, physical examination findings, documented genetic alleles) that have not been connected previously. To accomplish this goal, a system would have to be designed that could cross-reference new findings to diagnoses, identify potentially new diagnoses, and know which related findings to query the electronic health record (EHR) for, and then bring these potentially new diagnoses to the radiologist's attention. This can form a virtuous cycle, where EHR entities can prompt the radiologist to look for possibly related findings, and findings can suggest the possibility of new diagnoses.

In summary, as a radiologist works on crafting a report for an examination, a suite of AI tools can assemble for them a sort of to-do list of issues to be addressed. This list could include questions prompted by the specific question or history as contained in the order, but such a tool will become more useful the more it can incorporate other components of the clinical context. These components should include specific diagnoses that have been attached to the patient, as well as prior treatments a patient has received (eg, surgery, radiation therapy). In addition, many of the findings and recommendations described in prior radiology reports should be addressed in subsequent reports, even if only to note resolution. Finally, as the radiologist describes findings in their report or image analysis tools create putative new findings and encode them for the radiologist to consider including them in the report, further potential issues can be raised. Taken together, this process forms a sort of dynamic list of issues that the report should be addressing. As the radiologist adds content to the report, each new addition might address one of these open issues, or create new issues to address, or both. When a radiologist thinks their report is complete, they can see that all the relevant issues have been addressed and sign their report with confidence that their report is providing maximum value for patients and providers.

One new challenge that arises for radiologists as reporting transitions from pure text generation is the process of managing data flow from upstream sources into the patient's clinical data as represented in the EHR. AI-based image analysis tools will create data structures based on the features automatically extracted from pixel data. In fact, such AI-generated data elements content can leverage existent standards such as the CAR/DS through the ACR Assist initiative also for integration into radiology reporting systems.[11,16] A new important role for the radiologist as they interpret images and generate report data will be to review these data structures and determine which should be included in the data to be transmitted to the EHR. This inclusion can take the form of either sub rosa inclusion in only the data layer, but also might be included as natural language (or part of a table) in the findings section of the text report. An additional important step for the radiologist to carry out is to provide feedback on the generated data, where appropriate. That is, a radiologist might reject the finding (eg, if the AI tool has recognized an artifact) or correct some of the data parameters (eg, changing a measurement). In addition, an AI tool might not be able to create complete descriptions of the findings it recognizes, and the radiologist must complete the description with additional data elements. These combined data could be used to automatically generate elements to be included in the text report or remain within the data layer to be transmitted to the EHR as structured data.

For example, consider the case of an AI tool that automatically detects and partially characterizes adrenal lesions. The generated data from the output of this tool (including descriptors for the side of the lesion, its size, and its radiodensity) would be automatically fed into a CAR/DS tool integrated into the reporting environment. As the radiologists reports on a case where such a lesion has been detected automatically, they can be alerted to the putative lesion. They can then confirm the lesion is a true lesion (rather than artifact) and be prompted to confirm the measurements and enter additional information about the lesion (eg, whether it has specifically benign features or has documented stability from prior examinations). Based on this additional information, the CAR/DS tool can then propose both report text for the radiologist to insert into the report and propose guideline-compliant recommendations for further management of the lesion (Fig. 1). In addition, the complete structured data characterization of the lesion is stored, blending both AI-tool generated data and information elicited from the radiologist.

An additional aspect of this management of the data flow is that it can generate feedback for monitoring and continuous improvement of the relevant AI tools. Even data that are not included in the data layer of the result as transmitted to the EHR can be

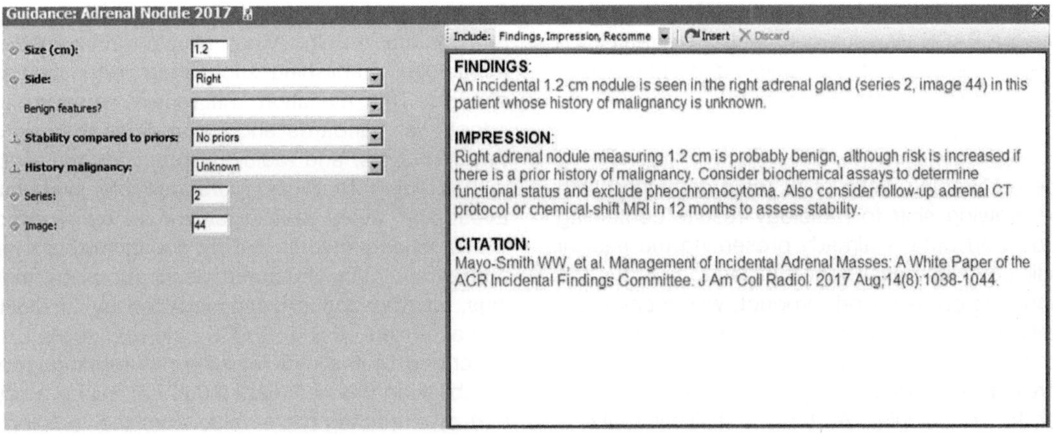

Guidance: Adrenal Nodule 2017
Size (cm): 1.2
Side: Right
Benign features?
Stability compared to priors: No priors
History malignancy: Unknown
Series: 2
Image: 44
Include: Findings, Impression, Recomme
Insert
Discard
FINDINGS:
An incidental 1.2 cm nodule is seen in the right adrenal gland (series 2, image 44) in this patient whose history of malignancy is unknown.
IMPRESSION:
Right adrenal nodule measuring 1.2 cm is probably benign, although risk is increased if there is a prior history of malignancy. Consider biochemical assays to determine functional status and exclude pheochromocytoma. Also consider follow-up adrenal CT protocol or chemical-shift MRI in 12 months to assess stability.
CITATION:
Mayo-Smith WW, et al. Management of Incidental Adrenal Masses: A White Paper of the ACR Incidental Findings Committee. J Am Coll Radiol. 2017 Aug;14(8):1038-1044.

Fig. 1. CAR/DS tool for incidentally detected adrenal nodules on a CT scan based on the ACR system. The reporting decision support tool can receive input both from an AI tool as well as from radiologists, and generate report text and propose guideline-compliant recommendations for further management of the lesion. The structured data—AI tool generated and from the radiologist—are recorded and can serve for various purposes such as monitoring and further improvements of relevant AI tools.

used to generate this feedback for monitoring and ongoing development. In fact, in some instances, the radiologist may be asked specific questions about AI-generated data to determine its correctness and utility including leveraging pixel AI output to assist on algorithm explainability (eg, allowing visualization of salience maps or key images such as the one used to derive the measurement of the largest axial diameter of a tumor from its automated segmentation). This feedback could serve for continuous optimization of ground truth and AI tools improvements over time.[17] A schematic representation of the data flow in such an AI-enabled radiology reporting process is summarized in Fig. 2. This points to the need to maintain a database of these structured data elements that would exist separate from the EHR, analogous to the image archive. Likely, the picture archiving and communication system (PACS) archiving function will come to include a separate area for maintaining pixel and structured data which is intended for tracking and feedback of AI tools and explicitly not for inclusion in the patient's medical record as represented in the EHR. For the AI-generated pixel data flagged for inclusion in the EHR based on radiologist feedback, a new generation of reporting

Scanner-generated
Technologist entered
Radiologist entered
AI tool extracted
Data Context
Data-Enabled
Reporting Environment
EHR
Registries

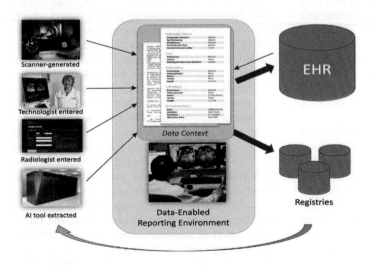

Fig. 2. Radiology reporting can become more focused on the management of structured data. Structured data can be generated automatically at the scanner, entered by technologists or radiologists, or automatically extracted by AI tools. Additional contextual data can be extracted from the EHR, possibly also with AI assistance. All of these form a reporting data context, which reporting software can leverage to provide assistance to the radiologist in creating and improving the report. In addition, as the radiologist uses the PACS viewer and dictates report text, structured descriptions of findings could be extracted and contribute to the data context. In this dynamic context, the radiologist both generates a natural language report and a data structure encoding radiologist-validated findings. This combined result can then be sent to the EHR as well as other databases, such as specialized clinical patient management systems (eg, for oncology practices) and research registries. Importantly, some of this captured structured data can be sent back to developers of AI tools for ongoing monitoring and improvement.

systems supporting structured pixel data synced with the PACS viewer would facilitate streamlined interactions between radiologists and AI output.

SUMMARY

The burgeoning wave of AI tools combined with the growing shift to radiology results containing structured data is already presenting the field of radiology with novel opportunities to improve the report, its primary work product, with many more tools and opportunities on the horizon. These improvements will be felt by radiologists, patient care teams, and increasingly, patients themselves. For the radiologist, AI tools will likely make a marked improvement to the actual process of interpreting and documenting radiology results. The application of AI has the potential to move the emphasis for radiologists from rote tasks of measuring and describing and onto more advanced cognitive tasks of analysis and synthesis. This will likely be through a combination of both tools that automatically detect and characterize findings and those which help the radiologist to identify important features of the patient's clinical history that might bear on the current report. For the teams caring for the patient, AI-assisted, data-oriented radiology reports can be more much more valuable in their care of the patient. For one, AI tools should help the report be more likely to answer not just the posed clinical question but other open clinical questions for the patient. Further, the data orientation based on reliable, automatically generated structured data allows radiology data to drive decision support and care pathways for providers, including registries and clinical management systems. Finally, as patients increasingly are able to access their medical records, the radiology report will need to become more accessible to them, and AI tools should be able to bring an accessible presentation of the radiology report tuned to each patient's circumstances.

However, as we move toward this new future, it is important to be aware of the challenges in deploying AI systems to assist radiologists in creating their reports. Addressing some of these challenges can begin even before reliable AI tools are available. First is the transition to more data-based radiology reporting. Clearly, there will have to be a robust infrastructure enabling fluid exchange of data between the various components of the radiology reporting process, including the EHR, the PACS viewer, various AI tools, and the voice-enabled report generation software. Emerging standards such as fast healthcare interoperability resources and the ACR/Radiological Society of North America common data element registry are forming what should prove instrumental in establishing such improved data exchange. This evolution will require vendors to adopt the standards and incorporate them into their products, and radiology practices to invest in upgrading to these more capable systems. Eventually, every radiologist should be working with a network of tools that are constantly creating and exchanging structured descriptions of findings, whether those being detected by AI tools, characterized using PACS viewer tools, or described by the radiologist in natural language. Establishing this new data plumbing will be a key part of extracting more value from the radiology report.

Even once this infrastructure is in place, radiologists will need to shift their actual reporting practices. The process of creating a data-enabled radiology report will differ significantly from the current text-oriented process. Rather than generating natural language as if dictating a letter, radiologists will be working to ensure that clinically useful data structures are being created (which could be used to automatically generate natural language descriptions). Given that these data will likely be used to drive downstream care of patients, it will be important for radiologists to extend their stewardship of the image acquisition process to include structured data generation as well. Radiologists will assess automatically generated data from AI tools and other sources and decide which structures should be included in the radiology result. They can then perform "three Cs" of data management: confirm, correct, and complete. Radiologists might be able to detect when there are errors in automatically generated data and either reject it or choose to include it, possibly with corrections; these should all send appropriate feedback to the data source. In addition, they can add additional information, possibly a categorization or other descriptive information, that an AI tool was unable to extract from the images. Eventually, the practice of radiology and the radiology report should evolve to place much less emphasis on the description of findings (which can be increasingly generated by software assistants based on automatically detected features), and much more emphasis on integrating the data being generated into the clinical context. The radiology report of the future could come to consist of a findings section including almost exclusively structured data rather than natural language descriptions followed by an impression synthesizing these findings with the patient's context.

To realize the fundamental shift in radiology practice promised by these new tools, reporting system software vendors will have to invent a whole new layer of technology to marry the data infrastructure with radiology practice. Specifically, radiology reporting software tools will have to change their nature fundamentally. Current generation reporting tools tend to take the form of a word processor with added voice recognition and some workflow integration features. A whole new way of working will be required to help radiologists with their new role of managing the flow of data from the pixel domain to the domain of structured clinical data. Part of this process will involve an accessible interface for managing and manipulating complex data structures. Generating a findings section should involve browsing appropriate data structures that have been automatically generated, either by AI image analysis or NLP tools, and structured annotations from a PACS viewer, and choosing those that should be included in the report to be sent to the EHR. As discussed elsewhere in this article, the radiologist would need to be able to correct and complete some of these descriptions; ideally, the reporting tool would prompt the radiologist and help them to step through this work. This process could become the primary method for radiologists to generate the findings section of their report. Perhaps, in addition, some elements of the impression section could be generated automatically by tools integrated into the reporting software based on the findings data, some of which will likely be AI based.[18] Again, the reporting software would likely need to prompt the radiologist to work through some of these steps and possibly perform important quality checks at this point.

AI tools have the potential to help drive a revolution in the radiology reporting process, both by providing specific kinds of assistance and an impetus for more data-oriented reporting. This work will necessarily entail a transformation of the reporting practice, technology, and product. The new practice of radiology reporting will likely be much more rewarding for radiologists, as more and more of the lower cognitive tasks of description and measurement can be performed by AI tools, leaving radiologists more time and cognitive bandwidth to synthesize and analyze the broader clinical picture (which other AI tools can help the radiologist better understand more rapidly). The report itself will likely increase dramatically in value, as it becomes more consistent and reliable and its embedded structured data can be used and reused in the context of other structured clinical data in the patient's record to drive more consistent, evidence-driven care.

CLINICS CARE POINTS

- Artificial intelligence tools can assist with radiology report consistency, ensure guideline-compliance, and facilitate longitudinal tracking.
- Radiologists will provide quality control of artificial intelligence-generated data.
- Artificial intelligence will allow radiologists to focus on advanced cognitive tasks while increasing the clinical value of reports.

DISCLOSURE

No direct sources of funding were used in the preparation for this article. The authors do not have any relevant conflicts of interest.

REFERENCES

1. Ganeshan D, Duong PAT, Probyn L, et al. Structured reporting in radiology. Acad Radiol 2018;25(1):66–73.
2. Oh SC, Cook TS, Kahn CE. PORTER: a prototype system for patient-oriented radiology reporting. J Digit Imaging 2016;29(4):450–4.
3. Martin-Carreras T, Kahn CE. Coverage and readability of information resources to help patients understand radiology reports. J Am Coll Radiol 2018;15(12):1681–6.
4. Goff DJ, Loehfelm TW. Automated radiology report summarization using an open-source natural language processing pipeline. J Digit Imaging 2018;31(2):185–92.
5. Bozkurt S, Alkim E, Banerjee I, et al. Automated detection of measurements and their descriptors in radiology reports using a hybrid natural language processing algorithm. J Digit Imaging 2019;32(4):544–53.
6. Banerjee I, Chen MC, Lungren MP, et al. Radiology report annotation using intelligent word embeddings: applied to multi-institutional chest CT cohort. J Biomed Inform 2018;77:11–20.
7. Pruitt P, Naidech A, Van Ornam J, et al. A natural language processing algorithm to extract characteristics of subdural hematoma from head CT reports. Emerg Radiol 2019;26(3):301–6.
8. Monshi MMA, Poon J, Chung V. Deep learning in generating radiology reports: a survey. Artif Intell Med 2020;106:101878.
9. Chen PH. Essential elements of natural language processing: what the radiologist should know. Acad Radiol 2020;27(1):6–12.

10. Sangwaiya MJ, Saini S, Blake MA, et al. Errare humanum est: frequency of laterality errors in radiology reports. Am J Roentgenol 2009;192(5):W239–44.

11. Alkasab TK, Bizzo BC, Berland LL, et al. Creation of an open framework for point-of-care computer-assisted reporting and decision support tools for radiologists. J Am Coll Radiol 2017;14(9):1184–9.

12. Scanslated. Available at: https://scanslated.com. Accessed February 16, 2021.

13. Kwak JJ, Tirumani SH, Van den Abbeele AD, et al. Cancer immunotherapy: imaging assessment of novel treatment response patterns and immune-related adverse events. Radiographics 2015;35(2):424–37.

14. Alessandrino F, Keraliya A, Lebovic J, et al. Intimate partner violence: a primer for radiologists to make the "invisible" visible. Radiographics 2020;40(7):2080–97.

15. Chen IY, Alsentzer E, Park H, et al. Intimate Partner Violence and Injury Prediction From Radiology Reports. Pac Symp Biocomput. 2021;26:55–66.

16. American College of Radiology (ACR). Assist. Available at: https://assist.acr.org/. Accessed February 6, 2021.

17. Pianykh OS, Langs G, Dewey M, et al. Continuous learning AI in radiology: implementation principles and early applications. Radiology 2020;297(1):6–14.

18. Rad AI. Available at: https://www.radai.com. Accessed February 16, 2021.

Artificial Intelligence for Quality Improvement in Radiology

Thomas W. Loehfelm, MD, PhD

KEYWORDS

• Informatics • Quality improvement • Operations • Metrics

KEY POINTS

- Realizing the potential of AI and informatics requires operational coordination and standardization across the imaging value chain and throughout the field
- Radiology quality definitions and metrics should incorporate more than just operational efficiencies as measured by turnaround times

INTRODUCTION

A common theme throughout this issue is the promise of artificial intelligence (AI) to impact nearly every step of the imaging value chain, from order placement to scheduling, image acquisition and reconstruction, worklist prioritization, diagnosis and interpretation, and reporting. Taken together, these efforts seek to improve the practice of diagnostic imaging, making radiology departments more precise and responsive, radiologists more accurate and efficient, and radiology reports more relevant and complete, culminating in improved patient outcomes and a more sustainable health care system.

Realizing these potential improvements will require substantially more strategic and operational coordination than in the past, as the various elements of the AI-enabled imaging value chain depend on and support upstream and downstream elements. Ensuring each component is based on nonproprietary standards, such as HL7 and DICOM, can mitigate some of the complexities of these intertwined workflows but still requires robust governance processes to identify deficiencies and react to change.

Measuring the improvements presents yet another challenge, in part because *defining* quality in radiology is complicated, in part because some elements of quality, such as diagnostic accuracy,

are difficult to generalize, and in part because there are often competing interests, each with a different definition of quality.

Perhaps the most commonly cited definition of quality in the radiology literature is from Hillman and colleagues[1] who stated:

Quality is the extent to which the right procedure is done in the right way at the right time, and the correct interpretation is accurately and quickly communicated to the patient and referring physician.

This definition of quality provides a good starting point and highlights the many links on the value chain that impact quality. This definition leaves open to interpretation or task-specific definition certain concepts relevant to AI in medical imaging, such as what "interpretation" means in this context, what constitutes "results," and what format "communication" takes. For example, population-health approaches to mining historical computed tomographic (CT) scans for disease risk factors, such as osteopenia or coronary artery calcium, are opportunities to extract value from historical diagnostic imaging studies, but our traditional mode of generating formatted plain text reports that are filed away in the electronic medical record (EMR) seems inadequate and antiquated for such a workflow with discrete data output.

UC Davis Medical Center, 4860 Y Street, Suite 3100, Sacramento, CA 95817, USA
E-mail address: twloehfelm@ucdavis.edu

Radiol Clin N Am 59 (2021) 1053–1062
https://doi.org/10.1016/j.rcl.2021.07.005
0033-8389/21/© 2021 Elsevier Inc. All rights reserved.

Many similar examples are conceivable, some that would exist outside of a traditional radiology report and some that may be generated in the context of a narrative report but, nevertheless, should be logged in a structured database for more efficient retrieval and processing. The infrastructure to create and store discrete data, either embedded within or in addition to plain text reports, is not yet widely adopted, but this is an area of active development.[2]

Kruskal and Larson[3] provide a general definition of value that is more malleable to the changing state of AI-driven radiology services: "The concept of value simply boils down to understanding the needs and desires of those whom an organization serves, and continuously working to improve how well those needs and desires are met". This conception of value puts the onus on each radiology group to identify their customers and work to understand their needs, and then develop the metrics and process controls to meet and exceed those needs consistently.

AI, and informatics tools more generally, are critical not only to driving quality improvement throughout the value chain but also in organizing and analyzing the data required to *demonstrate* that quality improvement.

OPERATIONAL QUALITY IMPROVEMENT

Informatics tools can improve both the accuracy and efficiency of operational workflows, including some tasks that precede image acquisition or reporting. One such task, the bane of existence for residents and fellows across the land, is examination protocoling—reviewing orders for diagnostic imaging studies, including free text examination indications as well as structured and unstructured data hiding in the nooks and crannies of the EMR, and then deciding on the appropriate series of patient preparatory and image acquisition steps to best address the clinical question. Machine learning methods that analyze free text examination indications and structured metadata, such as demographics, ordering service, and patient location, can automatically protocol neuroradiology MR imaging examinations with high accuracy.[4] Examination indications, however, are often incomplete or even discordant with contemporaneous clinical notes from the same providers,[5] highlighting the data quality chasms that still litter the EMR landscape and confound these clinical decision support and automated protocoling efforts. Successful and generalizable automated protocoling solutions will require highly integrated electronic health records (EHRs) that are actively designed to facilitate the accurate capture and transmission of clinical data, and to be successful those solutions will likely need access to a comprehensive data set, including EMR notes.

The LOINC/RSNA Radiology Playbook is the joint product of efforts by the RSNA and the Regenstrief Institute to standardize terminology of radiology procedures,[6] which is a key prerequisite for the development of AI tools that could influence radiology operations upstream of image acquisition in a generalizable way. The ongoing development of these standardized terminology resources is essential, and yet adoption of the playbooks seems to be lacking based on the fewer than 10 PubMed references to either the LOINC/RSNA Radiology Playbook or its predecessor, the RadLex Playbook, in the nearly 10 years since the RadLex Playbook was first referenced in 2012.[7]

Turnaround time (TAT), whether measured from order placement to final report, or examination complete to final report, is, for better or worse, one of the most common operational quality metrics in radiology. TAT expectations are built into most professional service agreements and are easy key performance indicators for hospital executive dashboards. With a mature informatics infrastructure, TATs between any steps of the process (Fig. 1) can be easily calculated from readily available timestamps.

More complicated metrics can be informative but require a nuanced understanding of and accounting for workflow. For example, academic radiology departments must balance workflow priorities of the medical center with their obligations to support resident education and autonomy. At my institution, senior residents work independently overnight generating preliminary interpretations for patients in the emergency room, which are then finalized the following day by an attending. Our Quality and Safety (Q&S) Committee defined a metric to ensure that we are reviewing those overnight preliminary reports in a timely manner—we set a target that 80% of preliminary reports should be finalized by 9:30 AM on weekdays and by noon on weekends. With this specific guidance from the Q&S Committee, our informatics group then developed a report for that metric for the bimonthly Q&S Committee meeting that distinguishes resident preliminary reports by radiology specialty, time of day, weekend versus weekday, and cross-sectional imaging versus radiography to address specific concerns of the various sections. This is an example of a radiology group working with the organization to identify a specific need (timely finalization of overnight preliminary reports) and then developing a metric to

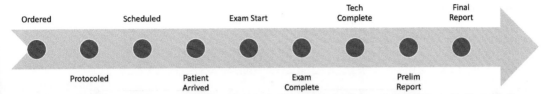

Fig. 1. An example of some of the milestones from order placement to final report submission. Turnaround times between any points on the chain may be useful to monitor specific quality initiatives and are commonly used to gauge radiology department efficiency. Although important, these metrics are incomplete assessments of radiology quality and should be augmented with more meaningful quality indicators when possible. Extracting value from turnaround times requires an understanding of radiology workflow and process controls to ensure data integrity.

monitor how well we are meeting that desire. The metric is informative and specific while preserving section chief autonomy in deciding how to construct a schedule and workflow priorities to meet the desired performance goal. An example report is shown in **Fig. 2**. Importantly it is the health care organization—not the informatics group—that determines what is *valuable*. It is sign of disorganization and a recipe for operational confusion to expect the informatics group alone to both define what is valuable and measure it—that process needs to be driven by department and organizational leaders.

Realizing the potential opportunity for AI and informatics tools to significantly impact the examination ordering, scheduling, and protocoling components of the imaging value chain will require a common and standardized terminology for those examinations and their composite steps. The LOINC/RSNA Radiology Playbook provides that structure but needs broader acceptance and adoption.

REPORT QUALITY IMPROVEMENT

Eberhardt and Heilbrun[8] derive the following radiology report value equation by extending the common health care adage that value equals quality health outcomes divided by cost, and defining *accuracy*, *utility*, *clarity*, *conciseness*, and *timeliness* as the dimensions of radiology report quality:

easy and objective to measure. This focus on TAT puts radiologists in a tenuous position with respect to hospital executive leaders, who, if they are metric driven, might come to see TAT as the *only* quality metric that matters in radiology because it is the only one readily available. Designing workflows specifically to minimize TAT negatively affects resident education in academic centers,[9] which could have pernicious effects on the field going forward.

Informatics methods can help to develop metrics complementary to TAT that offer a more complete solution to the report value equation. For example, clarity and conciseness are generally summarized as the *readability* of text, and this is usually expressed as the education level required to comprehend the text. So, a readability score of 8 implies that the text is comprehensible to readers with at least an eighth-grade education. Calculating a readability score, such as the most widely used Flesch-Kincaid Grade formula,[10] involves simple natural language processing techniques. Returning back to Eberhardt and Heilbrun's derivation of a radiology report value equation, the investigators include a sample report impression in an all-too-familiar verbose format, which they then rework to be more concise while retaining information content—the changes result in an improvement of 4 grade levels of readability **(Table 1)**.

$$Report\ Value\ (RV) = \frac{(Accurate + Useful) * (Clear + Concise + Timely)}{Cost}$$

Of these parameters, timeliness is the easiest to measure, and because of that most radiology groups include assessment of TAT in their quality reports. Although useful, too much quality and customer service improvement effort in radiology is focused on TAT simply because it is relatively

Note that the concise statement is not just a simplified version—it still includes appropriate medical terminology, for example, and still includes the evidence supporting the diagnosis of pneumoperitoneum. And striving for improved readability does not imply that other physicians

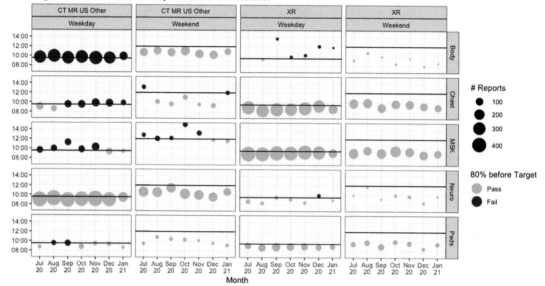

Fig. 2. A sample report monitoring compliance with a specific departmental Quality and Safety objective. The objective is specific to workflow at an academic medical center where timely finalization of resident overnight preliminary reports was considered a priority by hospital leadership. The radiology department set a target that 80% of overnight preliminary reports would be finalized by 9:30 AM on weekdays and by noon on weekends (*horizontal black line*). The graphs show the time when 80% of overnight prelims have been finalized as a dot whose size scales with the number of reports and whose color indicates success (green) or failure (red) in meeting the metric. Graphs are further distinguished by section, by modality, and by weekday type.

cannot comprehend a report written at a 12th-grade level. Rather it recognizes that there is *value* in clarity and conciseness, honoring the aphorism commonly attributed to Einstein that "everything should be as simple as it can be, but not simpler."[11]

With an informatics pipeline in place to catalog radiology reports and parse them into sections ("Indication," "Findings," "Impression," etc.), one can calculate the Flesch-Kincaid Grade level of impressions crafted by individual attendings and then compare readability for attendings working in the same section. For example, analyzing 51,000 report Impressions from ultrasound reports generated by Abdominal Imagers over a 3-year period at one institution shows that their average readability varies by 5 grade levels—the most readable radiologist produced Impressions at an 11.6th-grade level and the least readable radiologist at a 16.5th-grade level (**Fig. 3**; T.W. Loehfelm, unpublished).

Including readability metrics in addition to TAT would be a step toward a fairer assessment of radiology value, but they still fail to capture the most important facet of our work: providing accurate and useful diagnoses. Here too AI and informatics methods are being developed to monitor

diagnostic accuracy and utility. Although a fully generalizable solution to assessing accuracy and utility is out of reach for now and the foreseeable future, there are specific scenarios that are tractable now.

Table 1 Readablility of example radiology report Impression statements	Flesch-Kincaid Grade
Verbose There are several bowel loops in the left lower quadrant that may have a Rigler sign and some gas triangles or polygons, which is concerning for free intraperitoneal air	12.2
Concise The left lower quadrant air pattern is concerning for pneumoperitoneum	8.4

Adapted from Eberhardt SC, Heilbrun ME. Radiology report value equation. RadioGraphics 2018;38(6):1888–96.

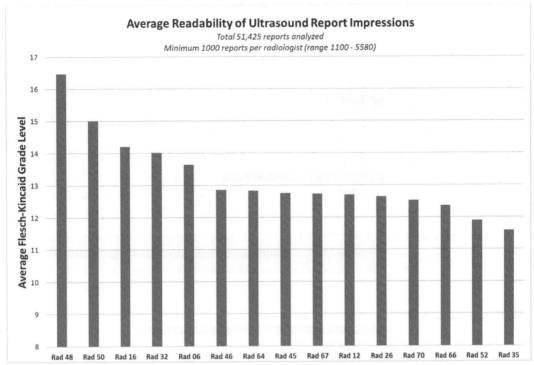

Fig. 3. The average readability of ultrasound report impressions generated by 15 radiologists at a single academic medical center over a 3-year period. Readability as estimated by the Flesh-Kincaid Grade Level of each impression varies by 5 grade levels—the least readable radiologist produced reports at a 16th-grade level and the most readable at an 11th-grade level.

Mammography is furthest ahead in this domain among the radiology specialties because of its early and universal adoption of standardized reporting and mandatory radiology-pathology correlation. The Breast Imaging Reporting and Data System (BI-RADS) was a landmark achievement for radiology, now in its fifth edition, and provides a common diagnosis and management framework that enables continuous practice improvement.[12] The American College of Radiology currently endorses 9 Reporting and Data Systems,[13] each one an opportunity to assess radiologist diagnostic accuracy.

For example, individual and group-level accuracy in interpreting pelvic MRIs performed for prostate cancer detection can be measured with good accuracy if the radiologists consistently report Prostate Imaging - Reporting and Data System (PI-RADS) score, the pathologists consistently report Gleason score, and appropriate informatics data processing pipelines are in place. The maximum PI-RADS score is automatically extracted from the radiology report, maximum Gleason score from a subsequent biopsy report, and clinically significant prostate cancer detection rate, the percentage of biopsies yielding Gleason 3 + 4 or higher, is calculated. Target ranges

can be set either by published expected detection rates or local convention, and outlier radiologists can be identified. "Undercallers" will show up as having *higher* cancer detection rates than expected (ie, cancer is found *more frequently than expected* for a given level of suspicion), and "overcallers" will show up as having *lower* cancer detection rates than expected (cancer is found *less frequently than expected* for a given level of suspicion). In the example dashboard in **Fig. 4**, the group (indicated by the thin vertical line) slightly *undercalls* PI-RADS 4—clinically significant prostate cancer is found in 57% of the biopsies of PI-RADS 4 patients when the expected rate is 15% to 50%. Whether this difference is important or not is up to each group to decide. Whether a single radiologist or a few are responsible for driving the metric can be determined by reviewing the corresponding dashboards for each member of the group—significant outliers can be identified for further training or mentorship.

Note that it is consistent use of risk stratification systems (PI-RADS and Gleason score in this case) that makes this possible. When radiologists can be encouraged to use a common risk stratification system, and when the imaging study is focused on such a specific clinical question, then the accuracy of the

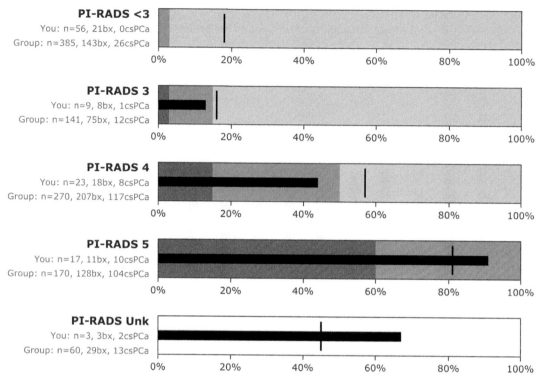

Fig. 4. Individual and group quality in interpreting prostate MR imaging as measured by the likelihood of finding clinically significant prostate cancer (csPCa; Gleason 3 + 4 or higher) on biopsy. Prostate MR imaging reports are grouped according to their highest PI-RADS assignment, and for each group the number of patients, number of biopsied patients, and number of patients with clinically significant prostate cancer are indicated for the specific user (*black bar*) and all other radiologists (the "group"; *thin vertical line*). Target ranges, determined by literature review and group preferences, are indicated by the grayscale of the background chart. The assumption is that clinically significant cancer should be found in about 15% of patients whose worst nodule is PI-RADS 3, 15% to 50% of patients whose worst nodule is PI-RADS 4, and greater than 60% of patients whose worst nodule is PI-RADS 5. Individuals whose performance falls considerably outside of those target ranges may benefit from retraining or mentorship in the application of PI-RADS.

radiologist can be fairly assessed. Similar dashboards are straightforward to create for mammography (BI-RADS) and thyroid ultrasound (TI-RADS).

It is considerably harder to design a generalizable automated system for monitoring diagnostic accuracy without the benefit of discrete risk stratification scores because of the immense variability in diagnoses that radiologists provide, the free text reporting style that those observations are trapped in, and the ambiguity of diagnoses that may never be proved by pathology or some other reference standard. We should not let perfect be the enemy of good though, and where we *can* monitor our performance, such as by correlating risk stratification from RADS classification with pathology results, we should.

Although not yet mature enough for generalized diagnostic accuracy assessment, automated radiology-pathology correlation tools can still provide tremendous value. Natural language processing software such as the Clinical Text Analysis and Knowledge Extraction System[14] can accurately extract anatomy, pathology, disease severity, and other clinically relevant concepts from unstructured free text reports, mapping those concepts to reference ontologies like SNOMED. Applying these sorts of tools to radiology and pathology report corpora effectively translates free text into discrete data and exposes the additional properties of and relations between concepts that are organized in the reference ontologies. These structured databases of translated free text reports can be used to automatically summarize radiology reports,[15] build peer learning educational resources,[16] and identify patient cohorts for machine-learning projects.[17] To work well these systems need to understand the structure, content, and temporal relationships of radiology and pathology reports and require robust operational infrastructure to manage data ingestion, processing, presentation, and secure access. An example of the process of using the Unified

Medical Language System semantic relationship *has_finding_site* to identify the relationship that exists between a radiology report that mentions "cholecystitis" in the Impression section and a pathology report with a specimen of "gallbladder" from the same patient is demonstrated in **Fig. 5**. Such systems are already useful for individual radiologist education, report searching, and peer review and have the potential to solve for the *Accuracy* variable in Eberhardt and Heilbrun's Radiology Report Value equation.

The final dimension of the report value equation that is so far unaddressed is *utility*—are our reports useful to the other physicians who rely on them to make diagnoses, determine next steps, and assess treatment response, and to the patients who seek to understand and actively manage their own health?

Some measures of utility can be discretized and measured automatically using some of the Natural Language Processing methods referenced earlier. Examples include assessing the completeness of information content for assessing tumor stage and status,[18] describing mammography observations *per* BI-RADS lexicon,[19] and assigning Lung-RADS classification.[20] Reports that are intended to provide these descriptions can be assumed to be *useful* if the report is assessed to be comprehensive relative to some reference standard of information content. This type of automatic utility metric is susceptible to the same limitations as the automatic diagnostic accuracy tools described in earlier discussion—they are feasible when there is a specific reference standard or disease process to focus on and when radiologists use consistent predictable terminology and constrained lexicons, but the more general case is currently intractable due to the extreme variety of uses for radiology services.

Tan and Krishnaraj (prepublished data, personal communication, 2021) have cut the Gordian knot to address the more general use case—to determine whether a report is useful, simply ask your customer if their needs were met. By embedding 5-star review mechanisms and soliciting comments directly in the EHR and patient portal, the investigators have opened direct lines of communication between the service provider and the customer and have solved for the *utility* variable of the value equation directly.

EXPANDING OUR REACH

As radiology becomes more data driven, both diagnostically and operationally, our field will be poised to leverage those information resources to expand the breadth of services we offer. We can not only generate diagnoses but also ensure appropriate follow-up steps, monitor radiology-pathology discordance to prompt reassessment, and help to identify gaps in service or inefficiencies in practice throughout the enterprise. As radiology

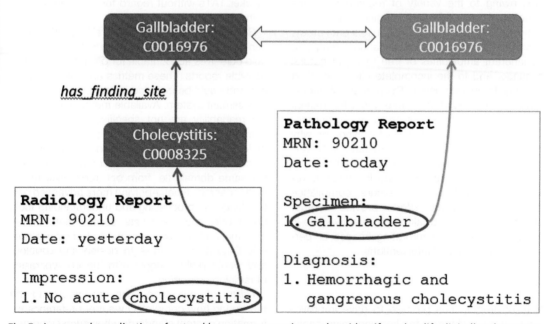

Fig. 5. An example application of natural language processing tools to identify and codify clinically relevant concepts in radiology and pathology reports. By referencing the "has_finding_site" relationship defined in SNOMED-CT, an NLP system can recognize that the radiology report that mentions *cholecystitis* is relevant to a gallbladder pathology specimen from the same patient.

services are so broad and fundamental to much of diagnostic medicine, we are uniquely positioned to monitor the full gamut of health care services. Our existing digital infrastructure coupled with the thoughtful and controlled inclusion of more advanced AI-driven digital advances can expand our reach and transform our reading rooms to health care journey command centers.

We can, for example, cross-reference our recommendations from tests like screening mammography and low-dose lung CT to EHR data resources to ensure that patients receive the appropriate and timely follow-up studies, identifying patients lost to follow-up, and engaging with them via patient portals or other direct communication. For these examples, as the department that both makes the recommendation and provides the follow-up service, we are best positioned to take ownership of the whole process, but this type of population health management is not widely adopted by radiology departments. As we develop more digital data resources and prioritize the *value* of the services we provide, we may identify more such opportunities to provide value beyond direct imaging services.

Although monitoring compliance with mammography or lung cancer screening recommendations is facilitated by the standardized risk-stratification systems available for those domains, the more general case of assessing compliance with various other radiologist recommendations is more complex, owing to the variety of recommendations made (eg, for a subsequent imaging examination, pathology correlation, comparison to a prior study, or correlation with clinical examination findings), to the inherent ambiguities of free text and natural language, and to the incomplete clinical context radiologists operate under. The readers of our reports nearly always know more about the patient than we do and may know of reasons why our recommendations should not be followed, or why they are moot given other circumstances. Nevertheless, many researchers have attempted to identify recommendations made in radiology reports and automatically measure compliance with them[21–24]—these efforts provide another inroad for radiology to take a more active role in patient care beyond interpreting images or performing image-guided interventions.

SUMMARY

AI holds tremendous promise to drive improvements at each stage of the imaging value chain. Realizing that potential requires mature informatics infrastructure and ongoing operational governance to ensure that each link of the chain effectively consumes and transmits information to upstream and downstream links. Measuring the improvement requires first that each radiology group identifies their customers, defines what "quality" and "value" means to them, and develops metrics that support the pursuit of improving quality and value.

Using the Radiology Report Value Equation from Eberhardt and Heilbrun as a reference framework, informatics tools can help to provide automated and objective assessments of report *accuracy*, *utility*, *clarity and conciseness* (ie, *readability*), and *timeliness*. Measuring and improving *any* of those elements requires operational management and infrastructure to ensure the data collected are reliable, comprehensive, and meaningful.

Timeliness metrics like TATs can be simple, such as measuring the average time between order placement and examination completion, or from examination completion to final report availability, or they can be complex, such as the example in **Fig. 2** of measuring the TAT of a specific subset of reports that depend on understanding and accounting for the complex workflows encountered in academic radiology departments. Radiology groups should be careful to not rely solely on TATs as the *only* dimension of quality and value simply because it is the easiest to measure—to do so minimizes our actual value and commoditizes our services in a way that makes us vulnerable to market forces that promise quicker TATs without regard for the other dimensions of quality.

Readability metrics from general linguistics fields can be applied to our reports as a first-pass effort to hold ourselves accountable for producing comprehensible reports. These metrics are easy to calculate and could be included in any radiology quality assessment system. Available methods of assessing readability are not specifically designed for biomedical texts, but although this deficiency might make comparisons to nonbiomedical domains inaccurate, it should not affect comparisons within the same domain (ie, from one radiologist to the next, or across time). Applying more advanced natural language processing and understanding tools could offer more accurate assessments of the grammar and syntax of our reports, but require specific linguistics expertise to design and develop, and would likely struggle with the idiosyncrasies of radiology reporting.

Utility of our work can be assessed by measuring how completely we meet reference information content standards when such standards are available, or more directly, by soliciting feedback directly from our clinical and patient customers. Striving to meet the needs of our customers will compel radiologists to work to identify those customers and their needs, which will necessitate the establishment of more robust and visible relationships with those customers. These efforts would directly align with the Imaging 3.0 initiative of the American College of Radiology.[25]

Accuracy of our work can be automatically measured for the subset of radiology studies that consistently use a risk-stratification system such as the various Reporting and Data Systems developed by the American College of Radiology and when pathology either applies a consistent grading system like the Gleason score for prostate cancer or when the range of pathology is sufficiently limited that it can be accurately extracted from the pathology report, such as for breast cancer and thyroid nodule diagnoses. More generalized assessments of accuracy are confounded by the immense variety of diagnoses that radiologists make, the free text reporting style used to encode the observations, and the lack of a reference standard for many diagnoses that are managed medically or for which pathology proof is otherwise not available. Nevertheless, tools to automatically correlate specific pathology reports to specific radiology reports are useful for education and research purposes even if they are not yet ready to support a generalizable diagnostic accuracy metric.

We need not assign a discrete score to *each* dimension of report value for *each* report generated, but we should start by acknowledging that simple TATs are a poor surrogate for quality and then embrace opportunities to measure and prove value across the other dimensions.

CLINICS CARE POINTS

- Structured radiology reports facilitate downstream value extraction.
- Metrics beyond turnaround time are required to properly demonstrate the true value of diagnostic imaging.
- Realizing and demonstrating the value of informatics methods to drive quality improvement requires robust infrastructure, governance, and alignment with institutional goals.

DISCLOSURE

Dr Loehfelm is the founder of PANORAD, LLC.

REFERENCES

1. Hillman BJ, Amis ES, Neiman HL. The future quality and safety of medical imaging: proceedings of the third annual ACR FORUM. J Am Coll Radiol 2004; 1(1):33–9.
2. Rubin DL, Kahn CE. Common data elements in radiology. Radiology 2016;283(3):837–44.
3. Kruskal JB, Larson DB. Strategies for radiology to thrive in the value era. Radiology 2018;289(1):3–7.
4. Brown AD, Marotta TR. Using machine learning for sequence-level automated MRI protocol selection in neuroradiology. J Am Med Inform Assoc 2018; 25(5):568–71.
5. Lacson R, Laroya R, Wang A, et al. Integrity of clinical information in computerized order requisitions for diagnostic imaging. J Am Med Inform Assoc 2018;25(12):1651–6.
6. Vreeman DJ, Abhyankar S, Wang KC, et al. The LOINC RSNA radiology playbook - a unified terminology for radiology procedures. J Am Med Inform Assoc 2018;25(7):885–93.
7. Kanal K, Zamora D, Price C, et al. SU-E-I-50: the ACR CT dose index registry: implementation challenges and preliminary data. Med Phys 2012;39(6 Part4):3636.
8. Eberhardt SC, Heilbrun ME. Radiology report value equation. Radiographics 2018;38(6):1888–96.
9. England E, Collins J, White RD, et al. Radiology report turnaround time: effect on resident education. Acad Radiol 2015;22(5):662–7.
10. Kincaid J, Fishburne R, Rogers R, et al. Derivation of new readability formulas (Automated Readability Index, Fog Count And Flesch Reading Ease Formula) for navy enlisted personnel. Institute for simulation and training [Internet]. 1975. Available at: https://stars.library.ucf.edu/istlibrary/56. Accessed August 20, 2021.
11. Prausnitz F. Roger sessions: how a "difficult" composer got that way. Illustrated edition. Oxford; New York: Oxford University Press; 2002.
12. Eghtedari M, Chong A, Rakow-Penner R, et al. Current status and future of BI-RADS in multimodality breast imaging, from the AJR special series on radiology reporting and data systems. AJR Am J Roentgenol 2021;216(4):860–73.
13. An JY, Unsdorfer KML, Weinreb JC. BI-RADS, C-RADS, CAD-RADS, LI-RADS, Lung-RADS, NI-RADS, O-RADS, PI-RADS, TI-RADS: reporting and data systems. Radiographics 2019;39(5):1435–6.
14. Savova GK, Masanz JJ, Ogren PV, et al. Mayo clinical text analysis and knowledge extraction system (cTAKES): architecture, component evaluation and applications. J Am Med Inform Assoc 2010;17(5): 507–13.
15. Goff DJ, Loehfelm TW. Automated radiology report summarization using an open-source natural

language processing pipeline. J Digit Imaging 2018; 31(2):185–92.

16. Filice RW. Radiology-pathology correlation to facilitate peer learning: an overview including recent artificial intelligence methods. J Am Coll Radiol 2019; 16(9, Part B):1279–85.

17. Tan WK, Hassanpour S, Heagerty PJ, et al. Comparison of natural language processing rules-based and machine-learning systems to identify lumbar spine imaging findings related to low back pain. Acad Radiol 2018;25(11):1422–32.

18. Cheng LTE, Zheng J, Savova GK, et al. Discerning tumor status from unstructured MRI reports–completeness of information in existing reports and utility of automated natural language processing. J Digit Imaging 2010;23(2):119–32.

19. Bozkurt S, Lipson JA, Senol U, et al. Automatic abstraction of imaging observations with their characteristics from mammography reports. J Am Med Inform Assoc 2015;22(e1):e81–92.

20. Beyer SE, McKee BJ, Regis SM, et al. Automatic Lung-RADS™ classification with a natural language

21. Cook TS, Lalevic D, Sloan C, et al. Implementation of an automated radiology recommendation-tracking engine for abdominal imaging findings of possible cancer. J Am Coll Radiol 2017;14(5):629–36.

22. Oliveira L, Tellis R, Qian Y, et al. Follow-up recommendation detection on radiology reports with incidental pulmonary nodules. Stud Health Technol Inform 2015;216:1028.

23. Yetisgen-Yildiz M, Gunn ML, Xia F, et al. Automatic identification of critical follow-up recommendation sentences in radiology reports. AMIA Annu Symp Proc 2011;2011:1593–602.

24. Dang PA, Kalra MK, Blake MA, et al. Extraction of recommendation features in radiology with natural language processing: exploratory study. AJR Am J Roentgenol 2008;191(2):313–20.

25. Ellenbogen PH. Imaging 3.0: what is it? J Am Coll Radiol 2013;10(4):229.

processing system. J Thorac Dis 2017;9(9): 3114–22.

Separating Hope from Hype
Artificial Intelligence Pitfalls and Challenges in Radiology

Jared Dunnmon, PhD

KEYWORDS

- Radiology • Artificial intelligence • Pitfalls and challenges

KEY POINTS

- AI systems can provide value to radiologists in several ways, ranging from reduced time on task to discovery of new knowledge.
- Potential challenges in deploying AI systems for radiology include myriad technical issues, difficulties mitigating algorithmic bias, and poor alignment between measured performance and clinical value.
- Promising directions to address these challenges include improved software engineering practices, close clinician involvement in model development, and robust postdeployment monitoring.

Although recent scientific studies suggest that artificial intelligence (AI) could provide value in many radiology applications, much of the hard engineering work required to consistently realize this value in practice remains to be done. In this article, we summarize the various ways in which AI can benefit radiology practice, identify key challenges that must be overcome for those benefits to be delivered, and discuss promising avenues by which these challenges can be addressed.

HOW CAN ARTIFICIAL INTELLIGENCE PROVIDE VALUE TO RADIOLOGISTS?

Although headlines often gravitate toward AI systems that claim to perform as well as or better than humans on a particular task, AI can provide value to radiologists in several specific ways. These include automated information extraction from imaging examinations, increased diagnostic certainty, decreased time on task, faster availability of results, reduced cost of care, better clinical outcomes, discovery of new knowledge, and improved patient access to radiological expertise.[1,2] While other chapters in this volume describe such applications in detail, we provide a brief overview here.

Leveraging information contained within an image to make prognostic and diagnostic decisions is a core component of radiology practice; AI systems can provide value to radiologists by enabling them to do so more effectively. For instance, although a clinician's diagnostic ability is defined by a combination of first principles knowledge and experience with specific cases, an AI system can leverage information contained in millions or billions of data points to refine how image features are mapped to prognostic or diagnostic outputs. Recent analyses of AI models trained on large radiology data sets demonstrate the potential not only to improve diagnostic sensitivity or specificity,[3,4] but also to yield novel image features that correspond more directly to the outcome of interest than those that comprise existing standards.[5] Furthermore, the fact that AI systems can perform such analysis with high levels of standardization across patients[5]—and without being vulnerable to fatigue or cognitive biases—can yield substantial value in the real world.[2,6] AI-based approaches can augment human analysis both by surfacing information that is not readily

Department of Biomedical Data Science, Stanford University, 1265 Welch Rd, Stanford, CA 94305, USA
E-mail address: jdunnmon@cs.stanford.edu

Radiol Clin N Am 59 (2021) 1063–1074
https://doi.org/10.1016/j.rcl.2021.07.006

apparent and by improving the utility of reconstructed images for human readers.[7]

AI systems can also provide value to radiologists by increasing the speed with which imaging results are processed and by reducing required clinician effort. Automated optimization of work-lists, for instance, can reduce time-to-treatment for life-threatening and severe conditions while still ensuring human review of all cases.[1,2,8,9] With appropriate algorithmic design and human factors engineering, the integration of AI-based triage and second read systems into clinical workflows holds the potential to decrease the time required per case. This would simultaneously increase patient access, lower costs, and improve outcomes by enabling radiologists to spend more of their time on cases that require substantial analysis.[1] Decreased time requirements would also help to alleviate the workforce shortage that radiology is expected to experience in the coming years as demand for services continues to increase.[1]

Finally, the consistent use of AI systems in radiology practice can yield new knowledge that improves patient care. The development of "radiomic" features that are not discernible by the human eye, but may nonetheless be predictive of outputs ranging from diagnosis to prognosis to treatment response, represents a particularly promising area of research.[10] AI can also play a supporting role in such tasks as patient selection, tumor tracking, and adverse event detection that can inform the clinical trials necessary to create new forms of diagnosis and treatment.[11]

AI systems that provide value in each of these ways have been conceptualized—and in some cases evaluated for clinical use—across a wide variety of applications, many of which have been detailed in this volume.[11] The balance of this article will describe important pitfalls in the development and deployment of these systems that must be addressed for AI systems to provide widespread value for radiologists.

WHAT CHALLENGES MUST BE OVERCOME FOR ARTIFICIAL INTELLIGENCE TO PROVIDE VALUE TO RADIOLOGISTS?

Translating the potential that academic studies and early clinical trials have shown into concrete improvements in radiology practice will require that researchers and practitioners alike be aware of the challenges that can accompany the development and deployment of AI systems in radiology applications. This section provides an overview of the major pitfalls that AI systems face in radiology, and the subsequent section will outline compelling approaches for addressing these challenges.

Meaningful Performance Measurement

The first, and perhaps most important challenge in developing an AI system for radiology is ensuring that the task of interest is sufficiently well-posed that performance can be meaningfully measured. Defining a suitable clinically relevant task is not always as easy as it might seem. Consider the example of chest x-ray (CXR) classification, a commonly studied application of AI. Much work in this area has focused on developing deep learning models that classify CXRs into 1 of the 14 different classes used in Rajpurkar and colleagues,[3] but it is clear that several of these classes (eg, atelectasis, consolidation, infiltration) can be inconsistently understood across different clinicians. As a result, models trained for this particular task may confuse these 3 classes, or may provide outputs with which certain clinicians would agree more than others. Such ambiguity in task definition reduces our ability to effectively measure performance.[12] Furthermore, it is critical to ensure that the measure of AI system performance is directly related to the outcome of interest. It is not immediately clear, for instance, that high levels of performance on a 14-class CXR abnormality classification task will translate into one of the types of value described previously (eg, reduced radiologist time, improved diagnostic certainty). In fact, one could argue that framing this task in a slightly different way—binary normal versus abnormal CXR triage for worklist prioritization[4,8]—could provide more direct clinical value because its place in the clinical workflow is clear, and metrics like turnaround time for high-priority cases can be immediately computed. Collaboration between radiology domain experts and AI developers will remain key to ensuring that AI systems are developed for tasks that are meaningful, and that performance is measured in ways that directly correlate with clinical value.

Even when a clinically useful task has been defined, inappropriately chosen performance metrics can hinder model development (see the Jayashree Kalpathy-Cramer and colleagues' article, "Basic AI Techniques: Evaluation of AI Performance," in this issue for more detail). Although sensitivity and specificity may be familiar to many clinicians, multiclass classification, segmentation, and reconstruction tasks are evaluated quite differently than binary classification, and metrics suitable to the task must be used. Equity considerations are also important in designing suitable metrics. For instance, it is often the case that deep learning models for classification perform well on classes that make up the most of the training set, but perform poorly on classes that are small. In some situations, this could be acceptable—in which case unweighted metrics are commonly used—but in others, it would not, meaning that class-weighted metrics should be reported. Furthermore, the common use of area under the receiver operating characteristic curve (AUROC) or area under the precision-recall curve as figures of merit should be viewed with caution; while useful in describing overall classification performance, these metrics can be misleading because they do not indicate how a model will perform at the specific operating points that must be chosen in practice.

In addition to computing an appropriate metric, evaluation procedures must be designed in a way that yields meaningful results. A common error is assuming that models that are internally validated—that is, that perform well on the same population on which they were developed—will continue to perform well when applied externally (ie, to a different population).[13] Evaluation data sets must represent the population on which a model is intended to be used, otherwise performance computed thereon will be misleading. When comparing multiple algorithms, performance should also be evaluated on a common data set to provide meaningful information.[14] Finally, a common pitfall in AI performance measurement occurs when the task schema is insufficiently granular to capture important variations in performance. A common example of this phenomenon—which has been termed "hidden stratification"[15]—occurs in classification problems when performance variation occurs due to a variable that the original data set curators did not consider.

As shown in **Fig. 1**, for instance, Oakden-Rayner and colleagues[15] recently demonstrated that while a common CXR classification model yields an overall AUROC value of 0.87 for detecting pneumothoraces, that performance increases to 0.95 on images that display a chest drain and drops to 0.77 on images that do not. Thus, if this model had been deployed in practice, it would have performed much worse on the very population—pneumothoraces without a chest drain—that would be of clinical interest. Similar issues can cause models to be biased and perform poorly on a given subclass (eg, non-Caucasian patients) because it just so happens that (a) that subclass makes up a minority of a data set and (b) the data set was not labeled with subclass information.

Creating Training Data Sets

Once an appropriate task and measurement metric have been defined, creating an AI system to perform that task generally requires constructing a data set on which a model will be trained. In supervised learning, which dominates current applications in radiology, this requires curating labeled training data. Unfortunately, the cost of creating these labeled data sets can limit the application of AI systems in clinical practice. Using the work of Gulshan and colleagues[16] as an example, 3 to 7 physicians, most of whom are licensed ophthalmologists, were reported to have graded every single one of 128,175 retinal fundus photographs. Conservatively assuming 3 labelers per image, 15 seconds per image, and a $100 per hour rate,

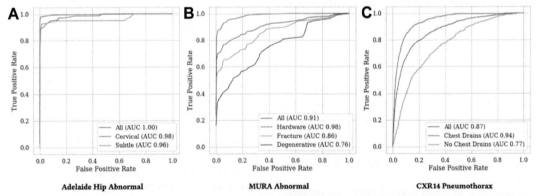

Fig. 1. ROC curves for subclasses of models trained on multiple data sets. (*A*) Model performance on different subclasses of the "abnormal" class for a model designed to detect abnormalities on radiographs from the Adelaide Hip Fracture data set. (*B*) Model performance on different subclasses of the "abnormal" class for a model designed to detect abnormalities in musculoskeletal radiographs from the MURA data set. (*C*) Model performance on different subclasses of the "pneumothorax" class for a multiclass CXR classification model designed to detect 14 different pathologies on the CXR-14 data set. (*From* Oakden-Rayner L, Dunnmon J, Carneiro G, Ré C. Hidden Stratification Causes Clinically Meaningful Failures in Machine Learning for Medical Imaging. Published online September 26, 2019. Accessed November 4, 2019. http://arxiv.org/abs/1909.12475.)

this comes out to a cost estimate in excess of $150,000 and 180 clinician-days for a single iteration of data labeling; in practice, multiple data labeling efforts are often necessary.

Importantly, even meticulously labeled training sets are not guaranteed to support models that generalize across different diseases, modalities, imaging systems, classification ontologies, clinical protocols, and medical guidelines, all of which change over time and with different application contexts.[5,13,17,18] This concept is known as *distribution shift*, and often causes model performance to degrade when used outside of the exact population on which the training set was constructed. This behavior has been observed in a variety of medical applications including pneumonia detection on CXR,[13] diabetic retinopathy detection on retinal fundus photographs,[18] and dermatology image classification,[17] and remains arguably the dominant challenge in applying AI systems in practice. Although various mechanisms for handling distribution shift exist, this problem cannot be considered solved, and mitigating it can remain a major cost driver for AI systems in radiology.

A final reason that the burden of creating training data sets can be problematic for AI systems in radiology is that it can lock in outdated standards of care or treatment protocols.[19] For instance, if an AI system for image triage was trained on a data set that did not contain cases from a newly discovered disease such as COVID-19, it could spuriously deprioritize individuals with those infections. Furthermore, continued use of models trained with expensive data sets that may someday reflect outmoded practice (eg, x-ray scoring systems that disadvantage marginalized patient subpopulations[5]) would result in patients receiving medical recommendations that are below the modern standard of clinical care. For radiologists, this issue may be particularly apparent for imaging protocols, which evolve over time and may be inconsistently implemented. As an example, widespread use of AI systems for computed tomographic (CT) analysis developed using a particular protocol for contrast timing may result in the continued use of that protocol even though it may be suboptimal for other reasons.[1]

In summary, creating appropriately representative labeled data sets is likely to remain a challenge for widespread use of AI systems in radiology, both because of the cost associated and the inherent difficulty of ensuring that a data set represents all important axes of variation, including variations caused by changes in radiology technology and practice in the future.

Mitigating Algorithmic Bias

A major challenge for both users and developers of clinical AI systems is ensuring that they do not create or amplify biases in the provision of care that would disadvantage particular groups of patients. In technical parlance, this involves building models that are "robust" to important variations in the patient population such as gender, ethnicity, socioeconomic status, and other protected factors. As described earlier, creating representative data sets for training and evaluation of AI models is an important component of mitigating model bias, and it is worth further discussing specific error modes that can lead to biased data sets. First, data from Electronic Health Records (EHRs) are often not meant for algorithm development, meaning that models developed using cohorts and labels drawn from EHRs may contain a variety of inherent biases such as those resulting from the use of billing codes rather than pathologic descriptions for diagnoses.[2] Second, because it can be difficult to access patient data (even for patients themselves), standard strategies for enrolling diverse populations in clinical development efforts can be difficult to apply.[1,2] Some health systems also suffer from selection bias, where information that would be useful for data labeling is only recorded for cases of particular academic or clinical interest. Furthermore, even with an appropriate cohort design, data may either be missing[20] or only available in certain segments of the population. A particularly striking example of this situation was highlighted recently by the work of Kaushal and colleagues,[21] which showed that most of the AI studies in imaging performed in the United States leveraged data from only 3 states. Prospective users of AI systems must be constantly vigilant for these types of data set curation issues that can result in biased algorithms.

Common training approaches that do not account for such issues as hidden stratification or class imbalance can also result in biased models. For instance, models are often trained to optimize average performance; such procedures result in models that perform well on majority classes (or subclasses) at the expense of less common groups in the population.

Finally, it is worth pointing out that unintended bias can also occur in algorithms aimed at improving elements of the image reconstruction process in volumetric imaging. For example, although both tomographic protocols and MR imaging could benefit from AI-based steps in the calibration, signal conditioning, denoising, and reconstruction processes, it is not always clear that mathematical transformations learned on a particular set of data or population will provide similar utility on other data sets.[7] Common axes of variation that should be considered in data set curation and algorithm design for such applications include scanner or hardware type, examination protocol, tracer type, patient characteristics, and other parameters that could affect image acquisition and reconstruction.

Measuring Correlation Instead of Causation

A particularly concerning pitfall in deep learning systems in particular has been their ability to make accurate predictions based on features that are correlated with the outcome, but which are *noncausal*. In radiology, examples include algorithms that predict severe disease when they recognize a portable scanner was used instead of a fixed x-ray machine (which would require the patient to be well enough to travel to the radiology department for the image), and those that rely on the presence of chest drains to predict pneumothorax.[13,15] In dermatology, a prime example is a recent algorithm that used the presence of surgical markings to recognize melanoma in dermoscopic images.[22] Because deep learning systems are usually optimized to maximize a specific performance metric without considering causality, they are prone to mistakes such as these, predicting outcomes based on confounding, noncausal features.

Technical and Engineering Issues

Even if the risks described to this point are appropriately mitigated, a variety of common technical issues can result in AI systems that do not perform as designed. One such problem is overfitting, which occurs when models perform well on a training set but poorly on a held-out evaluation set; this is often the result of insufficient regularization during training or distribution shift between training and evaluation sets. Data leakage between training and evaluation sets occurs when samples that are in the evaluation set also appear in the training set, and leads to overly optimistic performance metrics on the evaluation set because the model was exposed to very similar examples during training (and it can memorize them rather than learn generally useful image features). Although the exact same examples can be included in both sets by accident, a more subtle version of this same error can occur when examples from the same patient are included in both training and evaluation sets.

Poorly calibrated models can also be problematic. A "calibrated" model is one in which the quantitative values output from the model reflect true probabilities; for example, if a well-calibrated diagnostic algorithm predicts that each of 4 patients has a disease with 75% probability, one should expect that 3 of those 4 patients would actually have the disease. If a model is not calibrated, clinicians could erroneously interpret model outputs in a manner that would negatively affect patient care.

AI systems can also simply fail; because AI systems are a type of software, bugs are unfortunately a fact of life. In radiology applications, particularly important types of engineering errors include images that are corrupted in transmission/storage and cause erroneous predictions; preprocessing differences between data sets or institutions that result in distribution shift; or simple coding errors that cause model weights to be incorrectly loaded or output to be incorrectly computed. These errors can have real-world consequences, like a critically ill patient being deprioritized or benefits being withheld from needy individuals.[23]

Finally, for image enhancement and reconstruction applications, a major technical challenge involves ensuring that as AI algorithms generate images that are more suitable for human interpretation, they do not insert spurious information that was not in the original image. The difference between *imputation* (the recovery of lost or imperfectly acquired information), *enhancement* (making better use of existing information), and *hallucination* (the creation of information that was not in the original image) is often subtle, and it can be difficult even for domain experts to evaluate.[7] As this area of the field—sometimes referred to as "upstream AI"—matures further, it will be critical to develop robust metrics and evaluation procedures to ensure that AI-enabled image processing techniques can provide value by improving image analysis without inserting spurious information.

Postdeployment Monitoring

Postdeployment monitoring represents an additional challenge for the deployment of AI systems. To mitigate issues related to distribution shift and model bias—as well as to continuously evaluate whether a model is providing the anticipated operational benefit—it is critical that models be constantly under assessment while deployed. Various strategies for postdeployment monitoring exist, including manual human audits of model output, automated algorithmic evaluation of distribution shift or hidden stratification, out-of-distribution (OOD) sample detection, and continued evaluation protocols, but many academic studies that demonstrate the initial viability of an AI system do not consider how postdeployment monitoring should be implemented.[15] Furthermore, when considering whether to deploy a given AI system, the cost of continuous monitoring—which includes subject matter expert time, additional data curation, and even the expense of taking a model out of service if it begins performing poorly—must be considered.

Deployment Details

In addition to technical and functional issues, deploying AI algorithms in radiology practice raises several ethical, medicolegal, economic, and logistical questions that have not yet been convincingly resolved.

First, if an outside developer creates a model, it must be decided how liability from mistakes that occur in the course of practice should be divided among the radiologist, the algorithm developer, the device manufacturer, and other relevant parties.[6] Furthermore, it is often not clear how the model output is explained to a patient, whether patients should be informed that AI algorithms were used in their care, and what recourse might be available toward disputing treatment decisions made based on model output. These issues become even more fraught if models have been fine-tuned for a particular site or deployment environment, and may depend on whether a given model has been developed internally on custom or open-source tooling, has been developed internally using a commercial platform, or is provided via a software-as-a-service or model-as-a-service agreement.

Second, AI models and deployment hardware must be co-optimized to ensure that model execution time is sufficiently rapid to provide anticipated value. In particular, if users of models deployed to edge devices (eg, laptops, phones, etc.), on extremely large images (eg, volumetric scans), or in time-critical contexts like interventional radiology do not ensure that sufficient compute capability and network bandwidth are available to support proposed use cases, the resulting slow-down in computing model outputs could have negative clinical consequences. The alternative, however, may be the deployment of expensive new hardware at clinical sites or the use of cloud processing, each of which involves its own risks and benefits.

Third, for models to be used ethically, policies regarding the use of and access to patient data by the patients, the treatment center, and any external parties must be explicitly delineated. Unfortunately, in many contexts, public policy has not yet provided sufficient guidance for users to know exactly what procedures should be observed on this front.

Fourth, security considerations in deployment must be appropriately addressed. Were bad actors to gain access to a model or the training data, various attacks can be envisioned that could reveal patient's identity, interfere with treatment, or exfiltrate valuable data to which various parties (including the patient) have exclusive rights as well as expectations of privacy. Proposed AI deployments in radiology often do not fully consider the scope of potential attack vectors on both data and models, and do not explicitly guard against such attacks as data poisoning (affecting model performance by altering training data) or model inversion (reconstructing training data from model parameters). Remaining robust to these sorts of attacks is heavily related to post-deployment monitoring described earlier, and may benefit from specific approaches to model training and evaluation.[24]

User Trust

For AI to provide value in radiology practice, these systems must gain the confidence of both patients and clinicians. Concerns about the deleterious effects of automated assistance on radiologist performance, lack of interpretability in clinical decisions, and the potential for reinforcement of existing biases or outmoded practice must be overcome.[19,25] Automation bias is a serious problem wherein the very fact that human readers have algorithmic support causes them to trust the automated result even when it is flawed. Deep neural networks have well-documented difficulties establishing exactly what reasoning led to a given model output. The danger of introducing models that disadvantage particular patient groups is ever-present. As a result, to make effective and equitable use of AI in radiology, it is critical to design workflows that incorporate not only algorithmic input and broad clinical domain expertise, but also the individualized expertise that doctors have about the situation of each patient and the intimate knowledge that each patient has of their own body.[20]

Regulatory Approval

Deployment of AI algorithms for clinical use cases will rarely occur outside the bounds of governmentally stipulated regulatory structures. As a result, regulations for AI systems in radiology must be designed to balance potential improvements in patient care with the risks that such systems can pose if deployed incorrectly. Though both governmental agencies[26] and independent bodies[27,28] have recently made substantial progress toward defining constructive paths forward, the evolving regulatory environment will likely mean that certain applications will move faster than others (eg, computer-assisted detection vs computer-assisted diagnosis), and that it will be particularly important for clinicians to understand exactly what models can and cannot do before using them in practice. Although substantial discussion of regulation for clinical AI models is handled in a separate chapter, it suffices to say that clinicians intending to use AI in practice should remain up to date on regulations governing system use, processes for approval, and associated reporting requirements.

HOW CAN THESE CHALLENGES BE OVERCOME?

Although the challenges described earlier are substantial, technical and operational approaches to mitigate nearly all of them either exist or are in development. The degree to which AI algorithms can provide meaningful value in radiology practice will likely be determined by the effectiveness with which these techniques are implemented in practice and rigorously analyzed in the context of real-world operational data.

Meaningful Performance Measurement

Several concrete steps could help to improve the performance measurement of AI models in radiology.

First, common, widely available data sets suitable for evaluating performance on tasks of clinical interest should be constructed and continuously updated by objective bodies such as professional societies, academic consortia, or government agencies. Importantly, these evaluation data sets should be labeled in a way that closely reflects the intended workflow into which the model will be deployed, as opposed to using arbitrary academic schema. Existing efforts like data sets released by the Radiological Society of North America (RSNA), The Cancer Imaging Archive (TCIA), and others should be expanded.[14,29–31] Furthermore, each task of clinical interest should have evaluation data sets that are *frequently updated* so that models can be evaluated on the latest imaging technologies and not be allowed to overfit to a particular evaluation set.

Second, data sets should be labeled with important subclasses to enable analysis of potential model bias and reduce the impact of hidden stratification. Recent unsupervised methods can also be used to algorithmically identify subclasses of interest.[32]

Third, it may sometimes be beneficial to define the scope of model functionality more narrowly to enable sharper measurements of performance.[8,33] Instead of aiming for a single model that can generalize across data from different institutions (ie, multiple distributions), for instance, modelers could consider developing multiple different single-institution models and avoid having to constantly measure relative performance across potentially different populations. Conceptually, this idea resembles recent approaches from precision medicine.[33] If applied carefully, such a strategy could improve the utility of performance measurements for AI models in radiology.

Finally, assessing model performance on downstream clinical tasks—rather than on intermediate performance metrics like accuracy—will help to ensure that performance is measured in a way that is clinically meaningful. Ideally, direct comparison to existing baseline systems should be performed via randomized controlled trials wherein the AI system should be directly integrated into a clinician workflow and the downstream clinical outcome is measured.[25] The more realistic the setting is, and the closer that we can come to measuring *clinical value* rather than *algorithmic performance*, the more likely we are to arrive at a useful assessment of AI system utility.

Creating Training Data Sets

Recent technical progress on methods that can relieve the burden of creating and updating data sets has been promising. First, methods from *weak supervision* have enabled large data sets with weaker, noisier labels to support AI models that perform similarly to those trained on hand-labeled data sets of similar size.[34–36] Many of these methods directly leverage human expertise in a way that enables rapid relabeling and retraining to combat model performance and distribution shift issues. Automated, NLP-based labelers have also shown promise in building labeled data sets, though adapting them to new domains can be labor-intensive.[37,38]

Other technical approaches have focused on leveraging additional sources of signal within the model training process. Modern data augmentation techniques enable users to increase the effective size of training data sets by applying transformations to existing images without disrupting the meaningful features within those images. Common examples include applying rotations to labeled images or synonymy swaps to labeled text in language modeling tasks.[39,40] Multitask learning—building models that learn to perform multiple, related tasks simultaneously—can also help to decrease the number of labeled examples required by leveraging additional information from the data set. Transfer learning applies a similar approach, but usually involves 2 steps: (1) pretraining a model on a task that is related to the final task of interest and (2) fine-tuning that pretrained model by continuing to train it on the task of interest.[41] In medical computer vision applications, for instance, it is particularly common to use models that are pretrained on the ImageNet database as a starting point on which to train models for clinical use cases.[8,11,33,42,43] Recent approaches from self-supervision and contrastive learning that leverage large, unlabeled datasets for model pretraining have also shown promise in reducing the required size of labeled data sets.[44]

In clinical applications, another way that the data curation burden can be reduced is by standardizing protocols. Instead of having to train models over images acquired via a wide variety of protocols—for example, tube currents, voltages, and reconstruction settings in CT—it can be advantageous to train models obtained using a standard protocol and then ensure that such models are only applied to images obtained using that standard protocol. Similar to the precision medicine perspective presented earlier, this approach trades off generalizability for a narrow task definition.

Mitigating Algorithmic Bias

Combating algorithmic bias is one of the single most important tasks required to deploy AI models ethically and equitably within radiology practice. In addition to constructing training data in as non-biased a way as possible, there exist several additional approaches that can help to mitigate this problem.

First, a variety of training algorithms focused on reducing the worst-case subgroup performance—that is, ensuring that there exists no subgroup of data on which a model performs substantially worse than another—have been the focus of recent research.[32,45–47] As these and additional approaches for improving algorithmic fairness are developed, they should be considered for clinical translation.[48]

Second, because these training algorithms are often used during model development rather than model deployment, clinical users may rarely interact with them. However, clinical users will routinely be exposed to model output, and as a result, tooling designed to clearly and dynamically evaluate model robustness will become an increasingly important part of successful AI deployments in radiology.[49,50] Research and development studies focused on enabling clinical

users to reliably determine which model features are most responsible for a given output, to quickly assess model performance on a wide variety of subclasses or subgroups, and to rapidly evaluate the effect of such variations on clinical outcomes would improve our ability to deploy models equitably.

Finally, direct participation from physician and patient communities in model development and deployment can help to ensure that individuals are best served by these models in practice. Indeed, as pointed out by Esteva and colleagues in their recent review article,[11] community participation recently enabled the discovery of data set bias and identified demographics underserved by a model for population health management.[51] A similar case occurred when evaluating models for detecting diabetic retinopathy in Southeast Asia, where socioeconomic factors heavily impacted model efficacy.[18] If radiologists are able to deploy AI models in cooperation with their clinical communities—while ensuring that non-AI backups are used when appropriate—these capabilities stand a much better chance of having a clinical impact that is both positive and equitable.

Measuring Correlation Instead of Causation

Ensuring that models do not rely on confounding variables in making their predictions requires many of the same strategies described earlier. Model auditing by human actors can help to discover cases where models make the right prediction for the wrong reason. External validation can be a particularly helpful tool in ensuring that data set artifacts are not responsible for model performance. Encouraging models to respect important invariances via data augmentation strategies can further reduce the possibility of noncausal features driving model predictions. Finally, interpretability analyses such as heatmaps that identify which structures informed the algorithmic decisions[52] and other visualization methods can help radiologists to identify such behavior before it becomes a problem (**Fig. 2**).

Technical and Engineering Issues

Many of the technical issues described here should be identified and addressed by applying best practices from software engineering. Clearly defining testing strategies before model development, ensuring that systems are routinely tested during deployment, and integrating the entire data processing pipeline into those procedures can reduce the probability of unintended errors making their way into critical software paths. In radiology, the data processing pipeline includes

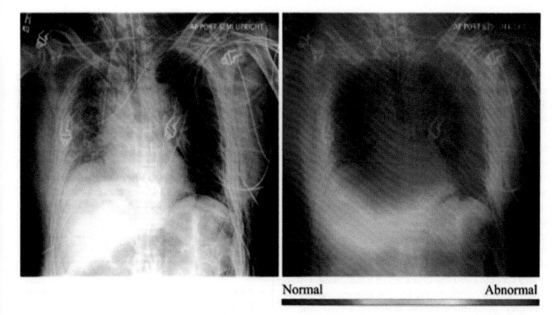

Normal   Abnormal

Fig. 2. Image (*left*) and class activation map (*right*) showing the area that most heavily influenced a neural network designed for binary radiograph triage to provide an "abnormal" prediction. Red indicates areas of relatively high contribution to an abnormal score, whereas blue areas indicate the opposite. (*From* Dunnmon JA, Yi D, Langlotz CP, Ré C, Rubin DL, Lungren MP. Assessment of Convolutional Neural Networks for Automated Classification of Chest Radiographs. *Radiology*. 2019;290(2):537-544.)

data ingestion from hardware, image reconstruction, transfer to and egress from a Picture Archiving and Communications System (PACS), conditioning operations such as histogram equalization, and model inference.

Postdeployment Monitoring

Postdeployment monitoring can be accomplished in several ways, as described by Oakden-Rayner and colleagues.[15] First, if clinicians are able to define subgroups or performance tests of interest before model development, tests based on these definitions can be implemented and continuously evaluated for anomalous behavior during deployment. Algorithmic auditing, where human experts periodically inspect model output to identify concerning trends, is often viable in cases where it is not possible to write a comprehensive set of tests before development. Finally, recently developed algorithmic measures for assessing worst-case subgroup performance can provide value by identifying poorly performing groups without human intervention.[32]

An important aspect of postdeployment monitoring is ensuring that cases on which the model was not intended to be executed—for instance, a lateral CXR for a model that was trained on frontal examinations—is not erroneously provided to a model for analysis. The increasing amount of research dedicated to the task of identifying samples that are outside the distribution on which a model was intended to operate, commonly called "out-of-distribution (OOD) detection," has provided encouraging evidence that OOD samples can be automatically identified and flagged. OOD detection should become a standard tool in postdeployment monitoring suites, and should inform both deployment practice and future model development.

Finally, consistent use of adverse event registers for AI systems in radiology could help to provide high-level monitoring for undesired outcomes. Such registers are standard practice for deployed medical products, and for AI systems would simply record any untoward medical occurrence that happened while that system was in use. Though they do not provide causal information, observational information from adverse event registers could be useful in postdeployment monitoring for broadly deployed AI systems in radiology.

Deployment Details

To address deployment challenges described earlier, additional development work is required on several fronts. On medicolegal issues of liability, responsibility, and data rights, the larger volumes of case law that should be expected in the near future should help to directly resolve some of these questions. On the hardware-software codesign front, effective systems engineering and modular design should become standard practice from model developers as the industry matures. Hospitals may ultimately desire to invest in their own inference hardware (eg, dedicated CPUs, GPUs, mobile devices), or even to run computation in a secure cloud environment; each of these decisions has advantages and disadvantages, and it is not clear what approach will become dominant. Finally, we expect a similar trend in model cybersecurity. As it becomes clear that both models and associated data have substantial economic value (and possibly legal protections), penetration testing and other traditional cybersecurity protocols will likely become an even more important part of medical information technology systems than they already are. Practitioners can improve the chances of a successful AI deployment by accounting for the associated engineering and compliance costs upfront, and ensuring that they weigh these costs against the expected value provided by the AI system.

User Trust

To improve user trust in AI systems for radiology, involving clinical and patient users in model and workflow development from the beginning is essential. To be able to use a system confidently in practice, clinician users must have trained with it, internalized its strengths and weaknesses, and become comfortable with both integrating its output into their decision processes and explaining those processes to patients. Like any clinical investigation, patient awareness and education will be paramount for effective engagement and improvement of care. Any improvements that can be made to model interpretability will assist clinician users in bridging this gap, and incorporating the possibility of a follow-up examination to confirm the predictions of an AI system would likely have positive outcomes in many cases. In the end, user trust will only be developed insomuch as the benefit of the AI systems for concrete clinical decisions can be directly observed by clinicians and clearly communicated to patients.

Regulatory Approval

Clinicians have an opportunity to work directly with the public policy community to create regulatory structures that incentivize innovation while maintaining appropriate safety standards. Linking regulatory guidance and approval to standardized reporting for model development and performance such as the SPIRIT-AI and CONSORT-AI guidelines would not only provide clarity for regulatory approvers, but also ensure that users of a given AI-based system are well-informed about exactly how it was developed, precisely what population it was intended for, and any other items that would be important for postdeployment monitoring and clinical use. Although much work in this area remains to be done, progress in recent years has been rapid, and we expect that the regulatory environment will continue to mature in the near future. Regulatory issues for AI systems in radiology are discussed in further detail in a separate H. Benjamin Harvey and Vrushab Gowda's article, "Regulatory Issues and Challenges to AI Adoption," in this issue.

CLINICS CARE POINTS

- Radiologists should think deeply about how to create workflows that do not force AI systems into a pre-existing role, but rather optimize human-machine teams.
- Clinicians who plan to use AI in practice should train extensively with it beforehand.
- When using AI models in the clinic, robust structures for post-deployment monitoring must be in place.
- AI-enabled workflows in radiology should always have a backup in case the AI system needs to be taken offline.

ACKNOWLEDGMENTS

The author is grateful to the following individuals for their helpful feedback on this work: Daniel Rubin, Matt Lungren, Luke Oakden-Rayner, Sarah Hooper, Khaled Saab, Neel Guha, Swetava Ganguli, and Adele Xu.

DISCLOSURE

The author has nothing to disclose.

REFERENCES

1. Thrall JH, Li X, Li Q, et al. Artificial Intelligence and Machine Learning in Radiology: Opportunities, Challenges, Pitfalls, and Criteria for Success. J Am Coll Radiol 2018;15:504–8.
2. Rajkomar A, Dean J, Kohane I. Machine Learning in Medicine. N Engl J Med 2019;380(14):1347–58.
3. Rajpurkar Id P, Jl Id, Ball RL, et al. Deep learning for chest radiograph diagnosis: A retrospective comparison of the CheXNeXt algorithm to practicing

radiologists. PLoS Med 2018. https://doi.org/10.1371/journal.pmed.1002686.

4. Tang YX, Tang YB, Peng Y, et al. Automated abnormality classification of chest radiographs using deep convolutional neural networks. NPJ Digit Med 2020;3(1). https://doi.org/10.1038/s41746-020-0273-z.

5. Pierson E, Cutler DM, Leskovec J, et al. An algorithmic approach to reducing unexplained pain disparities in underserved populations. Nat Med 2021; 27(1):136–40.

6. Chiwome L, Okojie OM, Rahman AKMJ, et al. Artificial Intelligence: Is It Armageddon for Breast Radiologists? Cureus 2020. https://doi.org/10.7759/cureus.8923.

7. Chaudhari AS, Sandino CM, Cole EK, et al. Prospective Deployment of Deep Learning in <scp>MRI</scp> : A Framework for Important Considerations, Challenges, and Recommendations for Best Practices. J Magn Reson Imaging 2020. https://doi.org/10.1002/jmri.27331. jmri.27331.

8. Dunnmon JA, Yi D, Langlotz CP, et al. Assessment of Convolutional Neural Networks for Automated Classification of Chest Radiographs. Radiology 2019; 290(2):537–44.

9. Titano JJ, Badgeley M, Schefflein J, et al. Automated deep-neural-network surveillance of cranial images for acute neurologic events. Nat Med 2018;24(9): 1337–41.

10. Lambin P, Leijenaar RTH, Deist TM, et al. Radiomics: The bridge between medical imaging and personalized medicine. Nat Rev Clin Oncol 2017.

11. Esteva A, Chou K, Yeung S, et al. Deep learning-enabled medical computer vision. NPJ Digit Med 2021;4(1):5. https://doi.org/10.1038/s41746-020-00376-2.

12. Exploring the ChestXray14 dataset: problems – Luke Oakden-Rayner. Available at: https://lukeoakdenrayner.wordpress.com/2017/12/18/the-chestxray14-dataset-problems/. Accessed January 24, 2018.

13. Zech JR, Badgeley MA, Liu M, et al. Variable generalization performance of a deep learning model to detect pneumonia in chest radiographs: A cross-sectional study. PLoS Med 2018;15(11): e1002683.

14. Sawyer Lee R, Dunnmon JA, He A, et al. Comparison of segmentation-free and segmentation-dependent computer-aided diagnosis of breast masses on a public mammography dataset. J Biomed Inform 2021;113:103656.

15. Oakden-Rayner L, Dunnmon J, Carneiro G, et al. Hidden stratification causes clinically meaningful failures in machine learning for medical imaging. Proceedings of the ACM conference on health, inference, and learning. 2020.

16. Gulshan V, Peng L, Coram M, et al. Development and Validation of a Deep Learning Algorithm for Detection of Diabetic Retinopathy in Retinal Fundus Photographs. JAMA 2016;316(22):2402.

17. Kamulegeya LH, Okello M, Bwanika JM, et al. Using artificial intelligence on dermatology conditions in Uganda: A case for diversity in training data sets for machine learning. bioRxiv 2019;826057. https://doi.org/10.1101/826057.

18. Beede E, Baylor E, Hersch F, et al. A Human-Centered Evaluation of a Deep Learning System Deployed in Clinics for the Detection of Diabetic Retinopathy. In: Conference on Human Factors in Computing Systems - Proceedings. Association for Computing Machinery; Honolulu, HI, April 25-30, 2020. p. 1-12. https://doi.org/10.1145/3313831.3376718.

19. Tsai TL, Fridsma DB, Gatti G. Computer decision support as a source of interpretation error: The case of electrocardiograms. J Am Med Inform Assoc 2003;10(5):478–83.

20. Thomas R. Medicine's Machine Learning Problem | Boston Review. Available at: https://bostonreview.net/science-nature/rachel-thomas-medicines-machine-learning-problem. Accessed January 9, 2021.

21. Kaushal A, Altman R, Langlotz C. Geographic distribution of US cohorts used to train deep learning algorithms. JAMA 2020;324(12):1212–3.

22. Winkler JK, Fink C, Toberer F, et al. Association between Surgical Skin Markings in Dermoscopic Images and Diagnostic Performance of a Deep Learning Convolutional Neural Network for Melanoma Recognition. JAMA Dermatol 2019;155(10):1135–41.

23. Lecher C. A healthcare algorithm started cutting care, and no one knew why - The Verge. Available at: https://www.theverge.com/2018/3/21/17144260/healthcare-medicaid-algorithm-arkansas-cerebral-palsy. Accessed January 18, 2021.

24. Cohen J, Rosenfeld E, Kolter JZ. Certified adversarial robustness via randomized smoothing. In: 36th International Conference on Machine Learning, ICML 2019. Long Beach, CA, June 10-15, 2019.

25. Challen R, Denny J, Pitt M, et al. Artificial intelligence, bias and clinical safety. BMJ Qual Saf 2019;28(3):231–7.

26. Harvey HB, Gowda V. How the FDA Regulates AI. Acad Radiol 2020;27(1):58-61. https://doi.org/10.1016/j.acra.2019.09.017.

27. Cruz Rivera S, Liu X, Chan AW, et al. Guidelines for clinical trial protocols for interventions involving artificial intelligence: the SPIRIT-AI extension. Nat Med 2020;26(9):1351–63.

28. Liu X, Cruz Rivera S, Moher D, et al. Reporting guidelines for clinical trial reports for interventions involving artificial intelligence: the CONSORT-AI extension. Nat Med 2020;26(9):1364–74.

29. Clark K, Vendt B, Smith K, et al. The cancer imaging archive (TCIA): Maintaining and operating a public information repository. J Digit Imaging 2013. https://doi.org/10.1007/s10278-013-9622-7.

30. Flanders AE, Prevedello LM, Shih G, et al. Construction of a Machine Learning Dataset through Collaboration: The RSNA 2019 Brain CT Hemorrhage Challenge. Radiol Artif Intell 2020. https://doi.org/10.1148/ryai.2020190211.

31. Johnson AEW, Pollard TJ, Berkowitz SJ, et al. MIMIC-CXR, a de-identified publicly available database of chest radiographs with free-text reports. Sci Data 2019. https://doi.org/10.1038/s41597-019-0322-0.

32. Sohoni N, Dunnmon JA, Angus G, et al. No Subclass Left Behind: Fine-Grained Robustness in Coarse-Grained Classification Problems. Advances in Neural Information Processing Systems 33 (2020).

33. Thrall JH, Fessell D, Pandharipande PV. Rethinking the Approach to Artificial Intelligence for Medical Image Analysis: The Case for Precision Diagnosis. J Am Coll Radiol 2021;18:174–9.

34. Ratner A, Bach SH, Ehrenberg H, et al. Snorkel: Rapid training data creation with weak supervision. Proc VLDB Endow 2017;11(3):269–82.

35. Dunnmon J, Ratner A, Khandwala N, et al. Cross-modal data programming enables rapid medical machine learning. Patterns, 1(2),100019.

36. Fries JA, Varma P, Chen VS, et al. Weakly supervised classification of aortic valve malformations using unlabeled cardiac MRI sequences. Nat Commun 2019;10(1):3111.

37. Irvin J, Rajpurkar P, Ko M, et al. CheXpert: A Large Chest Radiograph Dataset with Uncertainty Labels and Expert Comparison. Proc AAAI Conf Artif Intell 2019;33(01):590–7.

38. Peng Y, Wang X, Lu L, et al. NegBio: a high-performance tool for negation and uncertainty detection in radiology reports. Proc Am Med Inform Assoc Summits Transl Sci 2018;2017:188.

39. Ratner AJ, Ehrenberg H, Hussain Z, et al. Learning to compose domain-specific transformations for data augmentation. Adv Neural Inf Process Syst 2017;30:3236–46.

40. Cubuk ED, Zoph B, Mane D, Vasudevan V, Le Q V. Autoaugment: Learning augmentation strategies from data. In: Proceedings of the IEEE Computer Society Conference on Computer Vision and Pattern Recognition. Long Beach, CA, June 16-20, 2019. https://doi.org/10.1109/CVPR.2019.00020.

41. Eyuboglu S, Angus G, Patel BN, et al. Multi-task weak supervision enables anatomically-resolved abnormality detection in whole-body FDG-PET/CT. Nat Commun. 2021;12(1):1880. https://doi.org/10.1038/s41467-021-22018-1.

42. Jia D, Dong W, Socher R, et al. ImageNet: A large-scale hierarchical image database. IEEE CVPR 2009;248–55. https://doi.org/10.1109/CVPR.2009.5206848.

43. Esteva A, Kuprel B, Novoa RA, et al. Dermatologist-Level Classification of Skin Cancer with Deep Neural Networks. Nature 2017;542(7639):115–8.

44. Azizi S, Mustafa B, Ryan F, et al. Big self-supervised models advance medical image classification; 2021. arXiv:2101.05224.

45. Sagawa S, Koh PW, Hashimoto TB, et al. Distributionally Robust Neural Networks for Group Shifts: On the Importance of Regularization for Worst-Case Generalization. 2019. Available at: http://arxiv.org/abs/1911.08731. Accessed December 3, 2019.

46. Arjovsky M, Bottou L, Gulrajani I, et al. Invariant risk Minimization 2019. Available at: http://arxiv.org/abs/1907.02893. Accessed November 23, 2019.

47. Pfohl S, Marafino B, Coulet A, et al. Creating fair models of atherosclerotic cardiovascular disease risk. Proceedings of the 2019 AAAI/ACM Conference on AI, Ethics, and Society. 2019.

48. Chen IY, Joshi S, Ghassemi M. Treating health disparities with artificial intelligence. Nat Med 2020;26(1):16–7.

49. Mitchell M, Wu S, Zaldivar A, et al. Model cards for model reporting. In: FAT* 2019 - Proceedings of the 2019 Conference on Fairness, Accountability, and Transparency. Atlanta, GA, January 29-31, 2019. https://doi.org/10.1145/3287560.3287596.

50. Goel K, Rajani N, Vig J, et al. Robustness Gym: Unifying the NLP Evaluation Landscape. NAACL-HLT 2021, 42.

51. Obermeyer Z, Powers B, Vogeli C, et al. Dissecting racial bias in an algorithm used to manage the health of populations. Science 2019;366(6464):447–53.

52. Zhou B, Khosla A, Lapedriza A, et al. Learning Deep Features for Discriminative Localization. In: IEEE CVPR. ; 2016:2921-2929. Available at: https://www.cv-foundation.org/openaccess/content_cvpr_2016/papers/Zhou_Learning_Deep_Features_CVPR_2016_paper.pdf. Accessed March 30, 2018.

Regulatory Issues and Challenges to Artificial Intelligence Adoption

Harlan Benjamin Harvey, MD, JD[a],*, Vrushab Gowda, JD[b]

KEYWORDS

- AI • Regulatory issues • Liability • Health law • Risk management

KEY POINTS

- The FDA does not currently possess an AI-specific regulatory paradigm, but instead applies its risk stratification framework for medical devices.
- In the coming years, the FDA may turn to a total product lifecycle approach to regulating AI products, similar to cGMP.
- Integrating AI products into radiology workflow patterns may require changes to reimbursement, interoperability, data security, and training patterns.
- AI is only as robust as the data it trains upon; high-quality, diverse, and adequately labeled datasets are essential to its success.
- Questions of liability in a clinical AI context are complex and remain unresolved.

INTRODUCTION

The past decade has borne witness to a remarkable transformation—the evolution of artificial intelligence (AI) technology from engineering novelty to revolutionary instrument. Having emerged from a desultory "AI winter," it now proliferates across multiple industry segments and extends deep through supply chains, enabling innovations as far afield as high-frequency trading, autonomous vehicles, personality computing, and mass surveillance.[1]

Health care has not escaped its sweep; AI technologies are increasingly gaining traction from drug discovery to surgical planning, to the extent it has earned the moniker "the stethoscope of the 21st century."[2] These developments are of particular salience to radiology, a data-intensive field leveraging pattern recognition, prognostic estimation, spatial modeling, and disease surveillance. Indeed, more AI products have been approved in the United States for radiologic application than for use in any other medical specialty, and many of these innovations originate from within imaging departments themselves.[3,4]

Despite its promise, AI technology exists in its nascency and remains largely untested in the clinical space. This nature is both a cause and a consequence of the uncertain legal–regulatory milieu it faces. The following discussion aims to shed light on these challenges, tracing the various pathways toward the US Food and Drug Administration (FDA) approval, the future of federal oversight, privacy issues, ethical dilemmas, and practical considerations related to implementation in radiologist practice.

SURVEYING THE REGULATORY LANDSCAPE: AN ALPHABET SOUP
Existing Pathways

At present, the FDA adopts a functional approach to the review, approval, and postmarket surveillance of AI technologies; no purpose-built regulatory framework specific to AI as yet exists. These products are assessed through standard paradigms, which primarily consider their (1) risk profile and (2) intended clinical use in determining the appropriate level of scrutiny.

[a] Radiology, Massachusetts General Hospital, Harvard Medical School, 175 Cambridge Street, Suite 200, Boston, MA 02114, USA; [b] Harvard Law School, 1563 Massachusetts Avenue, Cambridge, MA 02138, USA
* Corresponding author.
E-mail address: hbharvey@mgh.harvard.edu

Radiol Clin N Am 59 (2021) 1075–1083
https://doi.org/10.1016/j.rcl.2021.07.007
0033-8389/21/© 2021 Elsevier Inc. All rights reserved.

The threshold question is whether or not a given AI-enabled product constitutes a medical device. In relevant part, the federal Food, Drug & Cosmetic Act defines this term as "an instrument . . . intended for use in the diagnosis. . .or in the cure, mitigation, treatment, or prevention of disease . . . which does not achieve its primary intended purposes through chemical action."[5] More specifically, the FDA incorporates by reference the International Medical Device Regulators Forum definition of Software as a Medical Device, which includes "software intended to be used for one or more medical purposes that perform these purposes without being part of a hardware medical device."[6] Should these conditions be met, 3 available pathways exist (ranging from class I to class III in increasing order of rigor) distinguished by the scope of patient risk exposure, each with differing data submission requirements. Premarket approval (to which most class III devices are subject) represents the most stringent classification; absent a showing to the contrary, this is the default level of review accorded to de novo applications and requires clinical studies to demonstrate safety and efficacy. A successful submission through this method confers FDA "approval" of the software in question.

Depending on the characteristics of the device, class I and II submissions may trigger the less comprehensive premarket notification, also known as 510(k). This process culminates in the device's FDA clearance, as opposed to approval; although devices processed via either pathway may be marketed, this distinction is critical for the purposes of accurate labeling. Premarket notification requires a showing of "substantial equivalence" to a previously approved predicate device, in many cases simplifying the application and review processes considerably. However, this designation is unlikely to applicable to many groundbreaking AI technologies that lack preapproved predicates owing to their novelty.[7] The FDA has spoken directly to its classification of radiologic image analyzers and distinguishes between computer-assisted detection and computer-assisted diagnosis devices. It defines the former as tools that "identify, mark, highlight, or in any other manner direct attention" to features of a radiologic study, rather than those that autonomously drive diagnosis or staging. Commensurately, the FDA has designated a number of computer-assisted detection products as class II devices while maintaining the heightened level of class III scrutiny for computer-assisted diagnosis technologies.[8]

The 21st Century Cures Act (hereafter "Cures Act") amends the Food, Drug & Cosmetic Act to establish a number of exemptions to the statutory definition of "device," and by extension, from the purview of FDA device regulation. Per its §3060(a), these include products (1) intended for administrative support, or used in (2) the maintenance of a healthy lifestyle, (3) electronic patient records, (4) storage or display of clinical data—and critically for radiology—(5) "unless the function is intended to acquire, process, or analyze a medical image . . . for the purpose of (i) displaying, analyzing, or printing medical information . . . (ii) supporting or providing recommendations to a health care professional about prevention, diagnosis, or treatment and . . . (iii) enabling such health care professional to *independently review* the basis for such recommendations to make a clinical diagnosis or treatment decision regarding an individual patient."[9]

The FDA has clarified the scope of these provisions in twin guidance documents, nonbinding policy statements delineating the FDA's interpretation of the law and articulating enforcement priorities. In Clinical Decision Support Software (CDS Draft Guidance), the FDA recognizes "independent review" as the critical operative term of the Cures Act's exemptions, establishing that health care professionals "be able to reach the same recommendation . . . without relying primarily on the software function" for the device to escape formal regulatory oversight. The FDA furthermore requires developers to disclose the "purpose or intended use of the software function, the intended user (eg, ultrasound technicians, vascular surgeons), the inputs used to generate the recommendation (eg, patient age and gender), and the rationale or support for the recommendation."[10] That said, it remains to be determined at the time of writing how the FDA will interpret the sufficiency of said "rationale or support" and whether regulatory bodies possess a legal "right to explanation."[11] Developers, for their part, may prove hesitant to reveal trade secrets in what is already a burgeoning, competitive market. However, failure to disclose these potentially sensitive details hazards classification of their product as a "device," outside of the ambit of the §3060(a) exceptions and subject to a substantial regulatory burden. Developers are thus confronted with a dilemma: either reveal proprietary details of their product for accelerated regulatory approval or rely on opacity to preserve their competitive advantage.[12] The situation is only further complicated in the cases of deep learning or "black box" algorithms, for which an accurate description of a continuously learning internal mechanism may prove a practical impossibility. Beyond mere compliance with the terms of the Cures Act, such technologies lay bare the shortcomings of existing regulatory regimes, conventional clinical trial design, and the current state of postmarket surveillance mechanisms as applied to sophisticated AI products.[13]

Through a second guidance document, Changes to Existing Medical Software Policies (Changes Guidance), the FDA recapitulates its principles of enforcement discretion with respect to the aforementioned exemptions. In brief, the FDA aims to focus its regulatory efforts on those products displaying patient-specific data and "alert[ing] a caregiver to take immediate clinical action" based on clinical parameters.[14]

Future Directions

The unique complexities of Software as a Medical Device products beckon novel approaches to regulation. This has not been lost on the FDA, which in 2017 established a pilot program for Software as a Medical Device precertification as part of its Digital Health Innovation Action Plan.[15] Known as Pre-Cert 1.0, it looks to features of the developer, rather than the product, in a total product lifecycle approach.[16] This derives inspiration from the current good manufacturing practices paradigm, which the FDA requires device manufacturers to comply with.[17] A number of service providers (to include Apple, Fitbit, and Verily, among others) currently participate, invited after having demonstrated "a robust culture of quality and organizational excellence, and a [commitment] to monitoring real-world performance."[16] The program continues as of 2020; however, it has not yet expanded beyond its 9 initial participants and the FDA acknowledges that its expansive breadth may require statutory authorization.[18] Nonetheless, it offers key insights into what a potential AI regulatory regime may resemble.

The FDA released its Proposed Regulatory Framework for Modifications to Artificial Intelligence/Machine Learning-Based Software as a Medical Device (Discussion Paper) in April 2019, presenting a wholly novel schema and seeking input thereof.[19] At its core, it underscores the inadequacy of existing regulatory architecture to govern continuously learning algorithms. Would an approved AI device require 510(k) clearance after each autodidactic "modification?"[20] When do said modifications translate into clinical significance? Which qualitative factors would be relied on in making this determination? Should devices be required to maintain logs of each decision path? At what point would an adaptive algorithm accumulate so many modifications that it may

no longer be credibly termed "substantially equivalent" to its previously approved form? Conventional frameworks largely leave these unanswered, although the FDA has provided some direction into answering the first of these questions, albeit within the limited context of locked algorithms.[7]

By contrast, the Discussion Paper advocates for a flexible total product lifecycle–based design control model borrowing from the Pre-Cert 1.0 program. It analyzes developer characteristics with an eye to establishing "good machine learning practices" and encourages cooperation with the FDA across the length of a product's lifespan. The FDA draws particular attention to the critical role of high-quality data, emphasizing consistency, generalizability, and the maintenance of distinctions between training, tuning, and test datasets. Performance data are to be shared routinely with the FDA, which in turn would be well-placed to provide dynamic regulatory assessments from development to postmarket performance monitoring.

Turning to features of the product itself, the Discussion Paper calls for a multiaxial approach to risk stratification incorporating the significance of the information the product offers to the health care decision, the state of the health care condition, and whether or not the algorithm involved is locked or adaptive. Developers are moreover to anticipate modifications ex ante and establish protocols to govern future algorithm change. These modifications would then be categorized into one or more of the following categories requiring tailored premarket review: (1) performance modifications with no change to input or intended use (eg, training on new datasets), (2) input modifications with no change to intended use (eg, developing interoperability, including new data types), and (3) modifications to intended use (eg, application to new patient populations or pathology). Such an approach aims to balance an appropriate degree of regulatory oversight with the flexibility necessary to encourage continued innovation.

IMPLEMENTATION CHALLENGES: THE GROWING PAINS OF ARTIFICIAL INTELLIGENCE EXPANSION
Investment and Integration

Securing regulatory approval is one matter, but adoption another entirely. This section concerns the practicalities of implementing AI technologies in real-world settings. For one, financial considerations hinder ready incorporation into existing infrastructure. A recent survey of hospitals and imaging centers confirms this finding, revealing cost as the primary impediment to adoption, followed by a "lack of strategic direction."[21] Software price tags only tell part of the story; factoring in the costs of annual licenses, servers, and the sophisticated hardware products necessary for deep learning applications, to say nothing of training and technical support service fees, complete AI packages could easily range into the hundreds of thousands of dollars.[22] It is unclear how this additional expense would figure in the broader payor environment. Would the costs of AI-enabled radiologic studies be passed on to patients—the final consumers in this picture? As a further twist, these present costs must be weighed against speculative and difficult-to-quantify future savings in the form of increased radiologist productivity, enhanced workflow efficiency, and the averted costs of downstream treatment. In addressing this issue and incentivizing the use of AI, there may be a role for novel reimbursement mechanisms to include new Current Procedural Terminology codes and modernized radiologist relative value unit schedules.[23,24]

Radiologic applications of AI moreover face a rapidly evolving landscape and remain in a relatively early stage of development. As a strategic matter, health care institutions may opt to wait until the field matures further and more advanced alternatives become available before incurring the costs of implementation. This tactic would enable them to exploit second-mover advantage rather than bear the risk of investing in first-generation products that may quickly approach obsolescence. The field also faces a plethora of competing products across the value chain, raising a number of interoperability concerns.[25] For example, image analysis, triaging, and report generation algorithms may derive from different developers, interface with different servers, and lack a common means of integrating with a given imaging department's workflow pattern. Establishment of a vendor-neutral framework is thus an integral step in avoiding process fragmentation and facilitating AI adoption. To this end, the Digital Imaging and Communications in Medicine Working Group 23 has been tasked with addressing interoperability challenges; once finalized, its recommendations may offer an avenue forward.[26] The state of existing AI-enabled imaging technology is moreover hampered by a marked user unfriendliness. It stands to benefit from streamlined user experience optimization, perhaps through full integration with picture archiving and communication systems, facilitating adoption, operator training, and troubleshooting.[27]

Paths to incorporating AI tools into existing image analysis protocols may assume a variety of forms. One study presented 5 options along a sliding scale toward increasing integration: (1) maintaining an AI-specific workstation electronically separate from picture archiving and communication systems; (2) establishing built-in image processing functions that automatically interface with picture archiving and communication systems; (3) deploying multiple programs in parallel, whose output is synthesized on a purpose-built integration framework; (4) investing in multiple, mutually interoperative AI products requiring no third-party platform for integration; and (5) full-spectrum integration directly linked to the electronic health record.[28] There is no one-size-fits-all approach to AI implementation; each of these options bears its own combination of advantages and drawbacks. Rather than treating this list as a spectrum of technological sophistication, it may be more appropriate to consider the specific resource demands of the institution contemplating AI expansion. The 5 options are suited to particular uses (eg, patient volume, deployment in imaging centers vs hospitals, general vs specialty practices) and impose variable capital requirements, both of which inform financial decision-making at the level of the individual group.

Clinical Validation

Clinical validity distinguishes mere technological curiosity from bona fide adjunct to patient care. Although a number of radiologic AI products have indeed proven revolutionary, this fact alone cannot be taken for granted. For instance, computer-assisted detection mammography became a nearly ubiquitous fixture of breast imaging in the first decade after FDA approval. Across the same span, a breakthrough study revealed that cancer detection sensitivity actually decreased among certain segments of radiologists who used this technique.[29] Although the outcome was likely multifactorial in origin, it suffices to demonstrate that AI technology, by itself, is no panacea. In a more modern iteration, rule-out algorithms display a number of similar shortcomings when applied to real-world clinical environments. For example, those designed for the rapid detection of intracerebral hemorrhage may function well for the task at hand, but neglect to account for the no less acute ramifications of a negative result, to include ischemic stroke or an inflammatory process.[30] Contemporary AI technologies reveal a limited ability to contextualize findings. They furthermore lack the capacity to approximate radiologist judgment calls regarding overdiagnosis; by their inherent overinclusive qualities, they may paradoxically contribute to a local increase, rather than a decrease, in medical expenditures.

At present, the development of radiologic AI applications is limited by the availability of use cases with well-annotated inputs and standardized outputs.[27] This issue turns on both the quality and quantity of data, although both are interrelated; high-quality output scales with data, particularly for deep learning algorithms.[31] Additionally, large training datasets are required for sensitive and specific detection of low-prevalence pathologies.[32] Yet consideration of volume does not necessarily reveal the full picture. This point is critical to note, because extrapolation from clinically unrepresentative datasets, however large, may introduce confounding variables and amplify noise.[31] The importance of a drive toward externally validated training datasets containing generalizable information can, therefore, not be understated. Worrisomely, a 2019 meta-analysis indicated that only 6% of published AI studies under review performed external validation.[33] These issues may in part find remedy by the establishment of open-source data repositories in the mold of the National Institutes of Health All of Us Research Program, drafting of multi-institutional data-sharing agreements, expansion of federated learning techniques, and research shift toward multicentric trials.[34–36] These agreements would stand to offer further usefulness from implementation of the FAIR Guiding Principles, which offer a scaffold for data stewardship through "findability, accessibility, interoperability, and reusability."[37]

Privacy and Ethical Issues

The sheer scale of patient data used in AI applications invites a number of concerns related to ownership, remuneration, privacy, and liability. At present, there is limited federal direction regarding the former. The Health Insurance Portability and Accountability Act establishes a patient right to inspection over their own medical records, but does not otherwise confer ownership rights.[38] Similarly, high court jurisprudence is largely silent on this matter; in the closest analog, the Supreme Court invalidated a Vermont statute prohibiting the commercial use of physicians' prescribing records on First Amendment grounds.[39] The issue has thus devolved upon the states, among whom only one—New Hampshire—expressly provides for patient ownership of data. Of the remaining states, 28 do not speak to control and the remaining 21 consider providers, or provider organizations, the ultimate owners of medical information.[40]

A well-cited Hastings Center study articulated a novel framework in which users as well as principals of a health care system bear the ethical imperative of improving it.[41] Some scholars have further expanded on this line of reasoning, contending that fiduciary duties are incumbent upon secondary users of clinical data (as distinguished from primary users who leverage patient information to provide patient care directly).[36,42] They establish a new theory of property envisioning these users as stewards of a public good, rather than proprietors outright, maintaining that it would be unethical to "sell" such data for profit. The theory does not explicitly require patient consent as a precondition for its use, given that downstream security measures are taken. Although seemingly heterodox, this is certainly not an isolated view in the bioethical community, particularly when consent would be impracticable or unduly burdensome to obtain.[43] In any event, federal regulations consider retrospective review of de-identified clinical data as exempt from traditional patient consent requirements, provided that the "information … is recorded by the investigator in such a manner that the identity of the human subjects cannot readily be ascertained directly or through identifiers linked to the subjects, the investigator does not contact the subjects, and the investigator will not re-identify subjects."[44] That said, federal waiver of the consent requirement may do little to thwart interlopers from attempting to re-identify anonymized medical information, particularly from digital reconstructions of imaging studies. The custodians of clinical data (AI developers, radiology centers, hospitals, and server administrators, among others) must therefore remain vigilant against any possible intrusions from malign, naïve, or lax actors.[45,46] Decentralized federated learning models and even blockchain solutions have been proposed to supplement traditional cybersecurity measures in protecting data integrity.[47]

There remains the risk that AI technologies would only benefit those whose data are accessed.[48] More concerningly, algorithmic bias bears the potential of amplifying racial and demographic disparities. Training datasets may not reflect the heterogeneity of pathology across institutional, state, and regional levels and are largely subject to a small pool of individuals' designations of ground truth. When deployed on a national scale, these AI applications may even unwittingly contribute to implicit discrimination.[49] These realities underscore the importance of maintaining large, robust datasets capturing the diversity inherent within the American health care system and establishing consensus guidelines for ground truth labeling. AI expansion within smaller, rural, or more modestly funded health care institutions presents additional complexities. These may either lack the wherewithal to purchase AI applications or, conversely, invest in AI as a means of expanding their imaging capabilities, but lack the physicians to exercise appropriate oversight. In this manner, its deployment may accentuate outcome disparities inadvertently. There is a significant niche for professional societies to establish guidelines on AI implementation in low-resource settings to dampen these untoward effects.

Liability

Radiologic applications of AI are born into an uncertain liability environment. Owing to both its technological complexity and the multitude of stakeholders involved in its deployment, traditional tort doctrine strains to provide satisfactory answers.[50] Radiologists, their employers in the health care system, and AI developers confront variable degrees of risk exposure and are in turn subject to various legal theories of liability, each of which will be discussed in turn.

As was the case before the advent of AI technologies, radiologists will continue to face medical professional liability under standard negligence principles. Plaintiffs in malpractice suits bear the burden of demonstrating (1) the existence of a duty [of care], (2) a breach of said duty, and (3) that damages were sustained (4) through a causal relationship between the latter 2 factors. Professional society standards and departmental protocols play a major role in establishing a court's treatment of (1) and (2). Proper integration of AI into radiology workflow patterns and careful drafting of protocol terms are therefore essential.

Health care systems may in turn encounter vicarious liability through the doctrine of *respondeat superior*, in which the faults of subordinates flow up the chain of agency to attach to principals. Translated into a clinical context, hospitals, imaging centers, and physician groups would thus be responsible for the malpractice of their employees' use of AI programs. Vicarious liability generally operates according to a "strict liability" basis, rather than on the negligence grounds outlined elsewhere in this article. One may think of this as a legal "on–off" switch, wherein a mere demonstration of harm suffices to trigger liability. Again, these concepts are neither particularly novel nor unique to AI.

The risk of AI developers, together with their interaction with the 2 previously discussed stakeholders, stares into legal *terra incognita*. It has been postulated that products liability frameworks would govern, although courts have generally not considered software as "products"

in a tangible sense.[51,52] There is reason to assume that this may change as AI technologies become increasingly embedded within physical platforms capable of causing bodily harm.[53] If this is so, a negligence framework would apply; however, questions of AI developer duty remain unanswered.[54] Which industry standards would be called on in the absence of an AI-specific framework? Are independent developers subject to different standards of care than multinational tech conglomerates? What of health care institutions who modify the programs they purchase or train them on new datasets? In this sense, AI technologies may prove victims of their own novelty, given the relative juvenescence of the field and sparse body of relevant case law from which to derive judicial precedent. It remains to be determined how courts will interpret fault and causation for continuously learning algorithms. Alternatively, AI developers could be held to principles of strict liability should plaintiffs assert that manufacturing defects inherent to the AI product itself caused their injuries.

These questions are further complicated by the apportionment of liability between these 3 sets of actors. For instance, a sued physician group may indemnify an AI developer in a malpractice suit and accordingly seek compensation. Plaintiffs may moreover sue any one or a combination of these 3 stakeholders in their own right. Qualitatively, AI technology pushes the frontiers of contemporary tort theory, raising novel issues of control, foreseeability, and *ex ante* quantifications of the magnitude and probability of harm in manners substantially more complicated than with human actors alone.

CLINICS CARE POINTS

- Not all clinical AI products require FDA approval; those used for administrative support or record management may be exempt.

- Radiology departments and clinics should seek to integrate AI technologies with PACS and the EHR.

- Radiologists should receive training in the basics of AI deployment and troubleshooting.

- Physicians, administrators, and support personnel must take measures to maintain the security, confidentiality, and robustness of patient data used in AI products.

- Radiologists and their employers should maintain standard operating procedures for clinical AI to reduce harm and mitigate liability exposure.

SUMMARY

AI tools used in radiology practice stand to revolutionize the field entirely. They have sustained a breakneck pace of development across the past 2 decades and retain continued scope for further improvement and clinical acceptance. Indeed, their capabilities are such that they prompt fears of machines supplanting human radiologists, a concern that has to date proven overblown. AI technologies should be more appropriately viewed as high-yield supplements to radiologist practice, augmenting physician performance and minimizing the scope for human error. By the same token, algorithms are demonstrably more effective when subject to human oversight, confirming that human–machine combinations yield superior outcomes than either in isolation, in what has been dubbed Kasparov's law.[20,55] A variety of methods have been proposed for establishing a division of labor between man and machine, to include using radiologic AI devices in triaging roles for human overread, labor sharing for time-intensive routine processes, or in add-on capacities to confirm human findings.[56]

Across the field of radiology, AI technologies have found broad application in autonomously detecting pathologies, optimizing radiation dose, establishing more efficient use patterns, alleviating radiologist burnout, and enhancing access to imaging technologies.[57] They demonstrate great clinical promise, but their continued expansion demands that institutional innovations keep pace with technological ones. This is the central thesis of this article, which identifies a number of these issues and proposes potential means of addressing them. These innovations extend not only to modernized FDA regulatory frameworks, but also to updated imaging department protocols, the formation of secure and ethical data repositories, a developing AI jurisprudence, and evolving cultural norms among patients, physicians, payors, administrators, and ultimately radiologists themselves.

DISCLOSURE

The authors have nothing to disclose.

REFERENCES

1. Schuchmann S. History of the first AI winter. Towards Data Science; 2019. Available at: https://towardsdatascience.com/history-of-the-first-ai-winter-6f8c2186f80b. Accessed August 8, 2020.

2. The Medical Futurist. Artificial intelligence is the stethoscope of the 21st century. 2017. Available at: https://medicalfuturist.com/ibm-watson-is-the-stethoscope-of-the-21st-century. Accessed August 8, 2020.

3. The Medical Futurist. FDA approvals for smart algorithms in medicine in one giant infographic. 2019. Available at: https://medicalfuturist.com/fda-approvals-for-algorithms-in-medicine/. Accessed August 8, 2020.

4. Eric J. Topol high-performance medicine: the convergence of human and artificial intelligence. Nat Med 2019;25:44–56.

5. 21 U.S.C. §321(h).

6. U.S. Food and Drug Administration. Software as a Medical Device (SAMD): clinical evaluation. 2017. Available at: https://www.fda.gov/media/100714/download. Accessed August 8, 2020.

7. U.S. Food and Drug Administration. Clinical performance assessment: considerations for computer-assisted detection devices applied to radiology images and radiology device data in premarket notification (510(k)) submissions. 2020. Available at: https://www.fda.gov/media/77642/download. Accessed August 8, 2020.

8. Radiology devices; reclassification of medical image analyzers, 83 fed. Reg. 25598.

9. 21 U.S.C. §360j(o).

10. U.S. Food and Drug Administration. Clinical and patient decision support software: draft guidance for industry and food and drug administration staff. 2020. Available at: https://www.fda.gov/media/109618/download. Accessed August 8, 2020.

11. Selbst AD, Powles J. Meaningful information and the right to explanation. Int Data Privacy Law 2017;7(4):233–42.

12. Price WN. Big data and black-box medical algorithms. Sci Transl Med 2018;10(471):eaao5333.

13. Price WN. Black-box medicine. Harv J L Tech 2015;28:419–67.

14. U.S. Food and Drug Administration. Changes to existing medical software policies resulting from section 3060 of the 21st Century Cures Act. 2019. Available at: https://www.fda.gov/media/109622/download. Accessed August 8, 2020.

15. U.S. Food and Drug Administration. Digital health innovation action plan. Available at: https://www.fda.gov/media/106331/download. Accessed August 8, 2020.

16. U.S. Food and Drug Administration. Digital Health Software Precertification (Pre-Cert) program. 2019. Available at: https://www.fda.gov/medical-devices/digital-health/digital-health-software-precertification-pre-cert-program. Accessed August 8, 2020.

17. U.S. Food and Drug Administration. Current Good Manufacturing Practices (CGMPs) for food and dietary supplements. 2020. Available at: https://www.fda.gov/food/guidance-regulation-food-and-dietary-supplements/current-good-manufacturing-practices-cgmps-food-and-dietary-supplements. Accessed August 8, 2020.

18. Slabodkin G. FDA still trying to fine-tune pre-cert as pilot enters 2020. MedTech Dive; 2020. Available at: https://www.medtechdive.com/news/fda-pre-cert-software-device-pilot-enters-another-year/574822/. Accessed August 8, 2020.

19. U.S. Food and Drug Administration. Proposed regulatory framework for modifications to artificial intelligence/machine learning (AI/ML)-based software as a medical device (SaMD) - discussion paper and request for feedback. Available at: https://www.fda.gov/media/122535/download. Accessed August 8, 2020.

20. Gerke S, Babic B, Evgeniou T, et al. The need for a system view to regulate artificial intelligence/machine learning-based software as medical device. NPJ Digital Med 2020;3:53.

21. Waldron T. The future of the AI market: 2019 study results. Definitive Healthcare; 2019. Available at: https://blog.definitivehc.com/2019-artificial-intelligence-study. Accessed August 8, 2020.

22. Rouger M. The cost of AI in radiology: is it really worth it? European Society of Radiology: AI Blog. 2019. Available at: https://ai.myesr.org/healthcare/the-cost-of-ai-in-radiology-is-it-really-worth-it/. Accessed August 8, 2020.

23. Allen B. Tackling the economics of artificial intelligence. Am Coll Radiol Data Sci Inst. Available at: https://www.acrdsi.org/Blog/Tackling-the-Economics. Accessed August 8, 2020.

24. Walter M. How will radiology providers be reimbursed for investing in AI? Radiology Business. 2018. Available at: https://www.radiologybusiness.com/topics/policy/ai-radiology-reimbursements-cpt-codes-hopps. Accessed August 8, 2020.

25. Tang A, Tam R, Cadrin-Chênevert A, et al. Canadian association of radiologists white paper on artificial intelligence in radiology. Can Assoc Radiol J 2018; 69:120–35.

26. Digital Imaging and Communications in Medicine. WG-23: artificial intelligence/application hosting. Available at: https://www.dicomstandard.org/wgs/wg-23/. Accessed August 8, 2020.

27. Allen B Jr, Seltzer SE, Langlotz CP, et al. A road map for translational research on artificial intelligence in medical imaging: from the 2018 National Institutes of Health/RSNA/ACR/The Academy Workshop. J Am Coll Radiol 2019;16(9 Pt A): 1179–89.

28. Metz C. 5 options for integrating image-based AI into Your radiology workflow. Quantib; 2019. Available at: https://www.quantib.com/blog/5-options-for-integrating-image-based-ai-into-your-radiology-workflow. Accessed August 8, 2020.

29. Lehman CD, Wellman RD, Buist DS, et al. Diagnostic accuracy of digital screening mammography with and without computer-aided detection. JAMA Intern Med 2015;175(11):1828–37.

30. American College of Radiology and Radiological Society of North America. Subject: (Docket No. FDA-2019-N-5592) "public Workshop - evolving role of artificial intelligence in radiological imaging;" Comments of the American College of Radiology 2020. Available at: https://www.acr.org/-/media/ACR/NOINDEX/Advocacy/acr_rsna_comments_fda-ai-evolvingrole-ws_6-30-2020.pdf. Accessed August 8, 2020.

31. Hosny A, Parmar C, Quackenbush J, et al. Artificial intelligence in radiology. Nat Rev Cancer 2018; 18(8):500–10.

32. Pesapane F, Volonté C, Codari M, et al. Artificial intelligence as a medical device in radiology: ethical and regulatory issues in Europe and the United States. Insights Imaging 2018;9(5): 745–53.

33. Kim DW, Jang HY, Kim KW, et al. Design characteristics of studies reporting the performance of artificial intelligence algorithms for diagnostic analysis of medical images: results from recently published papers. Korean J Radiol 2019;20(3):405–10.

34. JASON. Artificial intelligence for health and health care. The MITRE Corporation; 2017. Available at: https://www.healthit.gov/sites/default/files/jsr-17-task-002_aiforhealthandhealthcare12122017.pdf. Accessed August 8, 2020.

35. National Institutes of Health. All of us research program. Available at: https://www.healthit.gov/sites/default/files/jsr-17-task-002_aiforhealthandhealthcare12122017.pdf. Accessed August 8, 2020.

36. Larson DB, Magnus DC, Lungren MP, et al. Ethics of using and sharing clinical imaging data for artificial intelligence: a proposed framework. Radiology 2020;295:675–82.

37. Wilkinson MD, Dumontier M, Aalbersberg IJ, et al. The FAIR guiding principles for scientific data management and stewardship. Sci Data 2016;3:160018.

38. Health Insurance Portability and Accountability Act of 1996. Public Law 104–191.

39. Sorrell v. IMS Health Inc., 564 U.S. 552 (2011).

40. Health Information & The Law. Who owns medical records: a 50 state comparison. 2015. Available at: http://www.healthinfolaw.org/comparative-analysis/who-owns-medical-records-50-state-comparison. Accessed August 8, 2020.

41. Faden RR. An ethics framework for a learning health care system: a departure from traditional research ethics and clinical ethics. Hastings Cent Rep 2013. Spec No:S16–S27.

42. Brady AP, Neri E. Artificial intelligence in radiology-ethical considerations. Diagnostics (Basel) 2020; 10(4):231.

43. Ballantyne A, Schaefer GO. Consent and the ethical duty to participate in health data research. J Med Ethics 2018;44(6):392–6.

44. 45 C.F.R. 46.104(d)(4).

45. Geis JR, Brady AP, Wu CC, et al. Ethics of artificial intelligence in radiology: summary of the joint European and North American Multisociety Statement. Radiology 2019;293(2):436–40.

46. Choi CQ. Medical imaging AI software is vulnerable to covert attacks. IEEE Spectrum; 2018. Available at: https://spectrum.ieee.org/the-human-os/biomedical/imaging/medical-imaging-ai-software-vulnerable-to-covert-attacks. Accessed August 8, 2020.

47. Gordon WJ, Catalini C. Blockchain technology for healthcare: facilitating the transition to patient-driven interoperability. Comput Struct Biotechnol J 2018;16:224–30.

48. Char DS, Shah NH, Magnus D. Implementing machine learning in health care - addressing ethical challenges. N Engl J Med 2018;378(11):981–3.

49. Buolamwini J, Gebru T. Gender shades: intersectional accuracy disparities in commercial gender classification. Proc Machine Learn Res 2018;81:1–15.

50. Sullivan HR, Schweikart SJ. Are current tort liability doctrines adequate for addressing injury caused by AI? AMA J Ethics 2019;21(2):E160–6.

51. Villasenor J. Products liability law as a way to address AI harms. Brookings; 2019. Available at: https://www.brookings.edu/research/products-liability-law-as-a-way-to-address-ai-harms/#:~:text=Manufacturers%20have%20an%20obligation%20to,the%20possibility%20of%20that%20outcome. Accessed August 8, 2020.

52. Restatement (Third) of Torts §19(a).

53. Harned Z, Lungren MP, Rajpurkar P. Comment, Machine Vision, Medical AI, and Malpractice. Harv. J.L. & Tech. Dig 2019. Available at: https://jolt.law.harvard.edu/digest/machine-vision-medical-ai-and-malpractice.

54. Kim S. Crashed software: assessing product liability for software defects in automated vehicles. Duke Law Tech Rev 2018;16:300–17.

55. Schaffter T, Buist DS, Lee CI, et al. Evaluation of combined artificial intelligence and radiologist assessment to interpret screening mammograms. JAMA Netw Open 2020;3(3):e200265.

56. Bossuyt PM, Irwig L, Craig J, et al. Comparative accuracy: assessing new tests against existing diagnostic pathways. BMJ 2006;332(7549):1089–92.

57. Pesapane F, Suter MB, Codari M, et al. Regulatory issues for artificial intelligence in radiology. In: Faintuch J, Faintuch S, editors. Precision medicine for investigators, practitioners and providers. London: Academic Press; 2020. p. 533–43.

Future Directions in Artificial Intelligence

Babak Saboury, MD, MPH[a,b,c], Michael Morris, MD, MS[a,b,d], Eliot Siegel, MD, FSIIM, FACR[e,f,*]

KEYWORDS

- Artificial intelligence • Radiology information architecture • Radiophenomics • Future of AI
- Autonomous AI

KEY POINTS

- Software architecture is likely to undergo a modern renaissance and provide radiologists and patients with more autonomy in how they use and interact with AI solutions.
- Larger medical image specific image databases for training and pre-trained neural networks for transfer learning are likely to emerge in the future.
- AI will not only impact the imaging evaluation workflow, but will also aid in operational logistics in the medical imaging center.
- Standards used to store and interact with medical imaging data such as DICOM will continue to evolve.

The future cannot be predicted, but futures can be invented.
> —(Dennis Gabor, awarded 1971 Nobel prize for inventing holography)

INTRODUCTION

Any attempt to predict the next 10 years, much less beyond, must keep in mind that just a decade ago, 2 of Geoffrey Hinton's University of Toronto graduate students achieved a major serendipitous conceptual leap forward in computer vision that was not anticipated by any futurists. Alex Krizhevsky realized that graphics processing units (graphics processing units were mostly associated then with video games) could profoundly speed up the execution of an algorithm invented in 1986 and subsequently improved by Hinton in the mid 2000s; the restricted Boltzmann machine. Subsequently, Alex's colleague, Ilya Sutskever, realized that this combination could be applied to the Stanford ImageNet challenge, which ultimately resulted in a landslide victory. They published the seminal paper, "Imagenet classification with deep convolutional neural networks" in 2012.[1] These deep convolutional neural networks have become so widely implemented that they have become what is now often generically referred to as artificial intelligence (AI).

Future predictions could similarly miss out on anticipating that type of game-changing leap forward, which could come in the form of new or previously described algorithms and existing or new hardware. Quantum computing could provide this type of quantum leap, but other major paradigm shifts are more likely in a 10-year time period,

---

B. Saboury and M. Morris contributed equally to this article and are considered co-first authors.

a Department of Radiology and Imaging Sciences, Clinical Center, National Institutes of Health, 9000 Rockville Pike, Building 10 Room 1C455, Bethesda, MD 20892, USA; b Department of Computer Science and Electrical Engineering, University of Maryland, Baltimore County, 1000 Hilltop Cir, Baltimore, MD 21250, USA; c Department of Radiology, Hospital of the University of Pennsylvania, 3400 Spruce Street, Philadelphia, PA 19104, USA; d Division of Clinical Informatics, Networking Health, 331 Oak Manor Drive STE 201, Glen Burnie, MD 21061, USA; e Department of Diagnostic Radiology and Nuclear Medicine, University of Maryland Medical Center, 22 South Greene Street, Baltimore, MD 20201, USA; f Department of Diagnostic Imaging, VA Maryland Healthcare System, 10 North Greene Street, Baltimore, MD 21201, USA

* Corresponding author. Department of Diagnostic Radiology and Nuclear Medicine, University of Maryland School of Medicine, University of Maryland Medical Center, 22 South Greene Street, Baltimore, MD 20201.
E-mail address: esiegel@som.umaryland.edu

Radiol Clin N Am 59 (2021) 1085–1095
https://doi.org/10.1016/j.rcl.2021.07.008

rendering the incremental and evolutionary predictions in this article obsolete. William Orton, President of Western Union's statement about the telephone in 1876 in which he asked, "why would any person want to use this ungainly and impractical device when he can send a messenger to the telegraph office," or Ken Olson, Chairman and Founder of Digital Equipment Corporation's statement that there "is no reason for any individual to have a computer in his home," come to mind when thinking about the potential folly of conjuring up predictions about the future that we are attempting in this article.

The status of AI in medical imaging in the next 10 years will depend on regulatory policy, reimbursement models, success in the incorporation of AI into routine workflow, development and adoption of standards versus platforms for AI applications, and the level of success in generalizing deep learning algorithms to different machines, geographies, and diverse patient populations to minimize bias. It will also depend on a major cultural change not only in the level of acceptance of computers in detection, diagnosis, and treatment, but also in knowing how to provide the added value of human wisdom and judgment. Finally, it is critical to improve our understanding of the pitfalls of deep learning and maintain a healthy and constructive skepticism as we explore the tremendous potential of the technology.

FUTURE REGULATORY ENVIRONMENT

At this time, there are 114 medical imaging software as a medical device products that have been cleared by the US Food and Drug Administration.[2] These developments are occurring at a rapidly accelerating pace from 2008 through 2020 with almost 70% of these receiving clearance in the past 2 years (**Fig. 1**).

In January 2021, the US Food and Drug Administration published an action plan for medical AI algorithms detailing its intention to publish "prespecifications," which address a fundamental change in the way in which algorithms are applied in clinical practice. These prespecifications describe how an AI application could change through learning, with feedback based on radiologist impressions as well as patient outcomes. This proposal for support for dynamic algorithms that could continuously adapt and improve would be a major game changer in AI and would revolutionize the way in which these algorithms are customized and improve with time.

Another impactful direction taken by the US Food and Drug Administration is the advancement

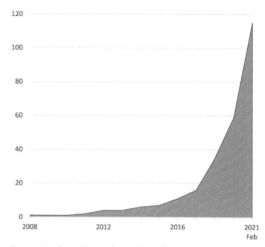

Fig. 1. AI algorithms cleared by the US Food and Drug Administration for medical Imaging showing exponential increase in clearances.

of pilots to evaluate real-world performance of these algorithms in clinical practice. This postmarket surveillance and the feedback garnered through these efforts will also have a major impact on how AI is regulated and consumed in the next several years.

THE PATIENT AS A DIRECT CONSUMER OF MEDICAL IMAGING ARTIFICIAL INTELLIGENCE
Nonradiologists Will Increasingly Have Access to and Rely on Artificial Intelligence Software

This shift is already happening with AI software designed to determine the likelihood that a patient has experienced an acute stroke owing to large vessel occlusion, with clinicians relying on the software to make a diagnosis to determine whether to expedite care for these patients. As these systems improve over the next few years, the relative added value of the radiologist in these types of cases will be called into question and their role in using their experience and judgment will be tested. At the end of 2018, there were an estimated 5 million subscriptions to AI dermatology applications with a projection of 7.2 million on smartphones by 2024.[3] Within a 10-year timeframe, patients will have access to an increasing number of radiology AI apps, including those that purport to detect and diagnose disease. Initially these AI applications will take the form of improved intelligent scheduling and translation of medical jargon for radiology reports. But eventually applications providing an analysis of MR imaging brain studies, knee MR imaging studies, computed tomography (CT) scans of the thorax for evaluation of lung nodules or chronic obstructive pulmonary disease, and many others will be available to consumers routinely. Once patients have access to their images in a format in which they can easily submit them to cloud AI providers, as is already done with smartphone cameras and skin cancer applications, there will be many additional regulatory concerns that will need to be addressed.

ARCHITECTURE OF THE FUTURE IN THE DELIVERY OF ARTIFICIAL INTELLIGENCE ALGORITHMS

Architecture is the stage on which we live our lives.

—*Mariam Kamara (architect)*

Despite almost 3 decades of experience with picture archiving and communication system (PACS) and filmless radiology, there has been surprisingly little change in the fundamental ways in which radiologists interact with their workstations and the largely monolithic model of having a single vendor supply their own proprietary suite of image review and visualization software, image storage, network and quantitative tools, and, in some cases, even speech recognition and reporting software. Although radiologists have supplemented these with third-party applications and products, these products rarely operate smoothly within the PACS workflow, although they can provide users with best of breed options for all these functions. These third-party applications typically require additional steps as well as additional physical workstations or monitors and are often time intensive and frustrating to use. Radiologists often prefer their own applications and workstation tools for different types of imaging studies, sometimes resulting in a warehouse of hardware and software solutions in the reading room environment. Access to clinical information through the electronic medical record is increasingly important as is access to all images in increasingly large health care networks.

The Academy for Radiology & Biomedical Imaging Research proposed a diagnostic cockpit, which is described as a "future-state digital platform to aggregate, organize, and simplify medical imaging results and patient-centric clinical data" to "help clinicians become 'diagnostic pilots' in detecting disease early, making accurate diagnosis, driving image-guided interventions, and improving downstream clinical management of patients."[4]

Today's working environment can be very confusing, cumbersome, and inaccessible to even the most sophisticated and cutting-edge radiologists.[5] Fundamental features such as hanging

protocols (automated set up of how one or more imaging studies are arranged on workstation monitors) are currently surprisingly primitive and brittle to minor changes in imaging sequences, number of monitors and other factors. Machine learning algorithms will be more generally used to re-engineer the "hanging protocol" challenge for PACS by replacing a rigid, highly structured set of rules with a predictive engine that watches radiologist behavior, more closely emulating the way in which a trainee learns the preferences of an attending radiologist. These algorithms will be optimized for a particular type of study, patient, and clinical indication incorporating the electronic medical record (**Box 1**).

AI applications in the future should be able to respond to and communicate with an "algorithm orchestrator" and with any component of a next generation radiology ecosystem through APIs based on agreed upon vendor-neutral and/or proprietary standards. Multiple apps and services will exist on a platform analogous to a smartphone operating system and marketplace (**Fig. 2**).[5]

In an analogous manner to streaming the song you like rather than the previous model of purchasing the whole CD with 2 songs you want and 16 you do not, radiologists and clinicians will be able to select best of breed applications that meet their specific needs for a specific study. A radiologist who is not specialized in a particular area could potentially perform at the level of a subspecialist with the correct AI applications.

In the vendor-neutral algorithm model, all components will be selected by an algorithm workflow orchestrator based on best of breed quality, reliability, and/or cost in a dynamic fashion. A more

---

Box 1
Radiologists should be able to

- Decide on how images should be reconstructed and visualized similar to pathologists determining preparation of a pathology specimen
- Decide about postreconstruction visualization tools and image processing and enhancement
- Implement radiomics quantification for specific indications
- Design their working–living space similar to the way surgeons can optimize their operating theater
- Freely shop in a marketplace to find a product that suits their individual needs and preferences and workflow

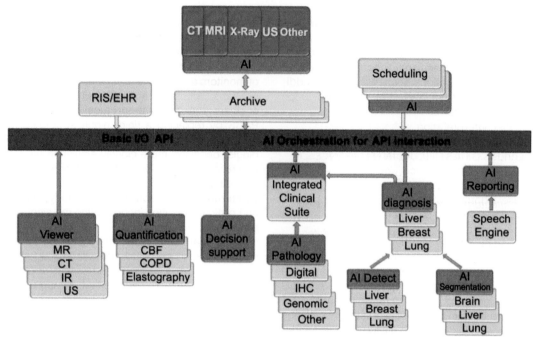

Fig. 2. Integrated Modular Architecture (Similar to Smartphone Apps/Appstore). The basic backbone I/O operating system serves as an AI orchestration engine that connects 1 or more archives and AI-enhanced workflow engines to multiple best of breed applications. These applications with their own AI capabilities can perform tasks such as viewing, quantification, decision support, and reporting. They could form integrated clinical suites that include AI-powered detection, diagnosis, segmentation, and genomic and pathology functionality. It is a large- and small-channel branched architecture. The main trunk (*red bar*) in this diagram provides API interfaces for all of the major components of the PACS system, plus multiple other functions, each with its own integrated, embedded AI. It is equivalent to horizontal integration with standard API interfaces. The components with integrated AI can be swapped in and swapped out using best of breed, without the need for dealing with cumbersome specialized interfaces. These AI applications can be used in various ensembles to integrate their functionality and enhances their overall performances and efficacy. Arrow legend: orange = DICOM; aqua = HL7 or Fast Health Interoperability Resources; blue = API. API, application programming interface; CBF, cerebral blood flow; COPD, chronic obstructive pulmonary disease; EHR, electronic health record; IHC, immune histochemistry; IR, interventional radiology; RIS, Radiology Information System; US, ultrasound. (*From* Radiology's Information Architecture Could Migrate to One Emulating That of Smartphones Dieter R. Enzmann, MD, W. Arnold, PhD, Edward Zaragoza, MD, Eliot Siegel, MD, Michael A. Pfeffer, MD Journal of the American ColCoreylege of Radiology 2020 171299-1306.)

dynamic, cost-effective, and interoperable storage infrastructure will facilitate exchange of medical images among various institutional clouds so that relevant comparison reports and images will be available when required. Radiologists will have the flexibility to select their preferred software for reviewing, analyzing, and reporting examinations, which will also enable smaller institutions or even individual radiologists the ability to level the playing field and have access to software and processing resources similar to those available currently at larger institutions.

Multifacility radiology and especially large national teleradiology groups are either incorporating or creating machine learning solutions to optimize case distribution to the radiologists. Two factors are typically considered in this optimization, namely, case urgency and radiologist specialization. Examples of the first include solutions for detecting certain critical findings on medical imaging examinations, such as intracerebral hemorrhage or stroke, pneumothorax, respiratory infections, and suspicious breast findings, and prioritizing these findings for review.[6–15] An example of the second approach is a workflow manager that claims a 15% increased efficiency of radiology interpretation and 82% subspecialist assigned reads.[16] An AI-driven complexity score could be used in the creation of a more sophisticated relative value unit assessment of radiologist productivity within a single group.

Ensembles of programs will be used to form a consensus of opinions or quantitative analysis and multiple programs could be used to complete various steps in the image interpretation process. For example, one could imagine an algorithm that could segment the adrenal glands, another that could analyze the distribution of density of pixels in this segmented region, still another that could compare contrast and noncontrast image, and still another that could create an a priori or post interpretation estimate of the odds of malignancy and determine the most likely diagnosis. These cooperative algorithms will become routine once advanced algorithm orchestration enabled platforms are available. These algorithm or workflow orchestration platforms will not only coordinate different applications, but also will allow interaction between the radiologist or clinician.

DATA FOR ARTIFICIAL INTELLIGENCE IN THE FUTURE

Initial attempts at creating de-identified public datasets such as The Cancer Imaging Archive[17] have been extraordinarily useful to the research and commercial communities; however, annotation of these images has been limited and the size of available datasets is considered to be relatively small.[18] Modifications to the DICOM standard and the adoption of annotation and mark-up standards such as the National Cancer Institute–sponsored Annotation and Image Mark-up initiative[19] have the potential to provide the needed foundation for easier cross-institutional exchange, decentralized repositories, and richer data labels and elements.

The current state of the art for security in digital imaging and for electronic patient records is substantially behind other sectors of the economy. Numerous vulnerabilities are inherent to not only deep learning imaging dataset aggregation efforts, but also in routine clinical practice with relatively insecure clinical data storage, a lack of audit of data access, the ability to inject or remove pathology in images without any ability to detect these changes, and the inherent security issues around physical media such as CDs, DVDs, and USB thumb drives.

A next-generation approach to the storage of DICOM images will begin to be implemented in the next several years owing to increasing security concerns over clinical and research imaging archives. DICOM was originally designed to enhance image accessibility with limited security functionality. The increasing use of blockchain and related technologies in other industries will finally come to health care medical records and specifically to medical imaging. Hash-based data structures known as Merkle trees can be used

for efficient data verification and are already used in peer-to-peer networks such as Tor, Bitcoin, and Git. These protocols will permit secure, fine grained access control of image exchange within and among health care facilities and will make it much more difficult to alter either DICOM tags or the pixels in a medical imaging study. These files will be interoperable with traditional DICOM storage and data exchange protocols, but will be optimized for performance and security, as well as the development of deep learning algorithms from stored medical images.

Federated machine learning models, which represent a class of distributed systems that rely on remote execution, will increasingly allow deep learning models to be trained on local data without having to upload the data from a facility's firewall, decreasing the risk of a patient privacy breech.[20] This method is viable, but not yet completely proven, for combining data from different institutions, machines, and geographic areas for a larger and more diverse database without the inherent issues related to sending studies outside of an institution's firewall. Challenges include coordinating a uniform methodology for data curation at multiple sites, and the lack of an agreement on how to update the central model state to achieve results comparable to those in which all the data were combined into a single dataset. Homomorphic encryption involves performing deep learning directly on encrypted data rather than using encryption merely for communication and storage of the data. Homomorphic encryption will result in much more secure multiparty computation. Secure encrypted processing hardware will become routine in computers and mobile devices such as next generations of smartphones to maintain encryption at these user edge devices.

Another promising technique that will become increasingly popular creates synthetic medical images from generative adversarial networks to potentially supply unlimited numbers of images that could be created from one or more image databases.

DEVELOPMENT OF NEW RADIOLOGY SPECIFIC NEURAL NETWORK ARCHITECTURES (BEYOND ImageNET)

Most of the current AI applications in medical imaging have relied on transfer learning from the widely used and popular visual database ImageNet.[21] This database is large and has been used for a wide variety of different computer vision applications in addition to medical imaging and has resulted in impressive advances for convolutional neural networks in image recognition tasks. In addition to not using medical images, but various objects such as animals and flowers and cars and others, there are other limitations to ImageNet for medical imaging applications, including the fact that it used just a single label description of images rather than multiple labels on an image. This latter multiple labeling is more applicable to medical images that frequently contain more than 1 feature on a single image. Large, coordinated efforts such as the recently created Medical Imaging and Data Resource Center and others may make tens of thousands of cases publicly accessible and could serve as a basis for adjunctive databases that are optimized for medical image deep learning.

In the future, labeling of these and other datasets could be incorporated directly into a radiologist's clinical workflow with improvements in annotation tools, incorporation of AI into viewer software, and with natural language generation. The use of structured DICOM (DICOM-SR)[22] or annotation image markup[23] for annotations over proprietary vendor-specific annotations may also help to realize this potential.

NON–PIXEL-BASED ARTIFICIAL INTELLIGENCE APPLICATIONS WILL BE DEVELOPED IN PARALLEL TO PIXEL-BASED ONES

Non–pixel-based applications using a variety of natural language understanding technologies will become widely implemented. Like the advances in human vision made possible by the 1.3 million pictures in the ImageNet annotated dataset, database-based models such as OpenAI's natural language processing model, GPT-3 are advancing natural language processing with more than 175 billion weighted connections between words.

The next generation of natural language processing and natural language understanding tools will be used to make radiology reports machine intelligible, given the fact that diagnostic imaging will be unlikely to make a full transition to structured reported within the next decade. Communication and follow-up of unexpected findings, synthesis of pertinent information from the electronic medical record for the radiologist, and automatic generation of an impression from the body of a report will use natural language understanding and will be ubiquitous within the decade. The extraction of a priori patient data from the electronic medical record will enable detection and decision support algorithms to provide more accurate and pertinent insights and these data will be made available to these AI algorithms.

The widespread use of liquid biopsies,[24] which use cell-free DNA, RNA, circulating tumor cells, and extracellular vesicles, has not yet occurred owing to a variety of pitfalls, including a lack of reproducibility and discordant results. Once these issues are addressed, it will become common to have patients referred for imaging who are found by liquid biopsy and/or genomic analysis to have substantially increased risks of having specific types or classes of cancer or other diseases. Cohen and colleagues[25] described a study with 10,006 women in which 31% of patients who were subsequently found to have cancer in 1 of 7 organs for which no standard screening is available, had a positive liquid biopsy. Additional workup to help localize these was done using PET/CT scans. The widespread use of liquid biopsies for screening will put increased pressure on imaging workflows, likely improving the efficiency of advanced imaging studies, which will have a higher pretest probability of an abnormal finding.

Another machine learning application will be to predict no-show rates for imaging examinations. This clinical scheduling issue has become even more of a challenge during the coronavirus disease 2019 (COVID-19) pandemic.

A recent AI approach to decrease no show rates resulted in a 17% decrease in the no-show rate within 6 months of implementation using predictive analytics.[26] These tools are even more important now than they were in the past and they will continue to be used with increasingly sophisticated and improving approaches. Tools for business optimization such as these may be the earliest opportunity for AI adoption in medical imaging because there is a clear return on investment. Future refinements could be used to predict the potential impact of overbooking patients for studies, determining which patients might need additional notification of appointments or assistance with transportation, predicted patient arrival times for those arriving before or after scheduled appointments, and even anticipatory rebooking of patients at highest risk for no shows. The pandemic has also accelerated the transition to remote diagnosis and the use of the cloud, which, in turn, has made cloud-based AI applications more acceptable to medical imaging facilities. Additionally, the scramble to obtain shared COVID-19–related imaging datasets has increased the engagement of the medical imaging scientific community with the clinical medicine community and brought about new collaborations. Through the increasing availability of shared resources for COVID-19 data as well as research funding for solutions to the pandemic, new collaborations have allowed radiologists to interface directly with computer scientists, data scientists, engineers, and industry to improve availability of AI resources for diagnosis and management of COVID-19.[27–30] This expansion of multidisciplinary collaborative science in support of the worldwide pandemic will open the door more permanently to more concerted and collaborative efforts.

Because teams of radiologists work remotely, there is an increasing need for workflow orchestration by PACS, VNA, and dedicated workflow vendors as well as a need to become even more efficient. We could be on the verge of an evolution/devolution of PACS into an AI-centric combination of independent modules for visualization, analysis, decision support, and reporting.

ARTIFICIAL INTELLIGENCE FOR THE ASSESSMENT AND IMPROVEMENT OF IMAGE QUALITY

There are currently very few objective methods to assess imaging examination quality with only relatively superficial reviews of image quality itself performed by accreditation organizations. The real-time assessment of medical image quality could become an important indicator for patient quality and safety data and even credentialing bodies in the future. Investigations have been performed to evaluate the use of AI to assess the quality of imaging acquisition at the point of care.[31] The examination could then be evaluated either after the study was completed or even during image acquisition to assess and optimize image quality.

There is a trade-off between image quality and parameters such as patient dose, image acquisition time, amount of contrast administered, and other factors. Using a combination of radiologist subjective ratings of overall image quality and indication-specific image quality as well as physics parameters such as image noise, target to background ratio, and contrast and spatial resolution, deep learning algorithms will be trained to predict radiologists' ratings for the quality of images. Another interesting parameter for image quality will be the performance of AI algorithms for a given imaging technique. An example of this would be evaluating the impact of lower dose CT scans of the thorax using lung nodule detection AI algorithms.[32]

ARTIFICIAL INTELLIGENCE AS A SCRIBE OR PERSONAL ASSISTANT

Medical scribes have been shown to improve relative value units and provider satisfaction.[33] Human assistants who serve as scribes are starting to be explored in diagnostic radiology as a means of improving efficiency where these assistants play multiple roles in optimizing the speed and quality of care and patient safety. With the use of these assistants, radiologists have been able to more than double throughput. This is largely due to the relative inefficiency of current case retrieval and hanging protocols and limitations of speech recognition technology. Studies performed at the Baltimore VA Medical Center in the 1990s found that only about 15%–20% of a radiologist's time was spent in the actual review of images; the remainder consisted of the time required for the gathering of patient history and study indication and review of prior reports, image retrieval and arrangement, dictation, and other workflow tasks. The potential for AI to take over a subset or all the functions of these radiology assistants/scribes is intriguing and could represent one of the highest returns on AI investment in diagnostic imaging.

ARTIFICIAL INTELLIGENCE FOR IMAGE ACQUISITION

One of the earliest and deepest implementations of AI is already occurring throughout the medical industry. AI as a means of optimization for image acquisition will continue to take advantage of the high level of redundancy in image acquisition systems, especially for MR imaging, CT scans, PET/CT scans, and nuclear medicine. Xu and colleagues[34] found that the inclusion of MR image contrasts into the inputs for AI models could result in acceptable image quality using as little as one 200th of the dataset comparable to taking 3 seconds of data from a 10-minute acquisition. One of the major CT providers uses a library of CT studies reconstructed with both statistical (reconstruction in seconds) reconstruction and model-based (reconstruction in hours) reconstruction to generate the much more resource intensive model-based reconstruction in seconds rather than hours. The implications for scanning time or dose reduction or image quality improvement are intriguing for all imaging modalities and multiple subsequent studies have demonstrated impressive results. Incorporation of deep learning will become ubiquitous in image reconstruction, but new pitfalls and artifacts will be introduced with a wide variety of different applications of deep learning.

FUTURE ARTIFICIAL INTELLIGENCE WILL TAKE PREVIOUS STUDIES INTO ACCOUNT

It has been suggested that a radiologist's best friend is the prior images. Unfortunately, virtually all of today's AI algorithms do not use information from prior studies nor do they create predictions based on trajectory of change over time. This factor represents a major deviation from routine radiology practice, where the goal of the radiologist is often to evaluate for significant interval change and use lack of change to suggest a benign etiology for a finding. Taking advantage of previous imaging studies performed hours or days before in the detection of stroke on a CT scan or previous mammograms in the detection of cancer could result in tremendous improvement in performance on these tasks.

DISEASE-BASED MULTIDISCIPLINARY CLINICAL PACKAGES

Analogous to a multidisciplinary conference of clinicians, multidisciplinary AI approaches could help in further guiding the diagnosis or management for complex pathology in a more patient-centered manner. In the future, basic capabilities such as the detection of lung nodules or intracranial bleeding will become more of a commodity application while instead there is more of an emphasis on a broad clinical package such as multiple sclerosis, chronic obstructive pulmonary disease, ischemia, heart disease, and others that include detection, diagnosis, quantification metrics, radiophenomics, change over time, and recommendations for treatment and follow-up.

AUTONOMOUS ARTIFICIAL INTELLIGENCE

AI algorithms continue to improve and approach or exceed the performance of a general or even specialty radiologist in certain well-defined areas. The first step toward this will be autonomous reading for a subset of studies of a particular type. This is an outgrowth of the current earlier stage of triage of worklists in which an AI program puts studies for example, of higher suspicion for intracranial bleed on a head CT scan at the top of a radiologist's worklist. The next logical step will be for AI to perform final reads, but only when it has a high level of confidence in its diagnosis.

Recently, there have been considerable improvements in the performance of algorithms used to detect malignancy in mammography. Kyono and colleagues[35] recently evaluated the use of deep learning in a dataset of more than 7000 women who were recalled for assessment as a part of the National Health Service screening program in the UK. They found that their AI algorithm could maintain a comparable with or better than human-level negative predictive value performance of 0.99 for an algorithm selected 34%

of mammograms when the prevalence of disease was 15% (the algorithm picked the 34% to interpret to achieve that negative predictive value) and could achieve that 0.99 negative predictive value negative predictive value for 91% of mammograms when the prevalence of disease was 1%. This ability to select studies highly likely to be negative will be used differently throughout the world. In countries such as the United States, for the foreseeable future and given regulatory and billing concerns, this will represent a triage mechanism to allow radiologists to review higher yield studies more carefully in comparison with a less comprehensive review of lower yield studies. In other countries, this technology will be more likely to be used to prescreen which studies are selected for human versus computer only interpretation.

Challenges posed by the adoption of AI in medical imaging have been well-described and include the patient care and ethical implications of bias in datasets selected to train AI algorithms, misapplication of AI based on a lack of understanding of the narrow focus of an algorithm, the use of AI to create false images with, for example, tumors removed or inserted into imaging studies, perceived or actual loss of value of human radiologists and threats to jobs, large-scale security breaches, and AI performing a different task than intended owing to the black box lack of visibility into what the AI system is actually doing. A current real threat is that the perception of AI as a threat itself is likely steering a subset of misinformed medical students away from the specialty of diagnostic imaging.[36]

NEXT-GENERATION TECHNOLOGIES IN ARTIFICIAL INTELLIGENCE

Deep learning will continue to evolve. The time-consuming and resource-intensive process of labeling data will encourage hybrid learning models in which one combines supervised and unsupervised learning. An example of this is the use of a semisupervised generative adversarial network achieving performance comparable with that required with hundreds of cases using only 25 samples.[37] This improvement is based on the idea that, in learning to discriminate between real and synthetic images, a generative adversarial network can learn structures without concrete labels. Composite learning seeks to combine knowledge from multiple models. Transfer learning is one example of this methodology, as are generative adversarial networks and adversarial learning in which the performance of one model can be represented in relationship to that of others. Ensemble methods that combine multiple algorithms designed to solve the same problem using different approaches are another example. Finally, reduced learning approaches are becoming more sophisticated in creating lightweight AI, which creates smaller neural networks without the loss of performance to effectively run deep learning algorithms on devices such as smartphones, portable radiographs, ultrasound examination, or MR imaging systems.

AI systems of the future will need to be less reliant on large numbers of training sets, be more easily understandable (explainable AI rather than black box), and will need to be more efficient in transferring learned knowledge. Alternatives and improvements such as adaptive resonance theory, also referred to as incremental learning, which does not require retraining to incorporate new learning; or cogency maximization, which is less computationally intensive and addresses the explainability issues with deep learning; and fuzzy sets systems, which allows data to be represented as probabilities rather than just true or false or as a set numeric value, represent future advances in deep learning.

BEYOND DEEP LEARNING AND ARTIFICIAL INTELLIGENCE

As Wang and Yeung observed in their seminal paper, Toward Bayesian Deep Learning: A Framework and Some Existing Methods,[38] next-generation AI systems will go beyond seeing, reading, and hearing to thinking. They foresee a Bayesian deep learning framework in the future and try to integrate them into a single probabilistic framework. This work will likely be a fruitful direction because so many tasks, especially in health care, require a combination of perception from neural networks, but also inference ability from probabilistic graphical models, which are described in this integrated framework. The combination of deep learning with Bayesian inferencing has the potential to significantly augment the utility of computers to help radiologists to not only observe but to also provide important insights to contribute impactfully for patient care.

SUMMARY

Dennis Gabor's observation that futures cannot be predicted, but futures can be invented, underscores the importance of radiologists serving as active players in the continuing evolution of AI in diagnostic imaging to enable us to determine our own future.

Ultimately, AI represents a tool with incredible potential for us to, once again, reinvent the practice of diagnostic imaging in a way that participates as fully as possible in the emerging health care ecosystem of data and decision support algorithms, to make us more efficient, reduce stress and burn-out, increased accuracy in diagnosis and follow-up recommendations, and improve communications and patient safety.

AI will undoubtedly make radiology more impactful and a more attractive specialty for potential trainees while making it an even more fascinating and wonderous subspecialty in health care.

CLINICS CARE POINTS

- The most important attribute of AI systems in medicine is their trustworthiness.
- Non-pixel based artificial intelligence applications will be developed in parallel to pixel-based ones.
- Radiologists must be actively involved in defining the future of AI in medical imaging.
- AI will undoubtedly make radiology more impactful and a more attractive specialty.

DISCLOSURE

The authors have nothing to disclose.

REFERENCES

1. Krizhevsky A, Sutskever I, Hinton GE. ImageNet classification with deep convolutional neural networks. In: Proceedings of the 25th International Conference on Neural Information Processing Systems - Volume 1. NIPS'12. Curran Associates Inc.; 2012:1097-1105. Available at: https://dl.acm.org/doi/10.5555/2999134.2999257. Accessed February 28, 2021.
2. Editorial Board: Keith Dreyer, Christoph Wald, Bibb Allen, Sheela Agarwal, Judy Gichoya, Jay Patti. FDA Cleared AI Algorithms. ACR Datascience Institute. Available at: https://models.acrdsi.org/. Accessed February 28, 2021.
3. Tintín V, Caiza J, Atencio H, et al. Artificial intelligence in mobile applications of dermatology: a systematic mapping study. In: First International Workshop on Applied Informatics for Economics, Society and Development (AIESD 2019). ; 2019:12-25. Available

at: http://ceur-ws.org/Vol-2486/icaiw_aiesd_2.pdf. Accessed February 28, 2021.

4. Krupinski E, Bronkalla M, Folio L, et al. Advancing the diagnostic cockpit of the future: an opportunity to improve diagnostic accuracy and efficiency. Acad Radiol 2019;26(4):579–81.

5. Enzmann DR, Arnold CW, Zaragoza E, et al. Radiology's information architecture could migrate to one emulating that of smartphones. J Am Coll Radiol 2020;17(10):1299–306.

6. Yi PH, Singh D, Harvey SC, et al. DeepCAT: deep computer-aided triage of screening mammography. J Digit Imaging 2021. https://doi.org/10.1007/s10278-020-00407-0.

7. Thrall JH, Fessell D, Pandharipande PV. Rethinking the approach to artificial intelligence for medical image analysis: the case for precision diagnosis. J Am Coll Radiol 2021;18(1 Pt B):174–9.

8. Dembrower K, Wåhlin E, Liu Y, et al. Effect of artificial intelligence-based triaging of breast cancer screening mammograms on cancer detection and radiologist workload: a retrospective simulation study. Lancet Digital Health 2020;2(9):e468–74.

9. Soun JE, Chow DS, Nagamine M, et al. Artificial intelligence and acute stroke imaging. AJNR Am J Neuroradiol 2021;42(1):2–11.

10. Wehbe RM, Sheng J, Dutta S, et al. DeepCOVID-XR: an artificial intelligence algorithm to detect COVID-19 on chest radiographs trained and tested on a large US clinical dataset. Radiology 2020;203511. https://doi.org/10.1148/radiol.2020203511.

11. Quiroz JC, Feng Y-Z, Cheng Z-Y, et al. Automated severity assessment of COVID-19 based on clinical and imaging data: algorithm development and validation. JMIR Med Inform 2021. https://doi.org/10.2196/24572.

12. Huang S-C, Pareek A, Zamanian R, et al. Multimodal fusion with deep neural networks for leveraging CT imaging and electronic health record: a case-study in pulmonary embolism detection. Sci Rep 2020; 10(1). https://doi.org/10.1038/s41598-020-78888-w.

13. Gupta R, Krishnam SP, Schaefer PW, et al. An East Coast perspective on artificial intelligence and machine learning: part 1. Neuroimaging Clin N Am 2020;30(4):459–66.

14. Gupta R, Krishnam SP, Schaefer PW, et al. An East Coast perspective on artificial intelligence and machine learning: part 2: ischemic stroke imaging and triage. Neuroimaging Clin N Am 2020;30(4):467–78.

15. Laserson J, Lantsman CD, Cohen-Sfady M, et al. TextRay: mining clinical reports to gain a broad understanding of chest x-rays. In: Frangi A, Schnabel J, Davatzikos C, et al, editors. Medical image computing and computer assisted intervention – MICCAI 2018. Switzerland: Springer International Publishing; 2018. p. 553–61. https://doi.org/10.1007/978-3-030-00934-2_62.

16. Deutsch AL. Managing multi-site workflow in the era of consolidation. Presented at the: HIMSS 2019 session #191; February 14, 2019; Orlando, FL. Available at: https://365.himss.org/sites/himss365/files/365/handouts/552576921/handout-191_FINAL.pdf. Accessed February 1, 2021.

17. Clark K, Vendt B, Smith K, et al. The Cancer Imaging Archive (TCIA): maintaining and operating a public information repository. J Digit Imaging 2013;26(6):1045–57.

18. Langlotz CP, Allen B, Erickson BJ, et al. A roadmap for foundational research on artificial intelligence in medical imaging: from the 2018 NIH/RSNA/ACR/The Academy Workshop. Radiology 2019;291(3):781–91.

19. Rubin DL, Willrett D, O'Connor MJ, et al. Automated tracking of quantitative assessments of tumor burden in clinical trials. Transl Oncol 2014;7(1):23–35.

20. Kaissis GA, Makowski MR, Rückert D, et al. Secure, privacy-preserving and federated machine learning in medical imaging. Nat Machine Intelligence 2020;2(6):305–11.

21. Deng J, Dong W, Socher R, Li L, Kai Li, Li Fei-Fei. ImageNet: A large-scale hierarchical image database. In: 2009 IEEE Conference on Computer Vision and Pattern Recognition. Miami (FL), June 20-25, 2009. p. 248-55. doi:10.1109/CVPR.2009.5206848.

22. Clunie DA. DICOM structured reporting. Bangor (PA): PixelMed Publishing; 2000. Available at: https://play.google.com/store/books/details?id=EVjOolUJNGUC.

23. Rubin DL, Mongkolwat P, Kleper V, et al. Annotation and image markup: accessing and interoperating with the semantic content in medical imaging. IEEE Intell Syst 2009;24(1):57–65.

24. Geeurickx E, Hendrix A. Targets, pitfalls and reference materials for liquid biopsy tests in cancer diagnostics. Mol Aspects Med 2020;72:100828.

25. Cohen JD, Li L, Wang Y, et al. Detection and localization of surgically resectable cancers with a multi-analyte blood test. Science 2018;359(6378):926–30.

26. Chong LR, Tsai KT, Lee LL, et al. Artificial intelligence predictive analytics in the management of outpatient MRI appointment no-shows. AJR Am J Roentgenol 2020;215(5):1155–62.

27. Mei X, Lee H-C, Diao K-Y, et al. Artificial intelligence–enabled rapid diagnosis of patients with COVID-19. Nat Med 2020;26(8):1224–8.

28. Medical Imaging and Data Resource Center. MIDRC. 2020. Available at: https://www.midrc.org/midrc-data. Accessed January 30, 2021.

29. Langlotz C. RSNA to collaborate on open-source COVID-19 medical image database. 2020. Available at: https://www.rsna.org/news/2020/july/covid-19-midrc. Accessed February 28, 2021.

30. MacDougall R. NIH Harnesses AI for COVID-19 diagnosis, treatment, and monitoring: collaborative network to enlist medical imaging and clinical data

sciences to reveal unique features of COVID-19 2020. Available at: https://www.nih.gov/news-events/news-releases/nih-harnesses-ai-covid-19-diagnosis-treatment-monitoring. Accessed February 28, 2021.

31. Kashyap S, Moradi M, Karargyris A, et al. Artificial intelligence for point of care radiograph quality assessment. In: Medical imaging 2019: computer-aided diagnosis, vol. 10950. San Diego (CA): International Society for Optics and Photonics; 2019. p. 109503K. https://doi.org/10.1117/12.2513092.

32. Lee JH, Grant BR, Chung JH, et al. Assessment of diagnostic image quality of computed tomography (CT) images of the lung using deep learning. In: Medical imaging 2018: physics of medical imaging, vol. 10573. Houston (TX): International Society for Optics and Photonics; 2018. p. 105731M. https://doi.org/10.1117/12.2292070.

33. Gottlieb M, Palter J, Westrick J, et al. Effect of medical scribes on throughput, revenue, and patient and provider satisfaction: a systematic review and meta-analysis. Ann Emerg Med 2021;77(2): 180–9.

34. Xu J, Gong E, Pauly J, et al. 200x low-dose PET reconstruction using deep learning. arXiv [csCV]. 2017. Available at: http://arxiv.org/abs/1712.04119. Accessed February 28, 2021.

35. Kyono T, Gilbert FJ, van der Schaar M. Improving workflow efficiency for mammography using machine learning. J Am Coll Radiol 2020;17(1 Pt A): 56–63.

36. Park CJ, Yi PH, Siegel EL. Medical student perspectives on the impact of artificial intelligence on the practice of medicine. Curr Probl Diagn Radiol 2020. https://doi.org/10.1067/j.cpradiol.2020.06.011.

37. Patel S, Kakadiya A, Mehta M, et al. Correlated discrete data generation using adversarial training. [csLG] arXiv 2018. Available at: http://arxiv.org/abs/1804.00925. Accessed February 28, 2021.

38. Wang H, Yeung D. Towards Bayesian deep learning: a framework and some existing methods. IEEE Trans Knowl Data Eng 2016;28(12): 3395–408.

UNITED STATES POSTAL SERVICE®
Statement of Ownership, Management, and Circulation
(All Periodicals Publications Except Requester Publications)

1. Publication Title	2. Publication Number	3. Filing Date
RADIOLOGIC CLINICS OF NORTH AMERICA	596 – 510	9/18/2021

4. Issue Frequency	5. Number of Issues Published Annually	6. Annual Subscription Price
JAN, MAR, MAY, JUL, SEP, NOV	6	$518.00

7. Complete Mailing Address of Known Office of Publication (Not printer) (Street, city, county, state, and ZIP+4®)

ELSEVIER INC.
230 Park Avenue, Suite 800
New York, NY 10169

Contact Person: Malathi Samayan
Telephone (Include area code): 91-44-4299-4507

8. Complete Mailing Address of Headquarters or General Business Office of Publisher (Not printer)

ELSEVIER INC.
230 Park Avenue, Suite 800
New York, NY 10169

9. Full Names and Complete Mailing Addresses of Publisher, Editor, and Managing Editor (Do not leave blank)

Publisher (Name and complete mailing address)

DOLORES MELONI, ELSEVIER INC.
1600 JOHN F KENNEDY BLVD. SUITE 1800
PHILADELPHIA, PA 19103-2899

Editor (Name and complete mailing address)

JOHN VASSALLO, ELSEVIER INC.
1600 JOHN F KENNEDY BLVD. SUITE 1800
PHILADELPHIA, PA 19103-2899

Managing Editor (Name and complete mailing address)

PATRICK MANLEY, ELSEVIER INC.
1600 JOHN F KENNEDY BLVD. SUITE 1800
PHILADELPHIA, PA 19103-2899

10. Owner (Do not leave blank. If the publication is owned by a corporation, give the name and address of the corporation immediately followed by the names and addresses of all stockholders owning or holding 1 percent or more of the total amount of stock. If not owned by a corporation, give the names and addresses of the individual owners. If owned by a partnership or other unincorporated firm, give its name and address as well as those of each individual owner. If the publication is published by a nonprofit organization, give its name and address.)

Full Name	Complete Mailing Address
WHOLLY OWNED SUBSIDIARY OF REED/ELSEVIER, US HOLDINGS	1600 JOHN F KENNEDY BLVD. SUITE 1800 PHILADELPHIA, PA 19103-2899

11. Known Bondholders, Mortgagees, and Other Security Holders Owning or Holding 1 Percent or More of Total Amount of Bonds, Mortgages, or Other Securities. If none, check box ► ☐ None

Full Name	Complete Mailing Address
N/A	

12. Tax Status (For completion by nonprofit organizations authorized to mail at nonprofit rates) (Check one)
The purpose, function, and nonprofit status of this organization and the exempt status for federal income tax purposes:
☒ Has Not Changed During Preceding 12 Months
☐ Has Changed During Preceding 12 Months (Publisher must submit explanation of change with this statement)

PS Form **3526**, July 2014 [Page 1 of 4 (see instructions page 4)] PSN: 7530-01-000-9631 PRIVACY NOTICE: See our privacy policy on www.usps.com.

---

13. Publication Title	14. Issue Date for Circulation Data Below
RADIOLOGIC CLINICS OF NORTH AMERICA	JULY 2021

15. Extent and Nature of Circulation		Average No. Copies Each Issue During Preceding 12 Months	No. Copies of Single Issue Published Nearest to Filing Date
a. Total Number of Copies (Net press run)		847	766
b. Paid Circulation (By Mail and Outside the Mail)	(1) Mailed Outside-County Paid Subscriptions Stated on PS Form 3541 (Include paid distribution above nominal rate, advertiser's proof copies, and exchange copies)	592	548
	(2) Mailed In-County Paid Subscriptions Stated on PS Form 3541 (Include paid distribution above nominal rate, advertiser's proof copies, and exchange copies)	0	0
	(3) Paid Distribution Outside the Mails Including Sales Through Dealers and Carriers, Street Vendors, Counter Sales, and Other Paid Distribution Outside USPS®	198	179
	(4) Paid Distribution by Other Classes of Mail Through the USPS (e.g., First-Class Mail®)	0	0
c. Total Paid Distribution (Sum of 15b (1), (2), (3), and (4)) ►		790	727
d. Free or Nominal Rate Distribution (By Mail and Outside the Mail)	(1) Free or Nominal Rate Outside-County Copies included on PS Form 3541	40	25
	(2) Free or Nominal Rate In-County Copies Included on PS Form 3541	0	0
	(3) Free or Nominal Rate Copies Mailed at Other Classes Through the USPS (e.g., First-Class Mail)	0	0
	(4) Free or Nominal Rate Distribution Outside the Mail (Carriers or other means)	40	25
e. Total Free or Nominal Rate Distribution (Sum of 15d (1), (2), (3) and (4)) ►		40	25
f. Total Distribution (Sum of 15c and 15e) ►		830	752
g. Copies not Distributed (See instructions to Publishers #4 (page #3)) ►		17	14
h. Total (Sum of 15f and g) ►		847	766
i. Percent Paid (15c divided by 15f times 100) ►		95.18%	96.67%

* If you are claiming electronic copies, go to line 16 on page 3. If you are not claiming electronic copies, skip to line 17 on page 3.

16. Electronic Copy Circulation	Average No. Copies Each Issue During Preceding 12 Months	No. Copies of Single Issue Published Nearest to Filing Date
a. Paid Electronic Copies ►		
b. Total Paid Print Copies (Line 15c) + Paid Electronic Copies (Line 16a) ►		
c. Total Print Distribution (Line 15f) + Paid Electronic Copies (Line 16a) ►		
d. Percent Paid (Both Print & Electronic Copies) (16b divided by 16c × 100) ►		

☒ I certify that 50% of all my distributed copies (electronic and print) are paid above a nominal price.

17. Publication of Statement of Ownership

☒ If the publication is a general publication, publication of this statement is required. Will be printed ☐ Publication not required.

in the NOVEMBER 2021 issue of this publication.

18. Signature and Title of Editor, Publisher, Business Manager, or Owner

Malathi Samayan *Malathi Samayan*   Date 9/18/2021

Malathi Samayan - Distribution Controller

I certify that all information furnished on this form is true and complete. I understand that anyone who furnishes false or misleading information on this form or who omits material or information requested on the form may be subject to criminal sanctions (including fines and imprisonment) and/or civil sanctions (including civil penalties).

PS Form **3526**, July 2014 (Page 3 of 4) PRIVACY NOTICE: See our privacy policy on www.usps.com

Moving?

Make sure your subscription moves with you!

To notify us of your new address, find your **Clinics Account Number** (located on your mailing label above your name), and contact customer service at:

Email: journalscustomerservice-usa@elsevier.com

800-654-2452 (subscribers in the U.S. & Canada)
314-447-8871 (subscribers outside of the U.S. & Canada)

Fax number: 314-447-8029

Elsevier Health Sciences Division
Subscription Customer Service
3251 Riverport Lane
Maryland Heights, MO 63043

*To ensure uninterrupted delivery of your subscription, please notify us at least 4 weeks in advance of move.

Printed and bound by CPI Group (UK) Ltd, Croydon, CR0 4YY

08/05/2025

01864700-0019